$8.00

$35.00 (5)

04/24
STAND PRICE
$5.00

Edward Jenner

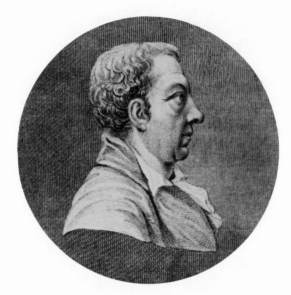

Edward Jenner portrait by John Drayton

Edward Jenner

THE CHELTENHAM YEARS

1795-1823

Being a Chronicle of the
Vaccination Campaign

BY

Paul Saunders

PREFACE BY WILLIAM LE FANU

University Press of New England
Hanover and London
1982

University Press of New England
Brandeis University
Brown University
Clark University
Dartmouth College
University of New Hampshire
University of Rhode Island
Tufts University
University of Vermont

Library of Congress Catalogue Card Number 81-51607
International Standard Book Number 0-87451-215-8

Printed in the United States of America

Library of Congress Cataloging in Publication data
will be found on the last printed page of this book.

To the memory of my mother
and my grandmother,
Madame Clara Sheppard Rotunda

While thus I rove through Chelta's flowing plain
And some faint embers of any youth remain
Shall not the muse her tuneful accents raise
And wake her slumb'ring lyre to sing thy praise
—John Anstey, 1803

CONTENTS

FOREWORD

Edward Jenner stands among the most renowned of the world's scientists. Although not so widely famous as his compatriots Newton and Darwin, he is remembered as one of the chief benefactors of human life. His faith that the discovery of vaccination would abolish smallpox from the earth was vindicated after nearly two hundred years: in October 1979 the World Health Organization announced that the terrible pandemic scourge had been eradicated from its last stronghold in the Horn of Africa by nine million vaccinations given in three years. Smallpox was conquered—not only there but on the African continent and throughout the world.

At the bicentenary of Jenner's birth in 1949 eminent authorities pointed to him as the begetter of several rapidly developing medical sciences. He had already been accepted in the last century, by the championship of Pasteur and Lister, as the pioneer of preventive medicine. He is also called the father of immunology. His vision and research had adumbrated the existence of viruses nearly a century before their precise identification opened a wide new field of knowledge, and in 1907 Clemens von Pirquet attributed his fertile and influential concept of allergy to inspiration from the work of "that man of genius, Jenner."

Despite Jenner's achievements and the acclaim voiced by his illustrious successors, so little is generally known of his life and work that even now hostile skepticism denigrates his reputation. Enough has been established to make his accomplishment impregnable, notwithstanding the mistakes recognized by his followers and which he himself took pains to rectify in the course of his work. There is room however for more information about his life.

Thirty years ago I published a survey of Jenner's writings, which proved its usefulness in tracing step by step the development of his thought and practice concerning smallpox and vaccination and demonstrating that his discovery was far from being "the lucky guess of a country surgeon." He had continually modified his opinions and his teaching between 1798 and 1822 when new evidence accrued, maintaining all the while the central truth of his discovery. Also discussed were his successful studies in natural history, which had already won him the regard of leading naturalists in England and abroad; scorned by his critics through several generations his findings have been corroborated by more sophisticated modern research.

Jenner's memory has not been neglected in the past three decades, as frequent papers on various aspects of his work proclaim. Attractive biographies by Dorothy Fisk and by Anthony Harding Rains have retold his story for the general public, while more recently the virologist Derrick Baxby has provided a judicial appraisal of the origins of vaccinia virus and Jenner's key position.

The main source of information about Jenner's career will always remain *The Life* by his friend John Baron. Much of Baron's book is fascinating, but it was unbalanced in arrangement and contained noticeable gaps in the narrative. In particular there is little information about the long years through which Jenner practiced in Cheltenham at the height of his powers and fame. This gap has now been filled. Paul Saunders is a long-time Cheltenham resident with an intimate knowledge of the town's history and a fine record as a fighter for the preservation of its architectural heritage. Through assiduous research in contemporary archives and publications he has discovered the leading part that Jenner played in the development of the intellectual and social life of Cheltenham during its most fashionable period, a role far beyond his professional work as its best-known physician. Saunders tells this story in a book full of human interest, for he has made himself familiar with the prominent residents and distinguished visitors who enlivened Cheltenham in the first quarter of the last century. He shows how Jenner attracted their friendship and engaged their interest as advocates in his vaccination crusade. He has added a record of abundant achievement to the chronicle of the last half, the most influential half, of Jenner's working life and expounds the interplay of local and national events and personalities in one of the most important movements in the never-ending pursuit of human health and well-being.

WILLIAM LE FANU

ACKNOWLEDGMENTS

I must express my special indebtedness to William Le Fanu, former Librarian of the Royal College of Surgeons and the world authority on Edward Jenner. His help and encouragement during the past ten years helped so much at times when the work I had embarked upon seemed almost hopeless. To Richard Wolfe, Curator at the Countway Library, Harvard Medical School, I owe a similar debt. His placing at my disposal the unrivalled resources of the library played a vital part in my researches. To Robert Goldwyn of the Harvard Medical School, a lifelong friend as well as medical scholar, and to Estralita Karsh of Ottawa, Canada, also a distinguished medical historian, I must express my deepest gratitude.

I would also like to thank the directors and staffs of the Widener Library at Harvard University, the Boston Public Library, the Dana Biomedical Library at Dartmouth Medical School, Hanover, New Hampshire, the Boston Atheneum, and the Cheltenham Public Library.

I must also thank Bernard Stradling, Gloucestershire County Librarian for granting me access to the Roland Austin Collection at Gloucester and all the other libraries under his jurisdiction. Special thanks are owed to Brian Smith of the Royal Commission on Historical Manuscripts, London, and former Director of the Records Office in Gloucester; David Addison, Director and Keeper of Fine Arts, Cheltenham Museum; Patricia Reynolds of the museum staff; and Rt. Hon. Lord Sherborne, who granted me permission to examine the Manorial Records in Gloucester.

To William Thomson, editor of *The Practitioner,* for publishing my article on Edward Jenner ten years ago, which had a great part in rousing international interest in the subject, and for his continued support ever since, I owe a particular debt of gratitude.

Two different lines of descent of the Jenner family represented by Lucille Bell (formerly Moore) and Zoë Jenner Phoenix have provided valuable help by sharing family lore and documents. I am indebted for the assistance through the years of Charles Parker of the *Gloucestershire Echo* and Noel Witcomb of the old *London Sun*.

I must also thank Mrs. Whyte-Boycott of Malvern, Worcestershire and Mr. R. C. Alcock of Charlton Kings, Gloucestershire, for the use of hitherto unknown letters of Edward Jenner. For the preparation of the final draft of the manuscript I am indebted to my nephew, Richard Saunders and his wife, Frederika, both of Washington, D.C. I must also mention the aid and encouragement I have received from my sons, Richard L. Saunders of Dartmouth College Medical School and Peter Saunders of Mansfield, Massachusetts, and of course the support all through these years of my wife, Jean M. Read Saunders. My devoted mother (1877–1981) failed, alas, to see the fruition of my work.

For services of various kinds I must thank Peter Pezzati, the distinguished painter, Lt. Col. Daniel McCarthy, and Joseph Mc-Veigh, all of Boston, and Mr. and Mrs. Richard Romaine of Groton, Massachusetts. Among all the friends and helpers in Cheltenham I must name, in particular, Thomas Overbury (and Mr. Jones of his staff), my friend the late Victor Moss, and R. M. Morgan, Headmaster of Cheltenham College, who graciously allowed me to photograph the little-known statue of Jenner in the College Chapel.

INTRODUCTION

The splendid old Georgian house at 8, St. George's Place, Cheltenham, where Edward Jenner lived from 1795 to 1820, was demolished by order of the Cheltenham Borough Council in September, 1969. In the process of trying to save the house I did a great deal of research to prove to the town fathers that it *was* the doctor's house, since their initial excuse was that he had not, indeed, lived there at all. In fact, they had placed a plaque on a house farther out of town and safely out of the way of developers' interests. As a result, one of the most important surviving medical shrines in the world was destroyed, and I was left with a vast quantity of hitherto unknown records of Jenner's life.

It was from this building, known as Jenner House, that the great pioneer conducted his campaign to rid the world of smallpox, and as the distinguished journalist Noel Witcomb put it, "he thereby saved more lives than have been lost in all the wars since the dawn of history."

In the eighteenth century, however, many more lives were lost by people being deliberately injected with the disease. Smallpox inoculation was based upon the theory that one could not have the disease twice. Through this inoculation, which was given in many hospitals and clinics established expressly for that purpose, smallpox could be contracted under every available medical and nursing safeguard. The patient, according to practitioners of inoculation, thus stood a better chance of surviving and achieving lifelong immunity if the attack did not prove fatal.

To Jenner, the idea of injecting so foul a disease into a healthy person was unthinkable, and he toiled for more than a quarter of a century to find an allied but relatively harmless malady that might be injected to immunize against smallpox. With his discovery of cowpox, Jenner's research met with success, and incidentally introduced a new medical term to describe injected substances—vaccine, from the Latin root of cowpox, *vaccinia*. But the great pioneer was more than a medical innovator.

Three years of research into contemporary Georgian newspaper files, manorial records, family papers, along with the cooperation of the Jenner family itself, revealed that the historical figure of Edward Jenner was a far cry from the one described in John Baron's 1838 biography, which has remained the definitive biographical work on Jenner. Baron was pressed into the role of reluctant biographer by the very proper Jenner family, who insisted that Jenner be portrayed as a cross between priest and welfare worker. What Baron neglected in his account was the social context of his subject. As a matter of fact, Jenner rode to victory amid the most licentious society in England and supported by a nobility of rakes and courtesans. As opposed to the vast amount of scholarship that has been produced on Jenner's medical contribution, virtually no original research since Baron has been done on his life. It was this dearth that prompted the late Dr. Henry Viets of Harvard to demand that I expand my disorganized mass of evidence into a book. "It crosses a new frontier in medical history," he insisted, and he went on to suggest the title that the book now bears. He also averred that by carefully screening off so many of the great ones of the earth who accepted Jenner as an equal, Baron had innocently contributed to the legend castigated by William Le Fanu, the greatest of Jennerian scholars, that Jenner was "an undistinguished country doctor who by lucky chance made known the preventive of smallpox for which the world was seeking." I trust that by having added a further seven years of research to the original three, we may now cross Henry Viets's new frontier and at last have a true picture of Edward Jenner.

Before he came to Cheltenham, Jenner's efforts to develop vaccination were almost at a standstill. Around his home in Berkeley, though he was appreciated as an excellent country doctor, no one encouraged him. His friends early deprecated what they considered his cowpox obsession, and for fear of ridicule he had to keep his ideas to himself. He confided to a close friend that he had discovered his smallpox preventive as early as 1780, and he inoculated his own infant son in 1789. Nevertheless, the years fled without any success in having his breakthrough taken seriously. Even toward the end of his Berkeley days, when it was obvious that he had an idea worth investigating, Jenner was still ignored both at home and in London. Never, perhaps, has a major advance in medicine had such rough passage to acceptance —particularly in the pioneer's own country—and Jenner was a poor man with no personal resources with which to combat the wealth and influence of his opponents. In fact, judging from the progress he made during a quarter of a century as a country doctor, it is possible to imagine vaccination being ignored or postponed to a more sympathetic age.

In 1795 Jenner came to Cheltenham, and it was most fortunate for posterity that, totally against the current in the rest of the country, the town took him to its aristocratic bosom. The story of his renaissance in Cheltenham is the focus of this book. His life there changed in every respect, and, most important, he was no longer fighting alone. But apart from professional potential, what a social transition the move represented! The grandeurs of Well Walk or the Cheltenham assembly rooms and salons were a million miles away from the muddy lanes and cottages of Berkeley. Instead of lumbering farmcarts, Jenner encountered chariots of prince or peer complete with outriders. The wealth and ostentation in dress and demeanor displayed a society concerned mainly with fashion and culture. England, cut off from Europe by the wars, aped the continental resorts, and its spas were attended by the richest aristocracy on earth. And since the rich can afford their vices, Cheltenham was very much the permissive society with the spontaneous generosity that so often goes with carefree morals.

Jenner's Cheltenham years, then, chronicle a great man mingling in the highest cultural and intellectual circles, and even taking a place as a leader of society. Cheltenham became his refuge when the populace of the country rejected him. The bankers and the belted earls, the actresses and the poets, the princes and the people took Jenner to their hearts and made his survival possible. The rakes and churchmen of the richest of Regency Spas agreed on one thing only: vaccination must prevail. Jenner seems to have met almost everyone who mattered, and his life was trans-

formed quickly and dramatically. Parliamentary grants to support
his research were obtained through the efforts of the Cheltenham coterie of peers, aided by the many great doctors who eventually flocked to Cheltenham to work near Jenner. His arch-
enemy Charles Creighton complained that the doctor's success
was due to "the powerful interests of the county of Gloucester in
Parliament and of the Berkeley family in particular." When the
Berkeleys moved the Berkeley Hunt to Cheltenham in 1809, neces-
sitating their living there in the winter as well as during the season,
this became doubly true. Whatever happened in any other part of
the country, Jenner now had his fortress.

   William Le Fanu has rightly observed that "Baron says little
of Jenner's social life." There were several key friendships during
Jenner's Cheltenham years that his biographer does not even
mention, or if the mere names *are* mentioned there are no details. People like John Hoppner, Michael Kelly, Lord Hardwick,
Joseph Farington, and Sir Isaac Heard, with their wide, fascinating circles, do not appear at all. James Moore, who probably
worked closer to Jenner in the vaccination drive than anyone
else, from 1803 onwards, is covered by the inclusion of many of
his letters, but not a word is said about his *brother,* Charles
Moore, who was the confidant and close friend of Sarah Siddons,
that keystone of the Jenner circle, and her tragic family who
spent a great deal of time in Cheltenham. John Angerstein is
briefly touched upon because of his chairmanship of the Royal
Jennerian Society, but not a word is said of his marriage into
the famous Lock family of Norbury, and how he was a friend of
Jenner's all through his life, visiting Cheltenham every season.
Samuel Lysons of Hempsted Court outside Gloucester is ignored
by Baron, and yet he was the brother-in-law of Charles Brandon
Trye, one of the greatest antiquarians of the day with constant
access to the royal family and who was, moreover, Jenner's patient. Nor is anything said of the celebrated General O'Hara who
introduced vaccination into Gibraltar and had a tempestuous
love affair with Mary Berry in Cheltenham, the same Mary Berry
who later travelled on the Continent with the Hardwicks, who
introduced vaccination into Ireland. But perhaps the biggest gap
is Baron's omission of the wide family relationships Jenner's

wife Catherine had with many of the vaccination pioneers—a phenomenon that explains so much of the Jenner record.

Looking over the Cheltenham list of arrivals of the Master of Ceremonies, one is surprised at the steady and changing stream of doctors who were considered of sufficient social stature to be included. The gradual development of the vaccination crusade made Cheltenham the Mecca of virtually everyone who played a role in the extermination of smallpox. Sooner or later they all got there—the doctors, soldiers, and statesmen from the ends of the earth. Abercromby, Hutchinson, Christie, O'Hara, Wellington, Wellesley, Crichton, and the rest returned from their far assignments to compare notes with those who had worked at home.

Jenner and vaccination are so completely interwoven that it is hard to think of him in any other context. Yet he became very much a key figure in society at large, not merely in medical circles. Although he mixed with influential people, perhaps no man ever met so many of the world's great with so little tangible benefit. He was on social terms with at least three of the royal dukes— sons of George III; he corresponded with Napoleon and the King of Spain; he was received by the monarchs of Russia, Prussia, and several other states; he collaborated with the composer Michael Kelly; and he argued natural history with Sir Joseph Banks. He enjoyed Rowland Hill's sermons and hobnobbed with the gayest libertines in England—Hertford, Berkeley, Egremont, among others. But, even with such a net spread widely beyond his own hearth, he loved his family before all else. Every new domestic event was an adventure—and the family ramifications were as broad as were his interests.

Jenner's life is inevitably an episodic record. Since his wife, Catherine, was virtually a permanent invalid, there was no regular social intercourse with other families, and throughout a great part of his life he hurried home every night. Because of her illness, they had little continuity of experience and little opportunity to plan an ongoing social life. Jenner was subject to every new development in the vaccination campaign as it rose and fell through the years. Outside his house, however, he was always alone on his social occasions.

"It is with relatives alone we feel that unity which allows us unreservedly to exchange thoughts," Jenner insisted; and it was the eroding of this precious family circle that made his later years so tragic. His zeal for vaccination was all he had left then, and he broke away completely from society occasions. He engaged in the Cheltenham Vaccination Conference in 1816, but he would not stay to meet the Duke of Wellington; he helped organize the Winter Relief Campaign of 1816–1817, but he would not attend the opening of the new Masonic Hall; he would visit vaccination supporter Matthew Baillie at Duntisbourn House, but not Governor Raffles at the Plough. He never received a knighthood, though many of the other vaccination pioneers did. I wonder if it would have been different if he had been in the line that welcomed George IV when he passed through Cheltenham in 1821? Loyalty to the tragic Queen Caroline was apparently still more important to Jenner than social advancement.

We find no evidence of one single all-important friend. The Parrys, father and son, came closest to this, but for the greater part of their lives they were in separate towns and met but seldom. It was a friendship stemming from treasured schoolday memories —not from continual and necessary companionship. The only constant in Jenner's life was his devotion to Catherine and to vaccination, and even this was jolted over its rough road by the vicissitudes created by the sorrows of bereavement and public ingratitude.

I have endeavored to set down the social milieu—the people with whom Jenner mixed, their family affairs, and their intrigues. I have dwelt upon the tragic impact of smallpox in the families of people he knew—poor little Miss Hicks and Catherine Pakenham (later Duchess of Wellington). We also look at a sampling of the cases that came before Jenner on the Cheltenham magistrates' bench, and his activity on the town council.

The regal living of the great society doctors never tempted Jenner to protect the vaccination discovery for his own profits. In this respect, he was the country doctor through all his splendid Cheltenham years, where the poor, condescendingly enough, respected him, and the rich loved him notwithstanding his rags.

Edward Jenner

✍ I ✍

The Country Doctor

1749-1794

Edward Jenner was the youngest of the six children—three boys and three girls—of Stephen Jenner, vicar of Berkeley, Gloucester-shire, where he was born on May 17, 1749. His mother was the daughter of the Reverend Henry Head, Prependary of Bristol Cathedral and a former vicar of Berkeley. Stephen Jenner, a man of some learning, was tutor to both the fifth Earl of Berkeley and his brother George—later Admiral Berkeley.[1] The early domestic link with this distinguished family played a great part in Jenner's life and it was George Berkeley who first pioneered the vaccination cause in Parliament.

The Jenners were traditionally a church family; both Edward's brothers, Stephen and Henry, went to Oxford to study for the ministry, and two of his three sisters married clergymen. The age gap between the children was so wide, however, that four of them were already grown-up by the time Edward was ready for school. We are told that the father was "a man of landed property" and he did, indeed, hold the lucrative parish of Rockhampton as well as Berkeley; but putting two sons through Oxford seems to have drained his resources, so that little was left for the youngest boy when both parents died within two months of each other, by December 1754. Shortly before their death, Henry had left Oxford[2] to become domestic chaplain to the Earl of Aylesbury.[3] Since this removed him far away from Berkeley it was left to the eldest, Stephen, as new head of the family, to take the five-year-old Edward under his care.

It is uncertain where Stephen and Edward lived for the next few years, since the vicarage at Berkeley was taken over by the

Reverend George Black early in the new year of 1755 and Rockhampton was occupied by the Reverend Edward Smith within days of Stephen Jenner's death. It is interesting that the little boy should have fallen to the custody of his brother, since his sister, Mary, married the Reverend Mr. Black and might easily have given the orphan a temporary home at the vicarage. As it was, Stephen contrived to cope for the next three years on the slender forty pounds stipend from the perpetual curacy of Stone and later what accrued to him as a fellow of Magdalen College.[4] He took his Master of Arts in 1756 and was ordained the same year. In 1757 the Reverend Mr. Smith, still a young man of twenty-seven, obligingly resigned the parish of Rockhampton and Stephen was appointed in his place. A somewhat saintly and dedicated man, the new rector of Rockhampton never married, but moved with his little brother into the rambling Georgian parsonage that became the Jenner family home for the next sixteen years. The rector's stipend was a comfortable hundred pounds per annum, and the glebe lands consisted of some twenty-seven acres of rich pasture and woodlands stretching all the way to the coast.

Rockhampton was a lonely, scattered parish of a mere twenty-two houses on the shore of the Severn Estuary and subject to disastrous high tides during the winter months.[5] In the spring and summer, however, it was an area of deep lanes and solitary water meadows—splendid country for the lover of nature. Here the child Jenner first developed his interest in habits of the smaller creatures of the countryside.[6] Here, too, during the long summer holidays he first developed his expertise on the fauna of the Bristol Channel, which the great surgeon John Hunter found so valuable in later years. But splendid as this pattern of life was for the holidays, it did not include the necessary element of formal education; there was no village school and scarcely any children of Jenner's age. So it was that, once they were comfortably settled in their new home, Stephen enrolled his young brother at Mr. Clissold's boarding school in Wotton-under-Edge. Edward was eight years old.

It is generally assumed that Jenner's interest in a cure for smallpox was partly a result of his own painful experience of smallpox inoculation as a child. Moreover, he left his home to go to school in the middle of the worst epidemic of the disease since 1723.

Scarcely a Gloucestershire parish escaped it. Every village and market town had its dreary death roll, and, the scarcely more merciful, newly pitted faces to mar the otherwise pleasant countryside.

Lady Mary Wortley Montague's inoculation system was popular in certain areas, and some doctors became rich as a result. In the small town of Wotton-under-Edge during the autumn preceding Jenner's arrival at Mr. Clissold's, at least one enterprising gentleman took advantage of the situation by opening a clinic. "Mr. Huntridge, Surgeon of Wotton-under-Edge," it was announced, "begs leave to acquaint the public that he is now fitting-up his Smallpox house at Tiely, a mile and a half distance from the town for the reception of patients to be inoculated; which patients may be admitted on the most moderate terms. The great success that has attended to his inoculation for the past sixteen years is well-known in the neighbourhood, he having inoculated last spring 446 out of which only four died; and he never had one die by inoculation before."[7] It would seem, however, that the enterprising surgeon's prosperity was short-lived, since his announcement was followed three weeks later by one from Squire Purnell and the churchwardens stating: "The Small Pox is entirely discharged from this town and parish." Undoubtedly, Mr. Purnell did not appreciate people being brought in to have their smallpox at Wotton-under-Edge. One of the Purnell girls, incidentally, whose family controlled most of the wool trade of the county, married the brother of Astley Cooper,[8] the celebrated surgeon, a few years later.

Although Wotton-under-Edge might have been emerging from the disease, the same could not be said of the rest of Gloucestershire. At periodic intervals through 1757, the parish officers of Cheltenham assured the outside world that the epidemic was over. "We whose names are underwritten do certify that the town of Cheltenham in Gloucestershire is now, and has been for six weeks past free of the smallpox." The efficacy of their statement was somewhat marred by the fact that they used the same wording on each new occasion. Actually the scourge was spreading and eventually every quarter of the county was affected. Stow-on-the-Wold, Tetbury, and Winchcombe were stricken, and the town of Newent in the

Forest-of-Dean lamented that the disease had "above a year past raged in this town and neighbourhood." In Tewkesbury it was said: "The smallpox for some time past hath raged in this borough."

The public authority did not approve much of inoculation—the deliberate introduction of the disease. At the Gloucester Assizes, March 21, 1758, it was proclaimed that "All manner of persons . . . entertaining, lodging and receiving strangers as well as those who shall be actually guilty of inoculating them, within the liberties of this city shall be proceeded against with the utmost rigours of the law."[9]

The hazards of smallpox notwithstanding, Wotton-under-Edge was a little metropolis compared with Rockhampton. There were children of Jenner's own age to mingle with at school, and the novel bustle of a market town to enjoy. Besides the butchers and bakers there was even a bookshop (a rare thing in a small country town), and behind it all the great escarpment of the Cotswolds to explore at will. But the young Jenner was something of a solitary and apparently made no friends. His first contacts with formal education resulted in a more orderly interest in natural history, and he was soon studying the lesser members of the animal kingdom with some depth and compassion.

In his maturity Jenner was fascinated by the creatures of the countryside; he wrote verses on the robin, the tomtit, the donkey, and the tiniest of all—the dormouse. In fact, it is this last animal that represents his earliest attempt at research of any kind. At the age of nine, while at Mr. Clissold's, he actually made a collection of the nests of the dormouse, which is, indeed, the only memorial of this year in his first school. But at least one other interest should be noted—the bookshop. The proprietor of this establishment, Joseph Bence,[10] was also a publisher in a very small way; yet he must have made a profound impression, since it was to this humble concern that Jenner returned, after being exposed for some years to the literary sophistication of London, with his first manuscript.

It is, indeed, possible that the especially bitter denunciation of smallpox inoculation in Wotton-under-Edge Jenner made toward the end of his life was on account of his brief residence in the town. In any event, the following year Stephen withdrew him from Mr. Clissold's and sent him to study with Dr. John Washbourne at Cirencester. Since this gentleman was a celebrated headmaster of Cirencester Grammar School, it has always been assumed that Jenner was enrolled directly in that institution. However, Washbourne did not take over the school until the retirement of his stepfather in 1765.[11] Mr. William Mathews, headmaster from 1756 to 1765, is not even mentioned in the Jenner family records, thus it is highly improbable that Jenner studied with him at the school.[12] If he was under the tutelage of Washbourne for his first seven years in Cirencester, it must have been as a private tutorial student—a common enough procedure in those days.

Unhappily, the smallpox epidemic manifested itself more severely in Cirencester than anywhere else in the country. When young Jenner arrived the streets were thronged with pock-marked survivors and the churchyard was steadily filling up with those who succumbed. The churchwardens announced despairingly: "The smallpox must in a short time be entirely over, *there being but few people remaining to have it.*" Nor were they inclined to be merciful to the inoculators. "Whosoever shall presume to bring any person or persons from any distant place or places, into this town (not belonging to this parish) having smallpox *or in order to have it here,* shall be prosecuted with the utmost rigour of the law."[13] Thus the shadow of inoculation followed the boy from his old school to his new one.

The first friend Jenner made in Cirencester was John Clinch, of an old Fairford family. He was destined for the church, but combined this intention with a profound interest in a medical career and did, indeed, end up a medical missionary. Two other boys, Caleb Parry and Charles Trye, entered the Grammar School with Jenner in 1765. They were both from church families and destined for medicine. Parry was the son of the local Presbyterian minister, a man of some literary distinction,[14] while Trye was the son of the rector of Leckhampton, near Cheltenham. These two schoolmates were some years younger than Jenner but of sufficient precocity to be his contemporaries in study. All four boys had a remarkable aptitude for biology; Jenner and Parry, however, shared a further interest and therefore the closest bond. Natural history was their first love and the country about Cirencester, where they made their early childhood forays, remained their favorite hunting ground, to which they frequently returned, for the rest of their lives.

When Dr. Washbourne formally became headmaster of the school in 1765, he soon revealed himself as something of an eccentric because he did not approve of day boys receiving a free education.[15] Since the foundation had been established for the precise purpose of delivering free instruction and since nonpaying scholars normally formed the majority of the student body, the new head's attitude was tantamount to the kiss of death for the school.

Dr. Washbourne would seem to have considered boarders from the country more profitable than town scholars who were accordingly discouraged, and the few that did offer themselves, besides being made to pay quite otherwise than free scholars used to pay, were by him excluded from the free school seats at church and put upon a very different footing from the boarding scholars who numbered between twenty and thirty.[16]

Manifestly, this policy did not go down very well with the local population, and it was obvious that the mercenary doctor's days were numbered. Young Parry—a town boy—was included among the pariahs, though the pew surcharge did not concern him since he attended his father's church. Nor did this early caste approach affect his relationship with his friend Jenner. On the contrary their common dedication to natural history provided the roots of Edward's scientific education while on the other hand, Dr. Washbourne's Greek and Latin lessons failed to penetrate.

It was probably the eagerness to obtain paying customers, as it were, that influenced the headmaster to accept Trye—a little boy of seven—in a student body that normally ranged from ten to eighteen years. The child was the offspring of an impoverished member of an extremely prominent Gloucestershire family. "He was distinguished as a boy of bright parts," it was said, "and soon acquired the common elements of education."[17] As a matter of fact, he became a brilliant classical scholar, far outstripping his older colleague, Jenner. Young Trye left in 1773, and the head dismissed what few boarders were left in 1780. Thus the school came to an inglorious if temporary closure.

Though it is clear that no parental money had been set aside for Jenner's education, his brother Stephen could possibly have financed him had a university career and the Church seemed appropriate. Stephen appears to have fared very well in terms of patronage and eventually, while maintaining the perpetual curacy of Stone, Gloucestershire, he acquired also the parish of Fettleton in Wiltshire. In any case, he was so selflessly devoted to his younger brother that he would have accepted almost any sacrifice to allow the boy a career of his choice. But Edward had not fared very well in the traditional disciplines at Cirencester and certainly had not achieved the required standard in the ancient tongues. Though he had learned little Latin and less Greek, the life of an orphan in an eighteenth-century boarding school had required him to find sources of free entertainment and interest in the countryside around him, precisely as he had to at home in Rockhampton. The cycle of the seasons and the changing colors of nature were the stuff of poetry, and as he matured he developed an even stronger aesthetic sense (curiously blended with scientific speculation), an interest in music, and a detestation of mathematics. After he had been home for more than a year, Edward was apprenticed by Stephen to Mr. John Ludlow, surgeon, of Chipping Sodbury.[18] Apprenticeship to an established doctor was the customary medical education at this time.

When Jenner went off to Chipping Sodbury to be a doctor, it was a completely new departure for the family, which had a long tradition of attendance at Oxford and study of the humanities. Fortunately, however, Jenner found both the subject and his tutor congenial, and he made rapid strides in his craft. The Ludlows were an old medical family with whom he developed a friendly relationship beyond the mere professional association. It was while he was training here that he first heard of cowpox being a relatively harmless substitute for smallpox. A dairymaid happened to be in the surgery on one occasion when the subject of the more serious disease came up, and she observed quickly, "I cannot have smallpox—I've already had cowpox."[19] This sowed a seed of curiosity in Jenner's mind that gradually flowered until the day in June, 1798, when the publication of his *Inquiry* materially altered the history of the world.

Indeed, the young man's early interest was almost inevitable.

The variola plague that had followed him through his schooldays
showed no sign of lessening—smallpox inoculation notwithstanding. During Jenner's apprenticeship, Charles Trye saw the disease
sweep down on the adjoining parish in Cheltenham in the warm
spring of 1769 and carry off a seventh of the population.[20] An
annual death toll of thirty-seven rose to nearly two hundred before the summer season set in and had a marked impact on the
number of visitors to the Wells. Nor were other parts of the
county exempt from the visitation; but the terrible disaster of
Cheltenham, where in addition to Trye so many of the Jenners'
friends lived, was very sobering. Much of Gloucestershire society,
including the Lysons, the Pruens, the Yorkes, the Berkeleys, the
Kingscotes, and, above all, the Aylesburys spent a considerable
part of their lives in this small watering place, which, with a declining population and shrinking income, bid fair to be ruined by
the perennial visits of the cursed plague. Perhaps this was the
phenomenon in the back of Jenner's mind that always made him
keep one foot, metaphorically speaking, in the Gloucestershire
countryside, even during the colorful and rewarding years he spent
in the capital.

Rockhampton seems to have never suffered from the disease;
probably the scattered nature of the parish and the bitter cold
winters were not conducive to incubation. Nor do we hear of any
visitation at Fettleton,[21] Stephen's other living in Wiltshire which
was owned by the Hicks family of Cheltenham. This last village
was a good fifty miles away from Rockhampton and probably not
visited very often by its incumbent. However, since it was in the
possession of the Jenners for so many years Edward must have
been there occasionally. Whatever the relationship of the Squire
Hicks with the Jenner family might have been, it is still the only
tenuous record we have of any friendship emanating from the
Jenners' sixteen years' pastorate of the two villages. Not a single
name of any acquaintance from Rockhampton itself is known, and
it is likely that Edward's long school holidays were spent in solitary communion with nature along the shores of the Severn Estuary. Nonetheless, if there was no human company neither was
there any human disease.

On attaining his majority in 1770, Jenner went to London to

complete his professional studies under the celebrated surgeon, John Hunter, at St. George's Hospital.[22] He actually lived with the Hunters in Jermyn Street, and soon became, so to speak, one of the family, even as he had at Sodbury. It was a friendship that lasted long after the termination of the apprenticeship until the great surgeon's death in 1793. The two London years spent working with Hunter were probably of more value to Jenner than any university course would have been. Hunter's household was an important center of intellectual and cultural debate, and the young man met many distinguished figures of the age whom he would never have met under the normal scheme of things. It was here that he was introduced to Sir Joseph Banks, who returned from his round-the-world voyage with Captain Cook in 1771.[23] Banks was very impressed with Jenner's profound interest in natural history and later offered him a place in Captain Cook's new expedition—an offer which was politely declined. It was probably at this time, also, that Jenner first met Everard Home, Mrs. Hunter's twelve-year-old brother and King's scholar at Westminster, who was to become president of the Royal College of Surgeons.[24] Yet another member of the family who became a lifelong friend was Matthew Baillie,[25] Hunter's nephew, who came to London in 1779 to study under John Hunter's brother, William.[26]

Not surprisingly, during Jenner's sojourn in London many things besides medicine influenced the young man's life. The Hunters had a splendid collection of paintings and, before she married, Mrs. Hunter had already achieved some celebrity in her own right, as Anne Home, the Scottish poet.[27] More important than this, however, was her interest in music, through which she exerted a powerful influence upon Jenner during his formative years when, among his other interests, he learned to play the violin and flute. Some time later the composer Haydn became a friend of the family's and Mrs. Hunter wrote many of the lyrics for his songs. She herself composed on occasion and is remembered today for at least one familiar air, "Lady Bothwell's Lament." Another friend of the family was Joseph Farington, the landscape painter, whose diary remains one of the most detailed records of the Jenner age.

In 1773, having completed his studies,[28] Jenner decided to return to Gloucestershire and follow the career of his heart—that of a country doctor. John Hunter did not wish him to leave but all his blandishments were in vain; the young man took the coach for the West Country and the simple life. He also took with him from Mrs. Hunter a deep knowledge of art and music that stayed with him for the rest of his days. Happy to have his brother back again, Stephen, who had never married, resigned the living of Rockhampton so that he might make a home for both of them in their native village of Berkeley. Meanwhile Hunter was not easily discouraged. Even after his pupil had settled into his new life, the great surgeon wrote and offered him a partnership for the modest investment of a thousand pounds—an offer that Jenner politely turned down.[29]

At this stage of his life Jenner, now twenty-four years old, seemed unlikely to make any particular impact in medicine. His friends in London, including John Hunter, esteemed him for his knowledge of natural history and for being a sincere young doctor. In one of Hunter's earliest letters, after Jenner's return to the countryside, the great surgeon urged him to study the habits of the cuckoo—a task upon which he embarked avidly. On the other hand, Jenner's interest in discovering a remedy for smallpox remained a secret with him for some years. Indeed it seemed that of the three brothers Henry was the most likely to bring a modest fame to the Jenner name. Not only did Lord Aylesbury give him the affluent parish of Little Bedwin in Wiltshire, but as domestic chaplain, the young clergyman spent the summers with the family in Cheltenham, where the Aylesburys were leaders of local society. It was here that Henry—not Edward—must have met and associated with several of the great noble families who later became the pioneers of the vaccination cause. If Stephen's devoted efforts to promote his younger brother's medical career have been inadequately recognized, Henry's have been largely ignored; but the latter's role as a bridge between the humble Jenners and the great ones of Cheltenham society should not be overlooked.

The year that Jenner concluded his apprenticeship with Hunter, Charles Trye was apprenticed to a surgeon in Worcester. A very precocious lad of fifteen, he had no difficulty in keeping abreast of his older schoolfellow, whose footsteps he eventually followed to the tutelage of the same distinguished surgeon in London. Trye's father had died in 1766 and his mother two years later; as a result he was thrown upon the charity of his kinsman Thomas Norwood in Cheltenham, where he spent the holidays. Trye and Jenner were orphans and both had been forced into medical apprenticeship after financial difficulties denied them a university education.

In more prosperous days the Tryes had owned the Hardwick estate just outside Gloucester, but in 1773 they sold it to the Yorke family, and when Sir Philip Yorke was elevated to the peerage in 1754 he took the name of Hardwick for his earldom. Fate decreed, however, that the family should follow the Tryes to Cheltenham, for in 1747 Catherine Dormer of Arle Court[30] willed that mansion to John Yorke, Lord Hardwick's third son, who had married her niece. This gave the family a town house in Cheltenham with the result that the third Lord Hardwick met Jenner in the earliest vaccination days and became one of the first supporters.

But the immediate concern of Jenner was the business of building up a country practice. The two other friends of his schooldays settled far from their Gloucestershire fields: Caleb Parry went to Edinburgh University and John Clinch, after ordination, to the almost unknown isle of Newfoundland. Jenner was a gregarious young man and was soon to discover new faces, among them Edward Gardner of Frampton-on-Severn, who had been to school with Thomas Chatterton and who also fancied himself as a poet of sorts, and Samuel Lysons, son of the rector of Rodmarton, who was related to the Tryes.

Although now officially established at his brother's house in Berkeley, Jenner appears to have had relatively little surgery work; rather he was actually a kind of journeyman doctor with an extremely wide range of practice. As Baron relates:

With some of his particular friends he often at this period of his life spent days in their houses especially in cases of sickness of a serious nature. In this way he made their home for a season his headquarters, and from thence went on visits to his patients in the surrounding districts. In a situation like the vale of Gloucester, this temporary journeying at a few miles distance from his own abode was not attended with much inconvenience from a professional point of view, and it was often a source of recreation and amusement to himself—and I may add of unmingled satisfaction to his friends.[31]

As a matter of fact, most of his observations and research for his work on the cuckoo was done at his Aunt Hooper's farm at Clapton. She was his father's sister, Deborah, and was very devoted to him.

Soon after Stephen resigned from Rockhampton, the living was given to his brother Henry to add to his charge of Little Bedwin.[32] It was a common practice in those days for the incumbent to draw the salary but for a curate in residence to actually do the work. This materially improved Henry's financial position, though his service with Lord Aylesbury forbade his spending much time in his new parish not many miles from Berkeley.

The year 1774 is the first in which any connection between Cheltenham and the Jenner family is found. It may be that Edward visited his friends Trye and Yorke there on earlier occasions, but in June of this year Henry's employers, the Aylesburys, actually made theater history. They discovered the great tragic actress Sarah Siddons[33] playing at the local theater, while, curiously enough, the town was celebrating the completion of an entire year without a single case of smallpox.[34] This remarkable woman whose name crops up so frequently in the Jenner circle should always be remembered for the fact that she first brought the Moore family to Cheltenham—thereby introducing, perhaps, the most important professional connection of Jenner's career.

After seeing her play but once, Lord Aylesbury brought the desperately poor young actress, eighteen years old and with an infant at her breast, to the attention of David Garrick, the most important theatrical figure of the age.[35] The saga of her subsequent rise is more like a fairy tale than real life. Garrick immediately sent his agent, Mr. King, to Cheltenham, and two days later Henry Bate, the great newspaper man, followed.[36] Sarah obtained her contract at Drury Lane and, incidentally, became devoted to Cheltenham and what was to become the Jenner circle for the rest of her life.

As her career developed Mrs. Siddons became increasingly attractive to younger men. Samuel Lysons[37] and his fellow law student at the Inner Temple, Charles Moore,[38] virtually devoted their lives to her service. The young—not as yet great—Gloucestershire painter, Thomas Lawrence,[39] also became deeply attached to her and remained so for the rest of his life. However, unlike the majority of the beautiful and talented women who were to compose so large a part of the Jenner circle, the great actress was of impeccable morality.

If Edward Jenner received a firsthand account of the business surrounding Sarah Siddons's discovery from his brother, he could scarcely have anticipated his own association with almost all these people in the years to come. Nor was he as concerned as his friends, who were far more ready to follow up the glamorous contacts emanating from Henry Jenner's association with the mighty.

In the meantime Jenner's practice was growing comfortably and patients were always hospitable to the easygoing young travelling surgeon as long as he kept off the subject of cowpox inoculation. The idea of direct smallpox injection died very hard in the countryside, and the phenomenon applied to doctors as well as to laymen. Nevertheless, Jenner carried on his researches unceasingly during the years from 1773 to 1795 spent in the country. He could still write to Hunter and occasionally mention his cowpox progress without fear of offending. Meetings at local inns with the few fellow country doctors provided a forum for exchange of views. Two separate clubs were formed at this time. One met at the Fleece Inn, at Rodborough near Stroud, which Jenner called the Medico Convivial Society. One that met at the Ship Inn, Alveston—a smuggler's hideout near Bristol—was called the Convivial-Medico. Occasionally friends who were not doctors were permitted to attend, and the latter part of the evening was always devoted to a dinner with an accent on the "convivial." All the same these occasions afforded valuable opportunities to talk about medicine and exchange ideas. Caleb Parry, who had set up practice in Bath, came to Rodborough when he could, and many of the early stages of his study of heart disease were presented to the company there. Jenner helped him considerably and might well have become a heart specialist himself had he not been so dedicated to seeking a cure for smallpox. An interesting member of the Alveston group was a surgeon of Thornbury named Fewster; interesting because he was later named by Jenner's enemies as the real discoverer of vaccination. As a matter of fact, he not only denied this himself, but at the time of publication of Jenner's *Inquiry* stated categorically that he saw no value in the system and preferred inoculation with smallpox. Sadly enough, Jenner's excessive concern with cowpox eventually irked his medical friends at Alveston so much that he was obliged to confine his observations to his few loyal supporters like Parry, Hunter, and Gardner.

In 1783 Jenner took Henry's son, also Henry, as apprentice and, as a result, had far more time for his cowpox research and his natural history. He appears to have worked the boy extremely hard. "His position was no sinecure," says Baron. "Besides attending to the numberless duties of a strictly professional nature, he found in other pursuits of his uncle many calls upon his time which he was obliged to answer. One of his occupations was to pay a daily morning visit to the nests which contained young cuckoos."[40] Jenner and his nephew formed a very good team, however, and when the cuckoo paper was ready to be read at the Royal Society, Jenner was only too glad to admit what valuable help he had received. Another project in which the boy helped was the study of the migration of birds, which was carried out mainly at Sannighar only a few miles down the Severn Estuary from Slimbridge, where the leading migratory waterfowl sanctuary in the country is now established.

By this time he was a prosperous country doctor with an excellent reputation in both natural history and medicine. Almost no one was interested in his cowpox research. Even Hunter looked upon him for another purpose: as an inexhaustible supply agent for creatures from the Bristol Channel. Dolphins, salmon, eels, seabirds—even a whale that washed up on high tide—were sent to London.[41] Sometimes Jenner's interests strayed beyond medicine and natural history, and in 1783 he arranged a balloon ascent at Berkeley Castle after hearing of Mongolfier's flight in France. No one flew in it, of course, but the poet Gardner affixed some verses to the bag, and they soared over the countryside where no verses had ever been before.

At this time Jenner made several important family connections. In 1784 a very precocious youth of sixteen joined Hunter's anatomy classes; his name was Astley Paston Cooper and he came of an old East Anglian family. Two years later his elder brother, Robert Bransby,[42] married the immensely wealthy wool heiress, Anne Purnell of Dursley, Gloucestershire, and the vast landed estates of the Purnells became the local headquarters of the Coopers. Francis Milman,[43] another distinguished London figure—he was head surgeon at Guy's Hospital—had himself married a Gloucestershire heiress some years previously. This brought him into the Cheltenham orbit and may well have been the occasion on which his well-known friendship with Jenner started. Trye in the meantime was courting Mary Lysons, whose two nephews were also showing signs of early fame. All these men were considerably younger than Jenner but seemed to be outstripping him in the race for recognition in their fields. Samuel Lysons, the younger of the doctor's nephews, while still studying law at the Inner Temple in a desultory manner, was already distinguishing himself as an antiquarian and was elected Fellow of the Society of Antiquarians in 1786. Eventually Jenner's patient, Lysons was an active young man but not physically strong.

In due course young Henry Jenner went off to London to study under Hunter, following in the footsteps of his uncle and the three other distinguished pupils, Astley Cooper, Matthew Baillie, and Charles Brandon Trye. Jenner himself was also in London early in 1787 to discuss vaccination with Hunter and to call on Sir Joseph Banks with whom he had been in sporadic correspondence ever since his apprenticeship years. Banks, also, depended upon him for the supply of information, if not actual specimens, of the fauna of the West of England. It was undoubtedly the influence of Banks that was responsible for Jenner's eventual election to the Royal Society in 1789, though not for his work in medicine but for his contributions to natural history. As he approached middle age, life seemed to be passing him by—at least as far as significant medical recognition was concerned.

Little is known of Jenner's romantic occasions. According to Baron he was crossed in love in 1778, at which time Hunter wrote him "a sympathetic but clumsy sort of letter." In 1788, however, when he was in his fortieth year, he married Catherine Kingscote,[44] a niece of the Countess of Suffolk. Though she was a sickly girl, it was, in the worldly sense, a splendid match. Her father was a rich man and connected with several noble houses. Moreover, the Suffolks were about to become the principal landowners of Cheltenham through their huge property investments in the town's development. After a rather long courtship the couple were married on March 6; they set up house in a rented cottage at Berkeley where Jenner, for the first time in his life, had a house of his own.

They had just about settled in, however, when news came of an event that was to change the whole pattern of their lives. At the beginning of the summer the King had an attack of a mental nature while at Windsor, and on his recovery the royal physician, Sir George Baker,[45] ordered him to Cheltenham Wells for an extended period of recuperation. His Majesty arrived on July 12, and the entire county of Gloucester tried to squeeze into the town, competing with the great national personages for the wholly inadequate accommodations available. The more influential figures of Jenner's still modest circle were in the forefront of all the social activities arranged to welcome the King, including Lord Aylesbury, Lord Berkeley, and Lord Ducie. Catherine's brother, Nigel Kingscote, took up residence in the town as did a relative of Sir Joseph Banks, Sir John D'Oyly. At long last it seemed as though Jenner's friends might pave a way for his ideas to reach the loftiest areas of influence. It was brother Henry, in Lord Aylesbury's suite, however, who found himself in the middle of the auspicious circle around the monarch made up of those who were to be the first pioneers of vaccination: the Duke of York, Lord Oxford, Lord Holland, Lord Kenmare, Michael Kelly, the composer, and the great comedy actress, Dorothy Jordan. Fanny Burney,[46] the Queen's dresser, was also present and must have known the Jenners, since she was a friend of Caleb Parry's, and her brother James had taken up the post with Sir Joseph Banks's South Seas expedition, on Jenner's turning it down in 1772.

If vaccination's first "royal" parent, Dorothy Jordan,[47] was not actually discovered in Cheltenham, certainly her fame was established there on this occasion. She appeared on July 23 for a four-day engagement, but so enthusiastic was the court's response that she stayed for the entire duration of the royal visit. Indeed her reception by the King was every bit as enthusiastic as Mrs. Siddons's by Lord Aylesbury. Two years later she became mistress of the King's second son, the Duke of Clarence,[48] later to become William IV, and mothered the first brood of royal children ever to be vaccinated.

After five weeks the King and his court returned to London. He did not reach Berkeley during his excursion to the local noble seats, but he came quite near when he dined with Jenner's friend and neighbor, Lord Ducie, at Woodchester. The royal visit, however, completely changed the social geography of the county. Cheltenham became the center of fashion and many people who had moved in during the King's residence decided to stay permanently, including some of Catherine Jenner's relatives. Whether Henry Jenner introduced his brother to any of the future vaccination pioneers at this time is uncertain. But after seeing the concentration of hundreds of the men who controlled British opinion at court during these five weeks in Cheltenham, it was apparent to Jenner that vaccination would have a much better chance by being exposed to a larger audience. Jenner at middle age still had to keep his cowpox research virtually to himself in Berkeley, even while his reputation as a naturalist made him something more than a local figure. Indeed, he kept his researches so discreet that vaccination figures very little in his surviving papers and letters before 1787;[49] yet by his own account he had formed his *basic conclusions* as far back as 1780 and his first *interest* during his apprenticeship with Dr. Ludlow some ten or twelve years before that.

Jenner, however, had other problems besides medicine at the time of the King's departure. Catherine was four months pregnant, and being of delicate constitution, she would have to be his main concern until her confinement. The baby was born on January 24 and named Edward after his father. Almost inevitably, John Hunter was the godfather, even though he did not come down to Berkeley for the christening. Ten months later in November, 1789, Jenner felt sufficiently confident of his new system to vaccinate his own son; not with cowpox serum, however, since he had not yet perfected a means for its extraction, but with swinepox matter.[50] A doctor friend, John Heathfield Hickes of Bristol—not to be confused with the Hicks of Fettleton—had been experimenting with this serum during the preceding year and had written a report on it in September.[51] He was, actually, Jenner's first *medical* ally of the vaccination cause in Gloucestershire, since neither Hunter nor Parry practiced in the county and Trye was at this time definitely unconvinced.

The year 1792 brought a number of things to a head locally which adversely affected Jenner's life. The Gloucestershire Medical Society, last of the little discussion groups that had meant so much to Jenner, quietly petered out. Caleb Parry was far too busy in his growing Bath practice to be helpful to Jenner, and Fewster, with his unsympathetic attitude to cowpox research, became an increasingly uncongenial companion. The purchase of Chantry Cottage,[52] a delightful retreat adjoining the village churchyard, gave Jenner the first property he had ever owned. But a decision to give up the surgical end of his practice so that he might concentrate on medicine scarcely helped to replace the purchase price. In fact a country doctor who did not operate was almost useless in a rural practice. Nor was his remaining source of income helped by Catherine's refusal to acknowledge the new "countess" at the castle.[53] It was apparent to virtually everyone that Lord Berkeley was not married to his mistress, but Catherine alone, of all the villagers, openly disapproved. Another problem was the fact that the low-lying fields along the Severn Estuary were not good for a person with tubercular tendencies—particularly in the summer months. Catherine was a young woman of the hills and was never very healthy away from them. In addition, young Henry, now an M.D., married a learned young woman named Susannah Pearce, which meant that he would need a rather larger share of his uncle's practice when he returned from London in the not-too-distant future.

On the other hand, possibilities for starting a medical practice in Cheltenham between 1788 and 1794 were almost perfect, since no one, as yet, seemed to have realized the potential of wealthy visitors. For some reason Sir George Baker had not attended His Majesty when the court was in residence, and the considerable amount of medical attention needed by the royal household was handled by a Dr. Clark, who was, in the manner of the day, previously described as "apothecary" in Moreau's 1783 Cheltenham guide. The field was wide open for a man of Jenner's ability, since none of the remaining promoted apothecaries represented any real challenge. However, if he wished to cater to the public who frequented the Wells, he would have to obtain a doctorate. His long association with John Hunter plus his fellowship of the Royal Society made this a relatively simple matter. On July 8, 1792, he was made *Doctor in Medicine* by the University of St. Andrews on the recommendation of Caleb Parry, M.D., of Bath and J. H. Hickes of Gloucester. It was a purchased degree in the common eighteenth-century pattern.[54]

Not very long afterwards Jenner met Thomas Fosbroke, the new curate of Horsley. Though more than twenty years the doctor's junior this young clergyman eventually became a close friend and provides a main authority for the details of Jenner's middle years. Unlike Jenner, Fosbroke was an excellent classical scholar, yet they had one thing in common—a love of poetry. It was, indeed, a joint literary effort by these two men that brought about Jenner's first contact with the Cheltenham literary scene. One of the leading social figures at the Spa was the learned Squire of Guiting Power—Powell Snell.[55] He was a wealthy, rather pompous but good-natured fellow, who fancied himself a writer and broke into indifferent verse whenever the occasion permitted. An older man than Jenner, he still cut a very gay figure in the 1790s. A production that he had written some years before, but only noticed by Jenner when Fosbroke appeared on the scene, simply invited parody.[56] In these lines from "To Laura," the hard-drinking, hard-riding squire portrays himself as a robin redbreast, who will, indeed, eat the marauding insects who annoy his love:

> "But now the earth throws off her mask,
>   And clouds portend no storm;
> To seize the fly's an easy task,
>   Or bolt the sluggish worm."[57]

To this the waggish Jenner wrote a witty reply, which Fosbroke translated into Latin. The joint effort was then sent to Snell; but far from being offended the poet became a friend of the doctor's and, in due course, a devoted supporter of vaccination. Such was the freemasonry of literary men.

It is possible that Jenner intended to move to Cheltenham on
the retirement of Dr. Clark in 1793, but his tendency to indolence
and the fact that Catherine became pregnant in the autumn delayed matters. Early in October Hunter died, only a month or two
after operating on Farington.[58] For Jenner, Hunter's death marked
not only the end of a friendship of nearly a quarter of a century,
but of a continuing and regular link with the London scene via
their correspondence. Inevitably his intellectual outlet now became
Cheltenham rather than the metropolis.

In 1794, after spending a year as a medical missionary in Newfoundland, Henry Jenner's young son George returned to England
and settled with his uncle in Berkeley. In addition Henry junior,
after finishing his apprenticeship (he was one of Hunter's last)
and qualifying in medicine, arrived with his young wife to resume
his place in the household. Jenner took Henry into partnership,
though the status of George was not defined. The resources of
the practice were being severely stretched by this time, and Henry
was not always an asset to the organization. By his uncle's own
definition, the young man developed into a kind of absentminded
genius whose social common sense did not always keep up with
his keen medical intellect. Be that as it may, he still cannot be
blamed for his part in involving Jenner in one of the most tragic—
not to say terrifying—experiences of his life. It simply happened
that he, of the trio, was on call that particular evening.

At six o'clock on April 17, 1794, a messenger came to the Jenner cottage asking that a doctor be sent to the hamlet of Swanley
on the Bristol road, where a traveller was seriously ill. Young
Henry accompanied the messenger to a small cottage where the
travelling party—consisting of a Mr. and Mrs. Reed, Mrs. Reed's
brother, James Watkins, and a youth named Robert Edgar—was
lodged. The young doctor found Mr. Reed in very poor condition indeed. He was sitting with his head in his hands trying to
staunch a scalp wound, which was bleeding freely, with his handkerchief. He also appeared to be suffering abdominal pain. According to Mrs. Reed, an attractive young woman much younger
than her husband, they had been on their way from Poole in
Dorset to Wales when Mr. Reed was taken ill and they had decided to rest at this cottage. They had been there two days and

his condition appeared to be getting worse. When Henry asked about the head wound the answers were very evasive, but the general idea was that he himself was responsible. The poor man seemed confused and suddenly began to vomit. "Was this brought on by the head pains?" Henry enquired, and was answered by a shake of the head. Reed had vomited before—possibly from drinking some soup that had stood all night in a pewter pot. This then was the strange situation that greeted the young surgeon when he arrived at the cottage. It is possible to piece together the background from evidence at the subsequent trial and entries in the *Annual Register* for 1794 and the *Gloucester Journal* in the week of the trial (April 18, 1796).[59]

Mrs. Reed had married her husband for purely financial reasons and was mainly concerned with obtaining his money as soon as possible and securing as a lover the youth Robert Edgar. William Reed, the husband, seems to have been extremely gullible, and after one or two bouts of sickness, undoubtedly brought about by his devoted wife, agreed to make a will leaving his estate, amounting to some £6,000, wholly to her. James Watkins, her brother and a complete scoundrel, maintained that he could persuade young Edgar to marry her if the husband's death could be contrived. It seems unlikely that the boy had any part in the murder plot, since he voluntarily told the whole story later on—a very risky business had he been guilty. Edgar apparently assumed that the victim was a very sick man and did not have long in this world. One or two attempts to poison the husband having failed, Mrs. Reed decided that a less subtle means might be more effective. Brother James, therefore, undertook the murder on condition that he was paid two hundred pounds. It was clear that nothing could be done in Poole where the family—and possibly even the situation—was known, so they decided to persuade Reed to make a trip into Wales. At some lonely spot on the journey it would surely be possible to achieve their purpose. Reed seems to have been unsuspicious right up to the end. He thought there was nothing strange about bringing the youth along with them, or even his wife's brother, for that matter. Perhaps the fact that Robert Edgar was a medical student made it seem reasonable for him to be in attendance, lest the "sick" Mr. Reed be stricken en

route. It was on reaching that lonely stretch of the Bristol-
Gloucester road just beyond the village of Stone that the plotters
decided that they had found the right place. On the night of
April 15, it was decided to halt at the cottage in Swanley, because
Mr. Reed was in need of rest. They seem to have had an arrangement with the inhabitants of the cottage to prepare their own
food, for Mrs. Reed promptly prepared her husband some poisoned soup, apparently a final effort before more drastic means
were employed. Again it failed. She then called upon her brother
to perform his mission as arranged. Watkins went to the sickroom
and belabored the invalid about the head, but did not succeed
in murdering him. Reed by this time must have been befuddled
from the abuse he was getting, and not really aware of the real
situation. Otherwise the murderers would never have risked the
long, drawn-out process. On the second day at the cottage, more
soup was provided, and a second beating, but this time the landlord, even though the victim himself said nothing, decided that
his lodger was very ill and needed a doctor.

After Henry Jenner's visit, Mrs. Reed persuaded her husband
to go to bed. When her brother entered the room, she told him
"the job was not completed" whereupon he went upstairs with a
broomstick and "struck the unfortunate man several times about
the head," leaving him for dead. As it turned out it was not the
blows that killed him but the belated effects of the poison. When
Henry appeared the next day he was very dissatisfied with the apparent cause of death. He fed some of the deceased's vomit to a
dog who lived at the cottage, and it died within minutes. He
consulted his uncle and murder was immediately suspected. In
the meantime, both Mrs. Reed and her brother absconded, but
young Edgar stayed behind and told as much of the story as he
could to the authorities. Dr. Jenner (Edward) seems to have
taken over at this point, since he was the senior partner in the
practice, and he analyzed the contents of the victim's stomach. He
found evidence of arsenic or mercury poisoning, but not trusting
to this alone, he gave some of the contents to a dog that died as
promptly as the other one had. Charles Brandon Trye also investigated the situation, and the three unanimously decided that
the victim had died from poisoning and not from the head in-

juries. At the inquest a verdict of willful murder was brought against Mrs. Reed and her brother. The brother was never taken. He fled to his father's house at Bishop's Frome, Herefordshire, where he shot himself. Mrs. Reed, however, was eventually arrested by the Bow Street runners, though it is not known how long after the crime. What is surprising is the fact that she was given bail—a most unusual thing in a murder case. She of course loaded all the blame on the conveniently deceased brother and even wrote to her husband's brother in London, commiserating him and condemning the "murderer." For some reason the machinery of prosecution took an inordinately long time, even for those days, and during the next eighteen months the woman may well have hoped that the case had been forgotten. Just after Christmas in 1795, however, she was again taken into custody and committed for trial at Gloucester Assizes.

Jenner's domestic and professional problems were not helped by the fact that the murder of Mr. Reed came almost simultaneously with the conclusion of Catherine's second pregnancy. Fortunately her confinements had been without complication, but the addition of a girl child—much as she was welcomed—did mean yet another strain on the family budget. Little Catherine Jenner was born in the spring of 1794 when the pinch of Jenner's restricted practice was already being felt. To be sure there was now more time for cowpox experiments but the successful culmination still seemed far off and public interest even farther. Jenner also continued to do a certain amount of writing, as he had ever since he came to Berkeley, but little of it was ever published. His pamphlet, *Emetic Tartar,* was printed and sold by Bence, the bookseller of Wotton-under-Edge, in 1783, but caused little comment. His other pamphlet was merely the offprint of the paper printed in the Philosophical Transactions of the Royal Society and entitled *Observations on the Natural History of the Cuckoo.* It was this work that secured his election to the society in February, 1789. Within the next three years it was translated into French and Italian and gave its author a respectable international recognition in the field of natural history. Interestingly enough, Jenner's observations on the cuckoo, at first rejected by leading English scholars, have been completely vindicated by modern research.[60] Another and much more ambitious work on the migration of birds occupied a great deal of his leisure during these Berkeley years but was never published in his lifetime.

By the summer of 1794 arrangements were completed whereby the Berkeley practice could be carried on in Jenner's absence. George and Henry were becoming known to an increasing circle of patients and in some respects better adjusted to local opinion than their uncle. It also appears that Henry senior, with the rest of his family, was staying at the village at this time.

Then, after the heat of the summer, typhus—the scourge of the Berkeley flatlands—attacked the area. Jenner himself was dangerously ill, but the household of Henry was by far the worst hit. He lost his wife and infant daughter as well as one of the female servants. All the survivors in both families gradually improved through the winter though Jenner's life was despaired of for a considerable time. Caleb Parry came all the way from Bath; John Ludlow—his old tutor's son—from Corsham in Wiltshire, and a Dr. Hickes from Bristol. The battle was eventually won but it left the patient in a very weak condition well into the following year. It was obvious that work of any kind would be out of the question for some time, and plans for the future were temporarily shelved. However, his medical advisers decided that a thorough rest of indefinite length at Cheltenham would be of great benefit. The move, Thomas Fosbroke relates, was in no way related to starting a practice in the town but purely for a complete rest and change, "to withdraw himself from the pressure of recurring business."[61] It was well into the spring of 1795 before Jenner was able to travel, but at the end of March, with Catherine and the two children he set off for Cheltenham to take lodgings over a shop in the High Street.

To St. George's Place
1795-1797

When Jenner fell ill in the autumn of 1794 his researches into cowpox inoculation were virtually completed, but the winter and spring of 1794–95 were perforce occupied by recuperation rather than implementation of his ideas. During the previous fifteen years at Berkeley his work had been mainly in the field of naturally contracted cowpox and, to a lesser extent, the kindred maladies of swinepox and horsepox, or grease. He patiently plodded through a pattern of case histories in which people year after year escaped smallpox infection because they had previously contracted the lesser disease. But he had to clothe the bones of a countryside tradition with the flesh of scientific proof.

The first important step in what was then still human medicine had been the discovery that horses frequently infected cows with the common virus, and milkmaids invariably contracted cowpox through the hands from handling the udders. This simple-sounding deduction actually took years of lonely, unsupported research. The idea of injecting cowpox serum into the human system should have seemed a logical extension of smallpox inoculation, but in the early stages the process did not appear so simple. From the beginning Jenner was disenchanted with the practice of deliberate infection. Smallpox was such a terrifying curse to the eighteenth-century mind that being subjected to the disease even under the most favorable circumstances, and with every facility for its treatment at hand, was not always acceptable. Although having one's smallpox to order, as it were, was preferable to catching it unprepared, the death rate connected with inoculation was still high and the likelihood of permanent disfigurement even higher. On the other hand, after twenty-odd years of diligent research, Jenner had failed to uncover a single death from cowpox.

With it all, however, variolation—smallpox inoculation—had a wide and respectable following for over fifty years, mainly because of the influential people who supported it. Lady Mary Wortley Montague, who brought it back from Levant, had the highest connections in society. One very wealthy family, the Parkers of Saltram, devoted a great part of their vast resources to encourage its use, and Lord Borington, head of the clan in Jenner's day, was still completely dedicated.[1] An even greater figure, Lord Lansdowne, lent his patronage to no less a person than John Ingenhousz, the leading inoculator in Europe and former physician to the Emperor of Austria.[2] In fact this distinguished doctor eventually took up residence at Bowood, the Lansdowne seat in Wiltshire, where he died some years later. Nor was variolation purely an English phenomenon; it was widely practiced all over Europe as well as North America, and through all strata of society. It was this well-established system that the country doctor sought to topple at the time of his removal to Cheltenham in 1795.

Catherine's arrival in the town with her ailing spouse and two infant children was modest enough. Instead of a villa or hotel, as one might have expected from her rank and connections, lodgings were taken over a shop in the High Street. Save for the name of the thoroughfare, the exact location of the premises is unknown; but in any case, it would seem that they were only there for a very short period, since there is no shred of anecdote or tradition one would normally expect to find relating to the residence of so important a man. There is a slight clue in the remark of John Fosbroke[3] (Thomas's son) who states: "It is worthy of record that the house which he [Jenner] inhabited on his first settling in Cheltenham is situated opposite a drug shop in the lower part of the High Street, then considered a capital but now an inferior residence; afterwards he resided at 8, St. George's Place."[4] This would place him next door to the Nag's Head Inn, about a hundred yards below the fashionable Smith's Boarding House, but on the other side of the road. There was, indeed, a house on the corner of the present Swindon Street occupied successively by doctors through the nineteenth century and which

local people used to say was "probably" the first Cheltenham address of the Jenners. It could be that the High Street premises
were used during an earlier visit or during occasional professional
calls on Berkeley patients who were visiting the town, and that 8,
St. George's Place was only taken when he needed a permanent
home.

The younger Fosbroke does not give a date to Jenner's first
professional *visits* to Cheltenham, but he does mention that "for
some years he was the sole physician of note in the town."[5] This
would certainly not apply to 1795, but it could relate to the two
years after Dr. Clark's retirement in 1793. It should also be noted
that the terrace in St. George's Place, specifically described as being inhabited from the beginning by "families of the highest
distinction,"[6] was built in 1795, the year Jenner actually *settled*
in Cheltenham on either a seasonal or permanent basis. The
weight of evidence, then, seems to indicate that he was staying in
his High Street lodgings when the new terrace was completed,
whereupon he decided to set up his practice at number eight.
But before going into details about his settling in, it might be
well to look at the society into which he was about to be im-
mersed. Like most country doctors, Jenner was a relatively poor
man living in a world of small farmers and peasants. Save for the
village squire and a few scattered fellow medicos, his daily routine
was naturally among the humble and unlearned.

It is hard to tell just who amongst the many important families
he might have already met through his brother's connection with
the Aylesbury's, but the majority of the peers, bankers, and statesmen would be completely outside his terms of reference in the
normal scheme of things. Of particular interest was the considerable number of unusually attractive female intellectuals who frequented the Wells. Fanny Burney, who knew the place so well
before and up to the visit of the King, did not return after her
marriage to General D'Arblay, but her friends, the Berry sisters, were very much in evidence.[7] Agnes and Mary Berry, equally
the protégées of Horace Walpole (Lord Orford), were both
talented writers, though not in the first flush of youth. The Lock
girls from Norbury, also gifted as well as beautiful, formed, through
their family connections, part of a much wider constellation of an

attractive intelligentsia.[8] Sporadically reigning over this coterie
was that grand old dame of eighteenth-century society—the
Duchess of Leinster. Thomas Coutts, the banker, regularly
brought his covey of marriageable daughters. The bluestockings
were deserting Bath for Cheltenham, and a large proportion of
them became involved in what can be called the Jenner circle.

Coutts was a member of the old guard—those who had been
coming regularly to the Wells ever since Lord Aylesbury's first
appearance. Another protégé of Coutts was the minor poet William Bagshaw Stevens,[9] a regular summer resident who courted
the muse with Powell Snell. Young George Monk Berkeley,[10]
grandson of the philosopher and a more promising poet than
either of them, had died at the Wells only the previous summer.
He was a colleague of Lysons's and Charles Moore's at the Inner
Temple, and was greatly mourned by the literary set. Charles's
father, the famous physician-novelist Dr. John Moore,[11] was
medical advisor to half the society women at the Wells, though
he never seems to have followed them or his son thither. Just as
Sir George Baker had not attended the King to Cheltenham, so
old Dr. Moore—sour, irascible, and expensive—let the ladies of
a dozen noble houses pursue their follies or pleasures unsuper-
vised. The Berrys and the Locks were also under his care, though
—by and large—they were far more circumspect in their behavior
than their grander sisters. In London, as yet showing no indication
of his future fame as an international vaccination authority, his
other son, James Carrick Moore,[12] was building up a fashionable
practice that threatened to outshine his father's. At this point the
sole member of the Moore family in Cheltenham was the mouse-
like Charles—who wanted simply to be near Mrs. Siddons.

When the Jenners arrived the town was agog with the dramatic
closing stages of Warren Hastings's trial, which had been dragging
on for more than seven years. Since the great Indian statesman
came of an old Cheltenham family his acquittal on April 23
caused great rejoicing. The real hero of the hour was the relatively obscure barrister Edward Law, who brilliantly defeated the
formidable array for the prosecution.[13] Law was to become Baron
Ellenborough, Lord Chief Justice of England; he also became, as
we shall see, one of Jenner's falsest—not to say most ungrateful—

friends. At the time of the trial Lord Suffolk, Catherine's uncle, was possibly the biggest landowner in the town and, in collaboration with the lawyer Joseph Pitt, played an increasing part in its development.[14] There is no record of Lord Suffolk's having provided any direct assistance to Catherine upon her arrival in Cheltenham, unless perhaps he had a hand in the selection of a permanent residence. The land on which the doctor's future home was then being completed was owned by Pitt, who had recently bought a great deal of land from Suffolk "north and south of the High Street." Fortunately Catherine's other two relatives in the peerage, Lady Peyton and Lord Rous, who only started coming to Cheltenham when the Jenners settled there, were much warmer in their friendship and more generous in their patronage.[15] All in all it would not be too hard for Jenner, after a long rest, to build up a comfortable practice among these rich people should he be so inclined. Then would come the completion of the cowpox experiments and their announcement to a world of intellectuals rather than to an uncomprehending peasantry.

Jenner, however, was not the only one to see possibilities in the town's paucity of real doctors. That very same summer of 1795 another seeker after Dr. Clark's mantle arrived in the person of Dr. Thomas Newell—well-connected, well-qualified, and only thirty-three years old to Jenner's forty-six.[16] He was accompanied by his wife Lucrezia and their infant son born the year before. But no rooms over a shop for him! Since he was a fairly rich man, he took the De la Bere mansion in High Street until he decided upon a permanent residence. His presence did not lead to any unhappy rivalry, however. The two families settled down amicably and eventually occupied premises in the same street almost next door to each other. Perhaps it should be recorded that they differed in politics. Newell was an enthusiastic Conservative and Jenner was a Whig.

At this time Cheltenham was really a town of one street, with but one coach road—St. George's Place—leading off it. The royal visit, however, had resulted in social amenities out of all proportion to the town's size. The Assembly Rooms were built in the grand manner and the Theatre Royal, even after the King's departure, provided fare worthy of the capital. Not only were the greatest figures of the stage regular performers—Siddons, Kemble, Jordan, Kean were almost accepted as permanent residents—but for Jenner many contacts were made that would never have been possible outside London. Prince Hoare, at his peak as a playwright, certainly spent the 1795 season in Cheltenham where he probably met Jenner for the first time.[17] His *Three and the Deuce,* the first dramatic work ever written about Cheltenham, was produced at the Haymarket when he got back to London September 2. It is a typical eighteenth-century farce of life at a fashionable watering place and dwells in part upon the pretty girls who frequented the Wells.

Jenner's observations on the same subject are very similar, though Hoare makes no comment on their additional intellectual charm. It will be remembered that Joanna Baillie, Matthew's sister and one of the successful playwrights of her day, was practically a member of Dr. Hunter's household, and her psychological plays represent an early link between medicine and the drama. In his intimacy with the Hunters from 1770 to 1793, Jenner—avid conversationalist that he was—must have had many opportunities for discussions of psychodrama.

Such then, socially and geographically, was the haven chosen for Jenner's convalescence. He was still a sick man, and his prime needs were for rest and freedom from worry. By all the evidence, he paid little attention to what went on in the outside world—particularly the world of medicine—and was nurtured by Catherine in a protective cocoon of picture galleries, poetry, and music. Before the summer was over, Jenner would complete a whole year away from the stress of medical practice. Perhaps he had already forgotten the vaguely pending murder trial—but as it turned out everything had been going a little too easily.

His two nephews in Berkeley had taken over the complexities of a well-established professional practice much too boldly, almost as though they never really expected their uncle to return— or if he did, only as an invalid and not to be seriously reckoned with. So, while Jenner was setting out to rebuild his health in Cheltenham, the nephews were very busy indeed trying to undo his work at home. He had apparently made no arrangement for any kind of periodic report on the business as the rather astonishing events of the spring indicate. There is every reason to believe that Jenner had long since given up any serious consideration of smallpox inoculation, particularly since in 1789 he inoculated his son with swinepox serum and was only a year away from his first successful vaccination. Yet the two brothers in Berkeley apparently began smallpox inoculation the moment he left the village. "In the Spring of 1795 three hundred and nine persons were inoculated with the smallpox in the town of Berkeley by Henry and George Jenner, all of which recovered." Thus ran the entry in the Berkeley Parish Registers.[18] The number is enormous for so small a place and might well have been an expression of the village's disapproval of Jenner's vaccination research. It is significant that such a mass operation when it became known was completely ignored by the family and never mentioned by Jenner himself. Perhaps George and Henry, like the other doctors in the area, were also worried by their uncle's obsession. It is a fact that years later Jenner referred to Henry as a fool.[19] It is ironic that in a county generally suspicious of smallpox inoculation, Berkeley was the site of a large number of inoculations.

But medicine, and even vaccination, had to be of secondary importance to Jenner for the time being. When the patient was completely recovered the fight would be resumed—but the immediate focus was on recovery and distraction. It was sad that in great part these pleasant distractions had to be undertaken alone. Though Mrs. Jenner obviously loved Cheltenham—all the evidence points to this—her name seldom appears in any record of the doctor's activities. She could undoubtedly walk gently in the sunshine as far as the Wells, sip the waters, and enjoy the colorful company about her. She could chat quietly with Edward and perhaps browse through one of the bookshops or art salons, but there it ended. Jenner was always alone. One can only assume that she was forbidden evening activities by the state of her health. She always had to be at home when the sun went down. Fortunately, however, the country around the town provided unlimited scope for driving, and she had many friends to visit if weather permitted. There were the Norwoods at Leckhampton Court (Trye's cousins) and Trye himself in Gloucester, where Catherine could eagerly examine the working of his newly established Charity for

the Relief of Poor Lying-in-Women. Then there were the Lysons
(Mrs. Trye's brothers) at Hempsted, only a few miles out, and
the Hicks at Witcombe Park, while new and interesting people
were arriving every day. Jenner, meanwhile, with no medical responsibilities to take up his time, rapidly carved himself a solid
position in local society.

The season was well advanced when one of the more colorful
military figures of the age came to Cheltenham immediately after
being released by the French. General Charles O'Hara was captured at the siege of Toulon and held prisoner in Paris all through
the Reign of Terror.[20] Farington relates in his diary: "Lysons (the
antiquary) was much with General O'Hara at Cheltenham and
heard him describe his condition while in France. At Lyons they
obliged him to remain near a guillotine while about forty persons were executed, most of them women; and some girls not
more than fifteen years of age."[21] There are many more para-
graphs of harrowing sadism that must have left the listeners
round-eyed or, in the case of Jenner, filled with horror tempered
by scientific interest. Lysons, O'Hara's companion on this occasion, was a water colorist and draftsman of ability. He illustrated
much of his antiquarian topographical work himself and has left
us pictures of many local landmarks as they were in Jenner's day.

The reason for O'Hara's hastening to Cheltenham immediately
following his release was to join the Berry sisters. He had made a
tentative engagement gesture with Mary before he had gone
away to the wars, and now he wished to make it official. It was
kept from the public, however, until some months later. This
coterie, already the friends of Lysons and Farington, was possibly
the link between Jenner and Charles James Fox, who came to
Cheltenham with his wife every season during the closing years
of his life. Fox lived at Vernon House, a tall Georgian building
that is still standing just off the Bath Road beside the Chelt.
Close as the Jenners and the Foxes ultimately became, I have
not been able to discover the actual time and circumstances of
their meeting save that it was in Cheltenham. I do not believe
that Fox was ever Jenner's patient. Lysons, on the other hand,
was of a rather delicate disposition and was eventually the patient of both Jenner and Matthew Baillie. As for General O'Hara,
he was gone again in September, and the next news Jenner had

of him was his energetic promotion of vaccination in his colony of Gibraltar three years later. His three weeks in Cheltenham had borne excellent fruit.

Though interested in all the arts, drawing and painting were not among Jenner's accomplishments (unless we include an "anatomical" sketch in a butcher's shop as art). But during this first summer at the Spa he was able to move with some celebrated figures in the art world the like of whom he had not seen since leaving John Hunter's house. He had been starved of this life for many years, and in his unusual state of temporary medical dissociation, he was drinking like a parched traveler at an oasis. It was a brilliant season, and everyone in England seemed to be on hand if only for a few days. Like as not he would never see some of these dashing people again, but the fleeting taste was still savored and enjoyed.

As we shall see, Jenner was greatly impressed by the efficacy of the mineral waters, but in these early years it was Baillie who played a dominant role in the rise of the Spa by sending the most distinguished patients there. He sent the Duke of Gloucester (George III's son-in-law) to Cheltenham at the turn of the century, and the prince was so impressed that he maintained a seasonal residence there for the rest of his life.[22] It was believed in those days that there was a certain complementary character between the waters of Cheltenham and Bath, and some doctors would recommend a course at one resort to be immediately followed by a course at the other. This relationship continued into the vaccination age when a number of Bath doctors, including Thomas Creaser and the younger Charles Parry, moved to Cheltenham permanently. Unlike Bath—and most other spas—Cheltenham waters were available all over the town. New wells were constantly being sunk and many varieties of mineral treatments were available. Of course the fashion gathered at the Royal Well— the original one—but speculators during the turn of the century made a great deal of money in opening rival ones. Even the Tryes had a mineral spring at Leckhampton Court, no doubt frequently patronized by the not-too-affluent Jenners. Failing that, the Jenners might have sampled Lord Hardwick's "purging spring" at Arle; and there was a similar one at the Hyde in Prestbury. In the latter village there was a delightful resort called the Grotto,

owned, at that time, by a Mr. Darke. It was a favorite spot of the
Jenners', being only two miles from the center of the town yet
having all the seclusion of the remotest countryside. It consisted
of "a pleasure garden, summer house, and grotto much frequented by breakfast, dinner or tea-drinking parties."[23]

Not all the people who came to Cheltenham after the King's
visit were fashionables, of course, and when Jenner arrived he
found several elderly men, part of the Bath-Cheltenham contingent, who came purely for the benefit from the waters. The celebrated author Christopher Anstey belonged in this category.[24] At
seventy-five, he was a fascinating old "period piece," arriving bag
and baggage with his family every summer. He was the eighteenth-
century "sipper of waters" and associate of doctors—a pedant but
an excellent versifier; a satirist but not cruel. His great work,
The New Bath Guide, is all about doctors and invalids and had
tremendous popularity. He was in Holy Orders but was a writer
beyond all else. In 1762 his earliest collaboration with the medical
world took place when in conjunction with a Dr. Roberts of
Bath he translated *Gray's Elegy* into Latin. The *Guide* followed
two years later and had such a phenomenal success that Dodsley,
the publisher, declared "that the profits on the sale were greater
than he had ever gained in the same period by any other book."
When Dodsley gave him two hundred pounds for the copyright,
Anstey promptly gave the money to the Bath Hospital. He quickly
became a great admirer of Jenner's. He was probably introduced
to him by Caleb Parry, and when they first met during that summer of 1795, the old poet was still very active and indeed had
just brought out another work. Anstey wrote light verse with
ease and fluency—much more polished than Powell Snell's but
somewhat in the same nature. In what must be the earliest lines
on Cheltenham by an established poet, he gave us, between 1780
and 1790, the following from "On the Recovery of a Young Lady
by the Use of the Cheltenham Waters":

> With pining sickness worn, her beauty fled,
> Hither my Charlotte's trembling steps I led,
> Meek and resigned from this salubrious Well
> She drank, and on the cup a blessing fell.[25]

Jenner's recovery—though not entirely due to the waters—was also a Cheltenham phenomenon. The complete change of his life pattern brought him from the brink of the grave, and his senses were for a few precious months happily able to dominate his intellect. His monumental contribution to medical science has often overshadowed his competency as a poet, musician, and art critic. These vital aesthetic interests were for the first time in his life his primary concern during the summer days of 1795. The years he had spent in London in the Hunter circle and the excursions he made there later did afford scope for certain cultural contacts, so that some of the faces he saw in the Cheltenham walks were not entirely new. Through Hunter he had met Philip Loutherburgh, the historical painter—a strange man, who came to England from Germany in 1771 primarily to paint theater scenes for Garrick.[26] Referring to Jenner, Farington tells us: "He knows Loutherburgh, and observed that he does not receive remarks on his work graciously. While Loutherburgh was painting one day John Hunter remarked that a certain part was too green: 'Not green enough!' said Loutherburgh, and dipping his pencil in the strongest green colour, put it on the canvas."[27] Nor was Jenner himself above blunt criticism if the spirit moved him. A comment of the younger Fosbroke's provides evidence of the doctor's interest in art, which continued to the end of his life.

His nephew, (Stephen) possessed talent for comic painting, and the superintendence of this youth's endeavours formed the amusement of his latter days. Of conception, originality and design in art, he possessed a good knowledge, as well as a correct eye and cultivated taste. An error in his nephew's colouring excited the following epigram:

> "What strange expressions fell from Peter Pindar's chops
>   The academic clouds he calls brass mops;
>   But (Stephen) fills us higher with surprise,
>   He throws long gravel walks across the skies."[28]

The attractions of a cultural and social nature with which Cheltenham abounded were matched by the more routine attractions any town had for a countryman. Jenner was fascinated by the butchers' shops of which there were six or seven. For him they were everchanging dissection exhibits, and he used to walk round with his great notebook in his hand making notes on certain cuts of meat and even doing quick sketches on the spot. If anything in particular interested him, he did not hesitate to enter the establishment and beg permission for a closer examination.[29] The apothecaries also held fascination for Jenner. At Mr. Cother's no less a personage than Savory, of Savory and Moore, had been apprenticed. This firm was already in Jenner's time a Bond Street landmark patronized by the highest in the land. But most of the Cheltenham apothecaries called themselves "doctors" following the King's visit.

The town medical officer or "Doctor to the Vestry" was Thomas Minster[30] who lived next door to the George Inn. He handled all the charity work and was later to have special duties in the vaccination program, treating certain poor children at five shillings a head. When he was appointed in 1793 he received a salary of eighteen pounds per annum with the stipulation, however, that "broken bones, smallpox and lying-in women were to be exempt from the said sum."[31] Dr. Hooper, who seems to have been the favorite of the fashionable set after Dr. Clark's retirement, lived in a regal style at the Great House in St. George's Place and, when King George III came to Cheltenham, it was along this quiet backwater that the royal cavalcade travelled on its drive to Fauconberg House.

Fanny Burney gives us our first description of Jenner's future home, St. George's Place:

When we arrived at Cheltenham which is almost all one long street, clean and well-paved we had to turn out of the public way about a quarter of a mile to proceed to Faunconberg Hall. It is indeed upon a most sweet spot surrounded by lofty hills beautifully variegated and abounded, for the principal object with the hills of Malvern.[32]

Walking from their quarters in Lower High Street, the Jenners would have passed along this thoroughfare every day on their way to the Wells. It is not surprising that as Jenner grew stronger he began to think about suitable premises in which to open a Cheltenham practice. On the left-hand side entering from the High Street was the fine terrace of four brand new houses. Perhaps, indeed, he even witnessed their completion. Their tall Georgian facades were graced with small iron balconies, and shallow steps led to wide front doors with delightful fanlights over them. There were a few other houses on either side of the road, but this terrace outshone them all. Almost opposite in 1795 was the group of buildings occupied by William Archer's livery stables. This well-known Cheltenham character was the great-grandfather of Fred Archer, whom so many called the greatest jockey in the world. Further down toward the Chelt was the old Friends' Meeting House, dating from 1660, where William Penn once preached. The four new houses are listed in the earliest Cheltenham directory as the leasehold of a Mr. Lambert, who also owned livery stables in the High Street. They were subleased, however, and there are no names of tenants listed.[33] Only when Jenner bought number eight, the one at the far end of the terrace, in 1804, was his name given at this address—the only address, incidentally, at which he was ever listed in Cheltenham. The fact that he himself never mentioned his lodgings in High Street might have been due to an eagerness to leave them. Good accommodation was very scarce in the town unless one could afford the Plough or George, and the doctor with his wife and two children certainly could not. In 1793 Moreau's *Tour to Cheltenham Royal Spa* laments: "A good general Boarding-Table seems to be much desired by the Company, and would certainly answer to any person, well-calculated, who may establish one."[34]

In all probability the motivation behind the move from lodgings to an independent residence was the decision in late summer to resume practice. Despite the fact that Thomas Fosbroke insists that the sojourn in Cheltenham was intended solely for recuperation and rest, as the months of lotus-eating went by, the poets and painters lost a little ground to Jenner's old love, medicine. It was not to cowpox inoculation that Jenner returned, however, but to a terminal case of dropsy. He had been away from practice for a whole year; it was inevitable that sooner or later in his continual social mingling, someone would seek his advice. As a matter of fact it was a fellow doctor—almost certainly Thomas Newell. As John Fosbroke put it: "There (in Cheltenham) practice as a natural result of high medical reputation was forced upon him"; a medical reputation apparently based on his conversation over the months, since he had attended no patients.[35] It was Jenner's

almost uncanny power of diagnosis that brought about his dramatic return to practice. (He could assess a person's condition in
many cases without examination—even in instances of obscure
and unsuspected diseases.) Called into consultation "by a learned
physician" with regard to a lady of fashion who was described as
"having a tendency to dropsy"—a disease for which the Cheltenham waters were a celebrated cure—Jenner was taken by his colleague to her house, where they found her up and dressed, sitting
on a sofa. She was, indeed, expecting company that evening. As
soon as Jenner saw her, he knew that she was dying; "a judgement
warranted by the expression on her countenance and other
moribund appearances to which he paid particular attention."
Apparently the other doctor did not take the opinion seriously.
When Jenner convinced him to the contrary, he then dissented
very forcefully "as to the indications of approaching dissolution,"
and they parted from the patient. The dire situation had grown
even more apparent during the time they were with her, however, and as they were leaving the house, "a female domestic
asked him (Jenner) what he thought of the mistress's state of
health." He told the poor girl with the bluntness he occasionally
showed that "it would not surprise him if she died within the
hour," but in any case he would call back then. When he returned
he was greeted by the same tearful maid who informed him that
her mistress had died at the exact time he had predicted. "This
incident," concluded Fosbroke, "was locally celebrated in a very
extensive degree."[36]

Though this celebrated resumption of general practice may
have been "forced" upon him, once launched Jenner entered into
it wholeheartedly and apparently did nothing in the way of cowpox research for the rest of the season. No sign exists of any letter or communication on the subject throughout his summer in
Cheltenham, nor is either Henry or George Jenner mentioned. On
the other hand, since all his research materials were in Berkeley,
the simple explanation of his conduct might have been his concern to make as much money as he could during the remainder of
the season—possibly so that he would be in a position to move
into the new house in St. George's Place. Besides the wealthy Dr.
Hooper, Jenner would now be the neighbor of Lord Faucon-

berg[37] at Bayshill Lodge, or at least he would be situated on the only thoroughfare that led to it. His lordship was one of the Grooms of the Chamber to the King, and what is more important, father-in-law of the Duke of Norfolk, who was to become such an important vaccination patron. Fauconberg's daughter, Lady Bellasye, was a rather wild girl; after bearing the Norfolk heir, she found herself a new lover—Lord Bingham, who became Earl of Lucan in 1799. The subsequent divorce had caused a great stir in the town the previous year, though it does not seem to have impaired Lady Bellasye's position in the highest circles, including the court.

If Jenner's expanding social connections and the commencement of a lucrative, fashionable practice turned him from his vaccination research for the time being, the permanent enemy, smallpox, nonetheless intruded into his summer idyll before the season was over. William Hicks, son of Sir Michael Hicks of Witcombe Park, had moved to Cheltenham from Bath the previous year and bought Belle Vue House, at the upper end of the High Street. Jenner knew the family well from the days when Stephen had been incumbent of their village of Fettleton.

William Hicks's financial position had greatly improved when his father had unexpectedly inherited the baronetcy in 1793, thus he was able to cut a prosperous figure when he arrived in the town with his wife and infant daughter. He was even selected to be officer-in-charge of the Cheltenham cavalry yeomanry at the end of the year—an event which his friend Powell Snell suitably commemorated in verse—though the appointment was scarcely in keeping with his modest physique or gentle temperament. Actually Hicks's life thus far had been one of tragedy and disappointment—nor did it improve significantly as the years went on. He was five years Jenner's junior but appeared much older and had a severe stutter. After his first wife died without leaving surviving issue, Hicks had married again at the age of thirty-nine. The young woman was "not pretty," but she presented him with a daughter, Ann Rachel, in 1794, just before they left Bath.[38] Initially there were some financial difficulties, even though the new wife came of a well-to-do family, but worse than that, soon after they settled in Cheltenham in 1795, the infant was stricken with smallpox. Jenner was certainly not practicing at the time, and though vaccination was still a year away, Ann Rachel did manage to survive. "Little Ann has recovered from the smallpox and looks very sprightly and clear from any humor,"[39] wrote her mother to the grandparents, but things were by no means as satisfactory as her statement suggested. If smallpox had not killed on this occasion, it had still destroyed. The child was stunted and, even if not pitted, tragically ugly. Later in the year, her maternal grandmother wrote that at the age of eighteen months Ann had not yet cut a tooth. Nor did she ever really recover her health. All through the years of her childhood she remained a pitiful case history of the lasting effect of smallpox. The piteous infant wreckage of a friend's child was a sobering reminder to Jenner of the urgency of his life's work.

It is probable that Jenner did not stay in Cheltenham right up to the end of the season in mid-November, since he does not mention the Cheltenham earthquake that took place on November 12.[40] As it happened, Jenner's return to Berkeley was a very melancholy occasion. The family had scarcely settled in when news came that Henry Jenner's third son, Lieutenant Stephen Jenner, had been drowned off Portland Bill when his troopship was wrecked in a storm on the way to the West Indies on November 18. Jenner's summer of rest, poetry, and music ended abruptly. The move to Cheltenham had gone off smoothly enough, to be sure. What had started out as a holiday for health reasons had developed into a prosperous new practice and precious patronage in the highest circles.

But Lieutenant Jenner's death was not the only counter blow. Scarcely was Jenner back in Berkeley when news came that the trial of Mrs. Reed was set down for the next Gloucester Assizes. The specter of this pending event must have intruded occasionally on those idyllic hours in Cheltenham, but in the spring, when Jenner was finally returning to his vital vaccination project, the specter became a grim reality. He was summoned to appear on March 28 to testify for the Crown against Mary Reed in what appeared to be a certain conviction and execution. In effect, he and Trye had the young woman's fate in their hands. Nor was she being tried merely for the murder, but, despite an Act of

Parliament passed four years before, she was charged with the more serious offense of petit treason for which the traditional penalty was to be drawn and burned at the stake. By far the commonest form of this crime was the poisoning of the husband by the wife. Indeed, in Jenner's own lifetime Ann Williams had been burned in Gloucester for killing her husband, and[41] as recently as 1789, a Mrs. Murphy had been strangled and burned in front of the debtor's door at Newgate for the petit treason of coining. To a person of Jenner's sensitivity, the crudities of the eighteenth-century penal code must have been horrifying, and Trye's situation was even worse. His home, Friar's Orchard, was almost within sight of Gloucester prison, where the wretched woman was incarcerated, and probably every day during the months of waiting the sight of those forbidding walls would remind him of the ordeal ahead.

If there was any alleviating factor in the matter, it was in the person of the judge himself, Sir Soulden Lawrence.[42] Although he was not renowned for his softness to the felons who came before him, he would possibly be patient with the two unfortunate doctors who were to be his main prosecution witnesses, since he was the son of Thomas Lawrence, President of the Royal College of Physicians from 1767 to 1774. As it happened the judge turned out to be unexpectedly—and untypically—considerate.

The awful day of the Assizes arrived, a crisp March morning burgeoning with all the promise of the opening spring. The prisoner, dressed in white, arrived at the court in a sedan chair. Understandably enough, she looked very nervous but "well nourished and in good health" notwithstanding her three months in prison.[43] Her counsel, Mr. Briggs, was an able psychologist. From the beginning—since the evidence itself was so damning— he was determined to use the prisoner's youth and beauty as a vehicle to move both judge and jury. When she stood in the dock, a delicate lonely figure, she looked so pathetic that his lordship ordered a chair to be brought for her—and then the long, apparently hopeless ordeal began. Having so little concrete evidence for the defense, Briggs concentrated on trying to tear down that of the prosecution. After Henry had given his evidence, Jenner asked the Court's permission to cross-examine him. He wished to make it absolutely clear that he had studied every minute point before he himself testified. There was no question in his mind as to the wretched girl's guilt, but nevertheless he must not be her judge. He must merely state the detailed facts of that fatal day exactly as he had found them. Trye, an intensely religious man, was even more upset. He, too, had to choose between the law of evidence and the quality of mercy, but he had to say that it was a case of death by poisoning. He pointed out that he had been a surgeon for twelve years—perhaps to show that he was guided by experience and scientific reasoning rather than by the wish to condemn a sinner.

When Jenner entered the witness box, Briggs exerted great pressure to make him concede that the dead man could conceivably have died a natural death. But the witness in his quiet way was unswerving. Without being aggressive he merely reiterated with great patience that "he did not think that Mr. Reed had died a natural death." Jenner agreed with Trye. His unchanging version of events was factual and unemotional—but extremely damning for the accused. Briggs could do nothing with him and the judge solemnly noted down Jenner's concluding remarks: "Mr. Reed did not die of an injury to the head, nor of a natural cause, considering how soon after taking the soup the distemper took place. . . . Some poisonous substance was taken into the stomach. . . . He grounded his opinion on the dogs, taking in the other circumstances."[44]

The judge was determined that the case should be concluded that day, and after the testimony had droned on for ten wretched hours, darkness fell and he ordered candles to be lighted. Only the tireless application of Briggs kept the battle going on for so long—a merciless ordeal for the two unhappy doctors who had been so vitally involved. Their dread of the moment of sentence—and the ghastly nature of the sentence anticipated—must have been unbearable. But finally, the case was finished and each counsel addressed the jury. The judge's summation was long and detailed, almost as though he, too, had been apprehensive about the awful task he would have to perform when the jurors returned. He was not unduly hard on the prisoner as she sat there "pale and beautiful" hanging on to every word, but there was little he could say that would bring her any hope.

It was after midnight, the morn of March 29 when the jury returned. They had been out for an hour and a quarter. Entirely against the evidence they found the prisoner—not guilty!

Justice flouted or not—Jenner and Trye must have been greatly relieved. It is interesting to speculate just what would have been the effect on Jenner had the verdict gone the other way. If he had been the unwilling vehicle for the judicial extermination of this vibrant young life, it would surely have left its mark upon his subsequent career. But when he and Trye thankfully returned to Friar's Orchard to celebrate *their* escape, the prisoner, it seems, was in no sense chastened by *her* narrow escape. She was guilty, of course, and with her fortunate endowment of physical beauty pursued the same dangerous pattern of behavior for the remainder of her short life. The *Bristol Gazette* of September 15, 1803, reports: "Mrs. Reed, who was tried at Gloucester in the year 1796 on a charge of poisoning her husband died lately at Southampton, after acknowledging her guilt in that and another transaction of equal atrocity. No language can describe the severity of her feelings and contrition bordered even on despair."

With the conclusion of the Reed trial, the final barrier against uninterrupted research was removed, and Jenner was enabled to enter the final phase. Within six weeks he had a perfect cowpox pustule on the arm of a Berkeley girl named Sarah Nelmes. She has been generally described as a Berkeley milkmaid, but in fact she was of an old, highly respected local family and certainly no peasant.[45] Her father was a prosperous farmer and she probably assisted with the husbandry of the family acres. On May 14, just three days before his forty-seventh birthday, Jenner injected matter from this pustule into the arm of an eight-year-old boy, James Phipps. After giving it just over a fortnight to incubate, Jenner inoculated the child with smallpox serum on July 1. Three weeks later the arm was still clean. The first successful vaccination had taken place. Just thirty years of research had finally borne fruit, but there was no fanfare nor friends beside him when his point was proved. On July 19, Jenner wrote to Gardner, his poet friend, telling him of the great event. "Listen to the most delightful part of my story. The boy has since been inoculated for the smallpox which, as I ventured to predict, produced no effect."[46] As far as we

know, this was the first written announcement of vaccination and
it passed almost unnoticed. Jenner patiently returned to Cheltenham and his new circle of friends. He also wrote to Clinch in Newfoundland on August 5 and probably to Henry Cline[47] and the
Margravine of Anspach soon afterwards.[48]

This was, however, the end of vaccination for the time being.
There were no further research developments for the rest of the
year, and as far as we know, no more letters to proclaim Jenner's
joy to the world. The main fact was that he had proved his case
conclusively, particularly to himself. Of course the real campaign
to spread the practice could only come after his findings had been
published, but he could discuss and explain all this to the sympathetic company in Cheltenham while he organized his papers.
It apparently never occurred to Jenner that nobody would be interested in publishing the report. Indeed, the great inoculator at
Bowood, Dr. Ingenhousz, took a very bleak view of this assault on
variolation.

Blissfully unaware of the pending storm, Jenner settled in to his
summer general practice quite smoothly, and was content to wait
until the winter to complete his findings for the press. Nor was he
any longer a recuperating invalid; he was now a resident physician
and, accordingly, much concerned with the Spa's prosperity. The
maladies he saw around him were vastly different from those of
the countryside. To a great extent they were the complaints of the
rich, and he soon became expert in this new realm of medicine.
His connection with the town was probably why it eventually became a center for the cure of liver complaints, and also for people
who had contracted physical disabilities as a result of service with
the East India Company. In what I believe is the first medical
comment of a Cheltenham doctor relative to India Jenner said:

If we don't make diseases to remove those of the liver, nature sometimes does. From a simple pimple to a sore leg, local affections are
remedies for a diseased liver; and on those principles liver disease is
treated in the East Indies. In proportion to the quantity of diseases
accumulated about the liver will be the degree of spontaneous affections which shoots out on the skin from gouty erysipelas to venous inflammation of gout.[49]

Since liver complaints were the ones most successfully treated by the Cheltenham waters, his expertise in this area of medicine was a valuable adjunct to the Spa's attractions.

There is no question but what his taking up residence and his endorsement of the waters was of great public benefit during this initial period, and it is only fair to remember this when we consider Jenner's own debt to the only place that supported him from the very beginning. The younger Fosbroke, who grew up in or near the doctor's domestic circle, saw the simultaneous rise of Jenner and of the Spa firsthand and never felt that his idol was sufficiently appreciated. He, indeed, speaks on the matter very forcefully:

To eminent persons in medicine every place of public resort is greatly indebted. The gratitude of the town of Cheltenham is well deserved by those whose reputation or connection invites people of wealth to the place. No Physician who settles in a watering-place derives his support from the inhabitants, but the inhabitants may derive support from the physician. Hence the greater the reputation of an individual becomes, the deeper the bond of obligation owed by the place in which he resides. It is fit that the people should be reminded of these relations.[50]

The fact that the writer was a Cheltenham physician himself when he made these observations should of course be noted, but he was not the only one to speak of the town along these lines. Farington also comments on the benefits Cheltenham received from the great doctors: "Dr. Jenner has a great opinion of the Cheltenham Waters,—but they may be drunk imprudently which he sees in the countenances of many young ladies at the Well—about three thousand people have drunk them this season and not one who came for the benefit of them has died."[51] Jenner told him this on September 13, incidentally, when the season still had nearly two more months to run. And a full season it was. If the public reaction to the first vaccination had been less than enthusiastic, Jenner's relaxation after the event more than compensated. The town was again full of painters, poets, and musicians, with the Berry sisters, as usual, dominating the soirees; but perhaps the most entertaining of all was his new friend, the great Irish tenor Michael Kelly.[52]

Kelly was a seasonal resident at Cheltenham, where he wrote

stage music between his personal appearances at the Theatre Royal. It was during this summer that he first met Jenner. He was accompanied by the actress Anna Maria Crouch (whose husband had left her five years earlier), and they were a romantic couple, though past the first flush of youth. They were greatly loved by Cheltenham society. As the local guide tells us: "The musical talents of Kelly and Crouch are in the highest estimation and most liberally rewarded every season by the visitors." James Leigh Hunt has left us a delightful poet's description of this splendid pair. Kelly, he says, had "a flushed, handsome, good-humoured face with the hair about his ears." He goes on to describe how he had first heard them sing: "It should be added that Mrs. Crouch was a lovely woman as well as a beautiful singer, and that the two performers were in love."[53] And for Jenner the music lover, Kelly was the epitome of the Romantic Age. Mrs. Hunter, to be sure, had enjoyed the friendship and collaboration of Haydn, but had not Mozart himself chosen Kelly to sing Basilio in *The Marriage of Figaro*? This handsome man brought the spirit of Vienna to the Cheltenham groves. In 1795 it had been Prince Hoare, in 1796 Michael Kelly. Elizabeth Billington herself, who had taken Naples by storm at the San Carlo two years before, would follow in a year or so, and her composer, Francesco Bianchi, after her. It was indeed an expanding horizon for the country doctor.

Kelly, who "moved with the mightiest," was greatly impressed with Jenner. He observed during this summer of 1796: "I also had the advantage of originating a friendship with that great and worthy man and friend Dr. Jenner, who often did me the honour to take his dinner with me; he wrote a very excellent Bacchanalian song, for which I composed the music."[54]

The summer progressed in the typical Cheltenham manner. More important than anything, of course, was the fact that it suited Catherine's tubercular condition, and she enjoyed perhaps the first surcease from the disease since their marriage eight years before. Jenner had apparently written in glowing terms of his new residential pattern to his friend Clinch in Newfoundland. Answering the letter of August 5, Clinch replies: "I was happy to hear that your situation at Cheltenham was both agreeable and salutary to you and your good lady in point of health. I sincerely hope that your other inducements for making that spot your summer resort are in some degree answerable to your expectations."[55]

Among the other inducements, of course, was the attitude of the population—particularly those in medicine—toward Jenner's ideas. Cother became an enthusiastic vaccination man, as did Minster and Newell. Moreover, those who were not entirely in agreement were in no sense unfriendly. No longer was he discouraged as he had been in Berkeley from discussing the matter that dominated his life. Though Trye was unconvinced until the publication of Jenner's *Inquiry*, there was no parallel in Cheltenham to the hostility that existed elsewhere. The salons were the scenes for debate rather than battle. Farington was an excellent Boswell in these Cheltenham discourses.

It will be remembered that George III had been in Cheltenham after his first attack of insanity and had suffered a more severe attack after he left. Some people blamed the visit to the town; others said that he would have been healthier if he had stayed there. Jenner was always interested in mental health. "Dr. Jenner," wrote Farington on September 24, "has found that *in insane patients* he has moderated their violence by keeping them sick with tartar emetic. He observed that a person is more likely to take cold who suddenly removes from *cold to heat* than from *heat to cold*. Camphor water is an excellent medicine for nervous complaints."[56] Farington delighted in recording snippets of medical anecdote and, indeed, knew most of the great doctors; but it is Kelly who gives us the most rewarding record of his summer in Cheltenham with Jenner.

As it happened, the presence of the Irishman this season was not for professional reasons. Mrs. Crouch was not in particularly good health and had been recommended to take the waters. She and Kelly shared a delightful habitation called Wyatts Cottage, situated "in the midst of cornfields." It was rented in conjunction with a mutual friend, Colonel North, and here Jenner would walk of a summer evening to make a convivial fourth at dinner, but never, as mentioned, accompanied by his gentle wife. Colonel North was a brilliant conversationalist as Kelly observed: "I enjoyed his delightful society for in repartee and ready wit who was his equal?"

Cheltenham was a haven for sporting Irishmen at this time. The

Earl of Howth spent a great deal of time at Wyatts Cottage and fancied himself as something of an epicure. As Kelly himself tells us:

I went one morning to a poulterer's shop and found the noble Earl buying some poultry. I ordered the poulterer to send me home a fine goose, wished his lordship "Good Morning" and was walking home at a quick pace when I heard my name hallooed out; and turning round to see who was calling me, I saw his lordship in the middle of the High Street; his lordship shouted out with a determined Irish accent, "Kelly, Kelly, I say, Kelly, Corn your goose! I tell you now, do, Kelly, corn him! Keep him in salt four days and then boil him with a wisp of white cabbage; and by the powers, he'll be mighty fine eating!" I took his lordship's advice and found it a delicious dish.[57]

These festive occasions formed Jenner's introduction to the Irish peerage that was to form such a vital force in his later work.

The redoubtable earl was not without his own medical aspirations. Kelly reports the earl's prescription for a sore throat:

He told me he had a never-failing recipe for a sore throat; his directions were—just before going to bed to get scalding water, and the finest double-refined sugar, with two juicy lemons, and above all some old Jamaican rum, and when in bed take a good jorum of it as hot as possible.

"Why, my lord," said I, "your prescription seems to be nothing more than punch."

"And what is better sir for a sore throat than a good punch?" asked his lordship. "Good punch at night and copious gargles of old Port by day, would cure any mortal disease in life."[58]

The witty co-occupant of Kelly's cottage, Colonel North, was also overly fond of the bottle.

The Colonel was ordered by his medical adviser [Jenner?] while drinking the Cheltenham waters, not to exceed one pint of wine a day; he promised not to exceed his pint nor did he; but it was a Scotch pint, six of port or claret, which was his daily portion. White wine at dinner, he said, went for nothing, though he flirted with the best part of a bottle of old Madeira every day.[59]

Jenner himself possessed a strong sense of humor and very quick wit. He could be scathing when conversation appeared to drop beneath his standard. On one occasion, Fosbroke tells us, someone answered him in a mutter. "Are you a ventriloquist?" he demanded. When answered no, Jenner replied: "Then I am wrong, for I thought the voice came from the bowels."[60] Though quick, his humor was never cruel. He was as easygoing in his domestic life as he was in the outside world. A quick retort or waggish piece of impudence from a servant was even appreciated. As Fosbroke continues—not too approvingly: "By the conceit of the lower orders he was rather entertained than annoyed: his own menials, as usually happens to others, rarely consulted their master." Jenner himself admitted ruefully: "They seldom ask my advice until things come to extremes; they go to so-and-so, who has 'a desperate good receipt.' " On the topic of amateur medicine, despite the well-aired opinions of his friends, Jenner complained: "Contrary to my advice, an old woman rubbed over a scalded head with snuff; next day little Tommy died."[61] The bluntness of this comment is characteristic.

Although the poet Powell Snell later refers to Jenner as his learned friend, their degree of intimacy during these months following the discovery of vaccination is not known. However, the poet William Stevens, who arrived as usual with the Couttses in midseason, was certainly on congenial terms with the doctor by this time. Stevens was something of a scholar as well as a versifier and derived his living from the headmastership of Repton School— not a lucrative post in those days, but one that enabled him to spend his summers at Cheltenham Wells. Even at the age of forty he might have felt there was still a chance of patronage among the assembled nobility. And though it was fourteen years since his last book of verses had appeared, he did get the occasional article in the *Gentleman's Magazine*. Like old Mr. Anstey, Stevens was something of an authority on the poet Gray and claimed to have unpublished material by that writer. Jenner told Farington all about it. "Dr. Jenner," wrote the diarist, "showed us some lines which Dr. Stevens gave him as having been written by the poet Gray as part of his elegy written in a Country Churchyard, but were omitted." A literary discovery of this significance and in connection with Jenner should perhaps be noted:

> Some rural Lass with all-conquering charms
> Perhaps now moulders in the grassy bourne;
> Some Helen, vain to set the field in arms,
> Some Emma dead of gentle love forlorn.[62]

Not the very best Gray, perhaps, but very close to his style. Farington, incidentally, who made this diary entry in September, 1796, must have rewritten it later since Stevens did not receive his doctorate until the following year.

Jenner ultimately knew the Duke of Clarence very well, but during these early seasons at Cheltenham, he was initially drawn into the circle of the duke's mistress, Mrs. Jordan, and it is conceivable that he met the duke through her. In 1796 she had already been living with His Royal Highness for five years and had celebrated the event in August by giving birth to a daughter, Sophia, who was vaccinated in due course. Mrs. Jordan's medical adviser, Dr. Francis Knight, who was a friend of Cline's, was one of the few who were impressed by Phipps's vaccination.

Returning to the affairs of Jenner's literary-dramatic circle, however, it was also in the course of this summer that the daughter of one of his patients first appeared at Drury Lane. "This season," wrote Michael Kelly, "Harriot, Miss Mellon, made her first appearance. Mr. Sheridan had seen her the previous season at Strafford where she was acting. She was a handsome girl and much esteemed."[63] The romantic saga of this beautiful but penniless Cheltenham girl who married one of the richest men in the world will be dwelt upon later, since Jenner himself was obliquely involved.[64]

During the second part of this very important year in the doctor's life, vaccination research was again almost completely shelved. True, Jenner had proved his contentions through the successful inoculation of Phipps, but this had not prevented him from hastening back to Cheltenham immediately afterwards to resume his life of dilettantism, fashionable practice, and, most important of all, the animated, proselytizing conversation. Most likely, Jenner's behavior was all part of a clever strategy. When his thesis was published, it would be better to stem from the pen of a social lion and intellectual leader of Cheltenham society than from a respected but simple country doctor. Far better to operate from strength. As young Fosbroke observed:

In establishing the cause of vaccination Dr. Jenner showed the wisdom of one well-versed in the disposition of men and the knowledge of such modes of conviction as are most acceptable to the human mind. But had he not both *fortune, fame* and *high* alliance, his merit would have been crushed or faintly supported, envy would have stung him to death and more powerful ambition would have seized and appropriated his laurels.[65]

And how real the latter threat became in the ensuing years.

In the meantime the task of building himself a secure place in an ever widening society was most congenial. For his nonmedical friends not the least of Jenner's attractions was his wealth of anecdote relating to his own profession and its bitter rivalries. Acrimony among doctors can indeed rise to a feverish pitch, and jealousy roused through the most petty incidents. In a conversation with Farington toward autumn (September 13), Jenner himself gave a hitherto unknown sidelight to the feud between Hunter and Jesse Foot.[66] "Foot the surgeon became rancorous against John Hunter because the latter seemed to describe a Bougie which Foot had invented as not necessary. To revenge himself he wrote of Hunter with much malignancy and assisted many falsehoods." Interestingly enough, it was Jenner's friend, Trye, who in 1787 replied to this attack on their old master in *A Review of Jesse Foot's Observations on the Venereal Disease, (being a reply to his attack on Mr. John Hunter)*.

Kelly had to go to London in September to open the new theater season. Both he and his mistress were manifestly improved by their course of waters. He describes his taking leave of Jenner:

When I was about leaving Cheltenham I was lamenting to the doctor the loss of the Spa waters, which had done Mrs. Crouch and me so much essential service. He told me under an injunction of secrecy (which I have never violated in his lifetime) that I had no cause to lament the loss of the waters, "for depend upon it," said he, "the Cheltenham Salts which you can obtain from Mr. Paytherus, Chemist, in Bond Street, and of him alone, are to the full, as efficacious to health as the water from the Well. This," continued the excellent man, "is the candid opinion I give you. I should not wish to promulgate it as it might prejudice many industrious people by keeping company from the Spa, which I should be sorry should it be the case."[67]

Then leavetaking over, Kelly and his love boarded the mail coach for London, and Jenner walked quietly home to Catherine. Most of the great ones departed as the dark nights drew near, but there were still the doctors to talk to—Trye, Cother, Newell, Minster, and, perhaps, the more humble apothecaries also. Later as the first winds of winter came off the hills, the good doctor—with Catherine and the children—took the Bristol stage to Berkeley. He was well content with his first entirely professional season in Cheltenham, even though some of his younger friends were apparently reaching to much dizzier social heights.

Back in Berkeley, the glitter and sunshine of the Cheltenham summer gradually faded into the gray winter background of routine. The year of the discovery had turned out to be something of an anticlimax. No one outside of Cheltenham seemed concerned and, as far as can be gathered, only Cline and Lady Craven wrote to congratulate Jenner. Of course, the inoculation of Phipps was talked about, and the company at Cheltenham undoubtedly spread it abroad when they returned to town, but most reaction in the capital was guarded or downright hostile. The potential of the discovery to the livelihood of hundreds of fashionable doctors committed to their lucrative practice of inoculation was very serious indeed; but the really bitter attacks came after the publication. Save for Jenner's ever warmer assimilation into the literary and art circles of Cheltenham, the year 1796 had passed like any other. Fate decreed, however, that this increasing celebrity at the Wells must be hindered by the call of professional obligation. The complete loss of the year 1797 was the first of the brutal series of frustrations that were to dog him for the entire period of the vaccination crusade.[68] He met with repeated interruptions of a nature beyond his control. Patients always had to come first.

The winter of 1796–97 was severe, and the county temperature actually dropped to three below zero on New Year's Eve. In remote parts of the countryside people perished from the cold, and it appears that soon after Christmas, Jenner took Catherine and the children back to the comparative shelter of Cheltenham. Meanwhile he himself was forced by his medical commitments to move into Berkeley Castle.[69]

Lady Berkeley had had a serious relapse after her first legitimate confinement in October, and by the end of the year the postnatal effects had become so grave that her life was considered to be in danger. The earl begged Jenner to take up residence with the family until the crisis was over, and, as the family physician, he had little choice but to acquiesce. The lady and her progeny had been under his care ever since her lord had installed her at the castle ten years before, and Jenner had served the older members of the family—in particular Lady Craven, the earl's sister—ever since he had set up practice in the village. Of course, this development completely halted the progress of his vaccination research. Baron, who was not concerned with delineating Jenner's association with the demimonde, assures us that the reason for the blank year of 1797 was a shortage of cowpox serum.[70] He does not mention the year at the castle.

Mary Cole, who lived with Lord Berkeley for eleven years before their marriage, understandably became a lifelong friend of Jenner's over and above their professional association. She was one of the trio of beautiful daughters of a butcher in Gloucester. Whether she knew the young doctor before she moved into the castle is uncertain, but Lysons apparently knew her well. The three girls seem to have been equally generous with their favors, and while Mary was in service with a family in Kent, her sister lived in the Temple for three years with a fellow-student of Lysons's named Edge.[71] Going back a generation, it was even rumored that the nymphs' handsome mother had once been the mistress of the Duke of Clarence.

One of the most notorious rakes of his day, Berkeley was forty years old when he met the attractive domestic servant and there is no doubt but what he fell deeply in love. He took her back to his castle where she was known as Miss Tudor, and a son was born to them on January 6, 1786. Other children followed and Jenner calmly pursued his duty as family physician while the scandalized Catherine flatly refused to set foot in the home of their most valued patient. For her part, once ensconced in the baronial splendor of Berkeley, Mary Cole became the soul of rectitude and was soon respected and accepted by the entire tenantry for her kindness. Unfortunately, however, the same tolerance did not obtain with all the earl's relations and the young woman (twenty years her lord's junior) turned more and more toward her doctor as the years went by. When the pressure became too uncomfortable, the earl announced that they were really married after all. He even went so far as to forge the register in Berkeley Church showing the ceremony to have taken place in 1785, well before the birth of their first child. The rector who had "presided" was comfortably dead by this time, so there was no problem in that direction.[72] But no one, friends or enemies, believed the story; "Lady Berkeley" was accepted by the countryfolk because they loved her, not because they accepted her title. Catherine, however, neither loved nor accepted. Finally, on May 16, 1796, Lord Berkeley secretly married his mistress in London when she was four months with child. The complications of the ensuing birth grew sufficiently serious as winter set in so that it was obviously a matter for twenty-four-hour medical care. The repeated hemorrhages were more than her system could stand and Jenner, who had saved her sister-in-law's life in similar circumstances more than twenty years before, seemed to be the family's only hope.

It was at this critical point in Jenner's commitments that news of an even more tragic nature was brought to him. His brother, Stephen, the only father figure he had really known, was stricken and died on February 23. It is strange that he is mentioned so little in the family records, but perhaps his very humility was responsible for this. It is not only circumstantial evidence that reveals the selfless dedication of an able man who devoted his life to rearing his younger brother. Gardner, Baron, and Fosbroke were all fulsome in their praise. The first-mentioned published a rambling panegyric the following year in the pompous manner of the day; stripped of the dross of the piece, Stephen's virtues emerge quite clearly. "He was a man of excellent sense; of a retired turn of mind. . . . The most shining part of his character was a quiet, amiable modesty, which shrunk from everything bearing the most distant resemblance to ostentation. . . . His critical observations were peculiarly penetrative and judicious; and his learning and general abilities were much greater than his modesty would permit him to display." Fosbroke, a parson himself, more than echoed these sentiments. "I transcribe from Gardner's *Miscellanies*[73] the character of an excellent encumbent, which from personal knowledge I know to be just, and below, rather than above, the truth: he was, in short, what a clergyman ought to be—his whole soul wrapped in the virtuous and the amiable." So much for the man who brought up Edward Jenner—amiable, modest, virtuous, and learned. Another writer (who did not know him personally, however) remarks that he was "distinguished alike for his *learning and benevolence.*" Stephen's career before he retired in 1773 does suggest that his prospects were promising enough. Had he not been a Fellow of Magdalen College, Oxford, and held, in addition to the living of Rockhampton, the rectorship of Fettleton in Wiltshire and the perpetual curacy of Stone? The Jenners had a long tradition of church activity, and only Edward of the three boys had not been able to follow it. But Stephen, twenty years his brother's senior, elected to submerge his own ambition for the advance of medicine. He died a bachelor. For Jenner the wrench was severe. Stephen was his last family link with Berkeley, and many a poignant memory of his years of the country practice from his brother's cottage must have passed through his mind when he returned from the funeral to resume his bedside watch over Mary Berkeley.

Berkeley Castle, with its many specters and piercing winter cold, was not the best place to endure such an intimate and deep bereavement. Catherine's hand would have meant all the difference at this melancholy time, but there was not a path open to him but the one he took. His patient was in a very poor way and the Berkeleys had been his patients for a quarter of a century. No doubt, moved by the Mary Magdalen example, under the circumstances Catherine Jenner would have waived her resolution never to set foot in the castle had Jenner asked her, but he apparently respected her moral convictions too deeply to press it. I can find no record of her actually visiting the countess either during or after her illness. Jenner continued to watch in solitude.

Walking the echoing halls and galleries of the old fortress in the course of that long and lonely spring Jenner got to know the family as he never had before; in particular the waspish, spoilt firstborn of the alliance, William Fitzharding, who had inherited his mother's free and easy morals but not her kindness, and his father's dissolute habits but not his good nature. It was said at the

legitimacy trial many years later that the reason why the earl was
so frantic about the birth of the youngest child was because it was
to be his heir—thus tacitly proving that his other three boys were
illegitimate. But Jenner stoutly maintained that such was not the
case. There was never any suggestion that this child was anything
but a younger son. The earl's sole concern throughout that critical
year was his wife's survival; he already had a sufficiency of heirs.
Not that the doctor believed the secret marriage story—he admitted that he did not—but rightly or wrongly the earl looked
upon the wretched little firstborn, William Fitzharding, as his
successor. At the age of eleven this boy was sufficiently master of
his young brothers to influence their entire lives. As grown-ups, at
the time of the trial in 1811, they still insisted that the title should
go to the obviously illegitimate first-born. Nay, even the rightful
heir—cause of Jenner's long incarceration—refused to take up his
inheritance. About the only thing William Fitzharding cared
about as a youth were field sports (his interest in the opposite sex
came many years later) and he was profoundly influenced by reading a copy of Somerville's *Chase,* which he found in the castle library.[74] It was possibly the first book he ever read and might conceivably have been the last; but it is also conceivable that this long
period of surveillance by Jenner in his childhood made an impression on his character. In the eighteenth century the sickroom of a
parent was an awesome holy of holies, even to a problem child.
Arrogant and insufferably insolent all through his years of growing up, William Fitzharding never seems to have clashed with the
genial doctor, even when he must have been aware of Catherine's
manifest disinclination for his company. Though he eventually
followed Jenner to Cheltenham, and became the uncrowned ruler
of the town for the rest of his life, he never intruded upon the
doctor's domestic scene until after Catherine's death—and then
with a respect and caution most uncharacteristic. The closeness of
Jenner's attendance upon his patient is indicated in the statement
he made at the peerage trial. The castle, Jenner said, "was his
permanent residence save for one or two excursions during the entire year."[75] The excursions one presumes would be to visit his
family.

On the other hand, though Jenner was in no position to leave the bedside of his patient for any period of time, he did have areas of leisure that permitted him to organize his evidence and prepare his findings for publication as soon as the opportunity presented itself. In March he managed to make a brief visit to Thomas Westphaling's house at Rudhall, near Ross-on-Wye, where he went over his research material with his friends Paytherus, Worthington, Hicks, and Gardner. They all agreed that it should be written up and sent to Everard Home, with the request that he submit it to Sir Joseph Banks and the Royal Society. Jenner completed the paper by March 25, but he seems to have been delayed in getting it off to London. Possibly Lady Berkeley had a relapse, because it was actually four months before Jenner was able to dispatch it on July 10. The title of this first vaccination manuscript was *An Inquiry into Natural History Disease Known in Gloucestershire as the Cowpox*.[76] To say that the reception it received was apathetic would be an understatement. After Banks had perused it he passed it to Lord Somerville,[77] President of the Board of Agriculture, and then it was simply returned to the author without being read to the Royal Society. Strangely enough Jenner himself did not seem unduly upset at the rebuff, but it is still hard to understand Somerville's and Banks's behavior. It is possible that they were not impressed by the manner in which Jenner had presented his case. After all, the work had been done in the disjointed intervals he could snatch from his attendance in the sickroom. So he philosophically returned to his task of revision as best he could. If formal channels of medical research would not consider publication, the findings could always come out at the author's expense.

The cold rejection by the Royal Society was really a reflection of the general opinion in the medical establishments at large. Even after the vaccination of Phipps only a small circle of Jenner's personal friends had any faith in the system. To be sure, it would be hard to get any significant backing until his research was published for everyone to read, but a certain number of doctors did hear about the Phipps case and remained quite unmoved. Charles James Fox's physician, Benjamin Moseley, was one of the earliest to ridicule the system, but he was a strange medical fish, despite his paper qualifications.[78] Having spent a large part of his life practicing in the West Indies, Moseley made a fortune prescribing for planters who were rich in both money and gullibility. He believed in what sounds suspiciously like voodoo and made the surprising assertion to Farington "that weak men only became mad."[79] The diarist also mentioned old Dr. Moore, who, unfortunately, detested Fox, one of Jenner's most powerful supporters. After Moore died, however, his sons swung enthusiastically toward Fox's point of view as far as vaccination was concerned.

Even Charles Trye found the practice very questionable at first, despite his loyal regard for Jenner. He was probably worried at the moral—or theological—implication of deliberately injecting someone with a disease. But while Jenner was, as it were, in a state of animated suspension at the castle, Trye underwent a change in fortune as unpredicted as it was unappreciated. Only a month after Jenner had lost the "foster father" who had brought him up, Trye, in the strange parallel life pattern that seems to have followed the two men, lost his own "foster father"—cousin Henry Norwood. Nor was his deep grief at all countered by the fact that, bypassing the natural heir, the deceased left his entire estate to Trye. Among the papers found after Trye's death a piece of writing entitled, "Written after coming into possession of the Leckhampton Estate" reveals the unwilling heir's reaction:

A.D. 1797. On the 26th of March my kinsman died and by his Will dated February 27th, 1797, bequeathed me his Manor and estate of Leckhampton; which being added to the fortune with which it had already pleased God to bless my industry has placed me according to the ordinary course of human events in a state of affluence and independence. . . . Grant, oh merciful Father, that I so may use Thy bounty as not to abuse it; that I may enjoy it with moderation, not employing it in the gratification of my sensual desires: not wasting it in vice and vanity, but applying it to the glory of God, and the good of my fellow creatures. Let me not trust in the multitude of my riches.[80]

After the first impact Trye, nevertheless, settled down very nicely with his new wealth and landed status. To be sure, he continued his work at the Gloucester hospital and kept up his house in the city, but his ownership of Leckhampton Court and its hundreds of acres installed him as a leader of Cheltenham society. He also soon realized that the possession of wealth enabled him to promote the myriad and definitely "unsensual" desires he possessed for the betterment of society. Nor were his religious sentiments of a Calvinistic nature; in fact they were very unostentatious and personal. The building of roads, improvements in agriculture, and eventually the spreading of free vaccination were some of the things made possible by his possession of money. The pagan arts also had a high place in Trye's scheme of things and he became a patron of the Gloucester Music Meeting. Actually it was not his first association with the arts. At the outset of his career, he had almost been lost to medicine to the enrichment of the Royal Academy. When Trye had been in London with Hunter, he was brought to the notice of John Sheldon, then professor of anatomy at the academy, who gave the young man a position as assistant and very soon his lectures became almost as celebrated as his master's. By 1784 Trye's reputation was such that Sheldon offered him a partnership. To become, at the age of twenty-six, jointly responsible for anatomical studies at the Royal Academy might very understandably have gone to his head, and he was about to sign the contract when an offer of employment came from his native county. Just as Jenner had turned down Hunter's offer ten years before so did Trye on the threshold of fame turn his back on the world's art capital to pursue his medicine in a provincial hospital. To be sure, the post he accepted—senior surgeon at the Gloucester Infirmary—was an excellent one, but it did remove him from the center of things. Dr. Daniel Lysons, who had been for many years physician at the Gloucester institution, was the great-grandson of William Trye of Hardwick Court on the female side.[81] Charles Trye was great-grandson in the male descent, so it is likely that the family connection had some influence in the young man's choice. Eight years later Trye strengthened the connection by marrying Dr. Lysons's niece, Mary (Samuel's sister), and they set up housekeeping at Friar's Orchard in the heart of the city.

An interesting anecdote relates to a historical painting that belonged to Trye. He carefully concealed his profound religious feeling from his friends but still forced himself to observe certain moral standards in a rather extreme way. Consequently, when Trye was presented with a Renaissance portrait of his ancestor,

Charles Brandon, Duke of Suffolk—obviously of great intrinsic
value and historical interest—he had it hung in a bedroom so that
no one should see it and identify him with ducal lineage. It was
also revealed, after his death, that Trye retired for a brief period
of spiritual contemplation before every operation.[82]

The season that Jenner lost at Cheltenham was one of remarkable social activity. Many people were present who would have
been of estimable value to him and could probably have brought
about the immediate publication of his *Inquiry*. With Lysons,
Mrs. Siddons, and Moore, was Robert Raikes, the famous Gloucestershire publisher and his nephew Thomas—a wealthy London
banker and fashionable dandy. But the doctor seems to have become the forgotten man. Only Fosbroke and Gardner visited him
during these tedious months, and even when her ladyship was over
the crisis in late summer the earl pleaded that Jenner stay in residence. In August she was nearly her old self—a year after her confinement—and there would have been ample time for social occasions outside the sickroom had any of his friends been interested.
During what should have been a vital period in Jenner's research
—the year following his first vaccination—his correspondence was
virtually nil. After the letter from John Clinch in December that
commented on the move to Cheltenham, there is no record of
anyone having written to him until June. The fact that he wrote
no letters himself during this time could be conceivably because
he reserved every moment of free time away from his patient for
his manuscript, but it does not explain his *receiving* no letters, particularly since there was a great deal happening to his friends.
Charles Trye was elected a Fellow of the Royal Society in the
spring, and he turned over his Charity for Poor Women (suitably
endowed) to a committee of Gloucester burgesses. Of much more
interest, however, was the birth of a son to his friend Thomas Fosbroke. Jenner later took the youngster under his wing at a very
early age, and he became almost as his own child in the years that
followed. Fate was to decree that Jenner would not have a son who
would carry on his medical crusade, but this young man made a
loyal and devoted substitute when he grew to manhood.

Lord Berkeley, in his bluff, rather awkward manner, was deeply
grateful for his doctor's unselfish devotion to his patient during
her long illness and actually grew interested in the vaccination

cause beyond his usual cursory attitude. There would have been plenty of lonely hours when the anxious husband and the learned medico would be in each other's company, and it was probably during these months that the peer arranged for young Matthew Tierney to come up to the castle.[83] Tierney was the medical officer of the South Gloucestershire Militia under Lord Berkeley's command. As was common in those days, the young man was quite unqualified, and was using his post-apprenticeship period to gain experience while waiting to enter medical school at Edinburgh. Tierney was so impressed with Jenner that after meeting, he began vaccinating his men on his own responsibility long before the army gave any formal approval of the system—almost certainly the first mass vaccination to take place anywhere. In 1799 upon entering Edinburgh University, he was still burning with zeal over the new discovery, and was, of course, an extremely experienced practitioner. What was more remarkable was his conversion of the celebrated professor James Gregory.[84]

Tierney, though unqualified as a physician, considered himself an expert in the field of vaccination and was deeply concerned when he heard the professor denounce the system in the course of a lecture. Accordingly, he visited the man at his home afterwards and actually argued him into accepting the very practice he had immediately before condemned. Nor was the conversion superficial. Tierney was subsequently allowed to inoculate the professor's child with serum specially provided by Jenner. The incident was a remarkable example of youthful tenacity. What was of much greater importance, however, was that Gregory himself became the pioneer of vaccination in Scotland from which country so many doctors were to make their way to Cheltenham. As for Tierney, he moved to Glasgow where he obtained his M.D. with a dissertation entitled *De Variola Vaccine*. For him there were no initial years of struggle. After his return to Gloucestershire Lord Berkeley introduced him to the Prince of Wales, who appointed him Household Physician in Brighton. By far the most honored of all the vaccination pioneers, he also became something of an authority in the fashionable field of mineral springs and it was to him that William Gibney dedicated his *Medical Guide to the Cheltenham Waters* many years later in 1825.

Lady Berkeley made a complete and permanent recovery after

such dedicated medical care. Still a comparatively young woman, she presented her lord with four more children before his death and outlived him by thirty-five years. But Jenner had his own family responsibilities towards the end of his extended attendance at the castle. Catherine became pregnant after he had committed himself to her ladyship's side and gave birth to their third and last child in the spring. Fortunately it was an uncomplicated confinement, and they named the infant Robert Fitzharding after his grandfather Kingscote. The Kingscote connection was indeed growing more and more valuable with the turn of events in the social world. In 1796 Sir John Rous, M.P., brother-in-law to Catherine's brother Thomas, was elevated to the peerage as Baron Rous of Dennington, and his sister, Frances Peyton, soon became one of the earliest and keenest supporters of vaccination, dragging her noble brother along with her in the process. Since Thomas Kingscote married into that family in 1794, it is probable that Frances heard all about the new system long before its announcement to the world.[85] Nor was future support for Jenner in the House of Lords the only fruit of the Peyton marriage. A cousin, Sir John Saunders Sebright, later sat in the Commons for Hertford where he proved a very useful ally and incidentally filled the gap left in the lower house by the elevation of his kinsman to the Lords.

However, these events, important as they were to Jenner's cause, were still, as it were, in the family—and in this context the Berkeleys might also be included. But the circle was due to widen rapidly. The main curiosity about vaccination in the ranks of the peerage came only after the publication of the *Inquiry*, and Jenner has left us no record of when the spate of noble supporters first made itself apparent. He has left us one clue, however, even though he does not give a specific date. In a letter to the National Institute of France some years later, he referred to "My valued friend and patron, the Marquis of Hertford . . . who encouraged my scheme of vaccination *when in its infancy* and contending with the prejudice of the world."[86] This would suggest that Hertford stepped in right after the vaccination of Phipps, since after the publication noble and, indeed, royal patronage was at a discount— even though it was prestigious rather than financial. It is possible, of course, that the reference to vaccination's infancy could well refer to the years of struggle before 1796 when no one took the idea seriously. Two phenomena support this view. The Hertfords were distantly related to the Berkeleys, which would suggest an avenue of introduction before the vaccination of Phipps brought the doctor into the public eye, and secondly, they were in a sense a Cheltenham family. At the time of Jenner's birth they had occupied Sandywell House, a few miles outside the town, though by the time he had grown up they were only at the Wells in the season.[87] Their ancestral home was—and is—at Ragley Hall in Warwickshire. Jenner may have been introduced to them in 1795, though Catherine would not have been too enthusiastic since both the marquis and his wife had rather advanced social views. Nevertheless, when her ladyship became the mistress of the Prince of Wales a few years later, it probably did Jenner's cause no harm at all.

∽ III ∽

The Cheltenham Fortress
1798-1800

When Edward Jenner emerged from Berkeley Castle after a year of isolation, receptiveness to vaccination was more guarded, and a number of its critics had been left uncontradicted for many months. In effect, he had to begin all over again. Jenner had resumed his cowpox research while still at the castle. His vaccination materials and agricultural contacts were all about him in the parish, but the long dry summer and relatively mild winter had not provided sufficient mud for any new cowpox outbreaks among the cattle. It was well into spring before there was any return of the disease. Even then the serum was not too readily obtained, and Jenner was forced to use horsepox matter when he resumed operations in March—nearly two years after his inoculation of Phipps. He did eventually obtain some cowpox matter from a young boy who had contracted the disease naturally, and the genuine serum from this child's arm was perfect in every respect. In a series of operations Jenner took successive material from pustule to pustule for a period of several weeks. His patients, both children and adults, being all successfully infected from the single pustule, he inoculated his son Robert on April 12. However the vaccine did not take. After a chain of perfect injections on strangers, his own child—at the very end of the line—remained unprotected.[1]

Although another year was well on its way Phipps's successful vaccination had still not been officially published to the world and interest waned. Only one friend, Richard Worthington, took sufficient interest to suggest that he add a whole series of new case histories, embodying his research during the current spring, before submitting it to the printer. The version he had sent to

Everard Home ended, of course, with the Phipps case, which an unenthusiastic reader may have considered insufficient evidence. The revision of the paper was finished at Westphaling's house with the cooperation of Henry Hicks, Paytherus, and Worthington in addition to Westphaling himself. Caleb Parry does not seem to have been in evidence, though it was to him that Jenner dedicated the work when it was finished.

Tragically, with the discovery of vaccination on the very point of being announced to the world, Henry Jenner died on April 28 at the age of sixty-two. It is not even certain that Edward Jenner saw his brother before the end. He died at his vicarage in Burbage, Wiltshire, and Jenner took his manuscript up to London at the end of April. Henry's death ended Jenner's formal link with the Aylesburys, but by this time that valuable connection had done its part and Jenner was permanently ensconced in Cheltenham society.[2] The rest of the county, however, remained little moved by his experiments.

With the publication date only a few weeks away, Jenner was still far from happy with the support he was receiving. He lamented to Edward Gardner:

My experiments move on, but I have to do all single-handed. Not the least assistance from the quarter I had the most right to expect it!!— Bodily labour I disregard but pressures of the mind grow too heavy for me. Added to all my other cares, I am troubled by the reigning epidemic—Impecunity. You must be more attentive to me than you were during the last Cheltenham recess. I believe you came here only once and then on your way from Bristol.[3]

For some reason Gardner had not been in evidence during the preparation of the final version of the pamphlet—a marked contrast to his eager concern after the vaccination of Phipps.

Though Jenner arrived in London with his manuscript at the end of April, he took an unusually long time to arrange for the printing. It is conceivable that he still hoped to get a publisher to accept the work commercially, but if so his hope was in vain. After nearly two months of waiting, he contracted to have it printed, out of his own meager resources, by Sampson Low, of 7, Berwick Street, Soho. It must have appeared about the beginning of July since the date of his dedication to Caleb Parry is June 21, and its slender seventy-five pages would not have taken many days to run off. There was no fanfare when it finally appeared. *An Inquiry into the Causes and Effects of the Variola Vaccine of Cowpox* might be said to have slid rather than erupted into the world.[4] What doctors Jenner met from the expensive quarters in Grosvenor Square, which he had hopefully taken on his arrival in town, were either politely apathetic or amusedly hostile. Moseley and Ingenhousz, who had considerable influence in the medical establishment, were quite condescending in their scorn.[5] Had they been as offensively gross in their hostility as some of the later opponents of the system, Jenner's wit and courage would have coped much more easily. As it was, their attitude apparently influenced him more than the encouragement and patient advice offered by men like Cline and Sir Walter Farquhar. There was an aura of loneliness in this trip to London that incurred expenses he could ill afford. None of his friends accompanied him and there were all too few people in the capital to receive him. Nevertheless Jenner's behavior was somewhat quixotic, in light of the fact that he had come up to launch a book that represented his life's work. He gave the city just two weeks to accept it and then decided to come home. He had spent two months on expensive groundwork at Grosvenor Square but only two weeks to see if it would prosper once it came out. Disillusioned and homesick, he took the early morning mail coach from the Angel near St. Clements on July 14 and joined Catherine and the children in Cheltenham the same night. It had not been a very impressive storming of the capital.

But at least Jenner was among his friends when the public reaction to the tract was manifested. Trye read it exhaustively, and after a great deal of soul-searching, reversed his earlier stand and became a dedicated practitioner among the Leckhampton villagers. Jenner, Minster, and Newell were the spearheads of the movement in Cheltenham, and Jenner's house was constantly besieged by eager patients completely converted to the new system. Cother had bought a house in the nearby hamlet of Alstone the previous May from the apothecary, Hinds (by then known as Dr. Hinds), and since Cother lived there for the rest of his life it is reasonable to assume that in the pioneer period vaccination was also practiced at this house.[6] The local doctors at least were mobilizing to the cause.

On the surface the vaccination situation throughout the country changed very little as a result of the publication of the *Inquiry*. The same people opposed it, and for the same reasons. In fact, with one exception, the practice was still ignored outside Gloucestershire and Gloucestershire people. The exception, however, was a very significant one. Within a fortnight of the tract's appearance, in July, Cline inaugurated vaccination at St. Thomas's Hospital, London. In the other great centers—Edinburgh and Dublin—there was no noticeable reaction at all.[7]

What Jenner did not realize was that there were already forces at work—particularly in highest brackets of the social order—that would within the year make his cause viable. Not only the loyal Cheltenham peers, Sherborne and Berkeley, but even higher up. Dr. E. F. Knight, the Duke of Clarence's physician, was in correspondence with Jenner early in September even though he did not actually come to Cheltenham, and all the necessary arrangements were made for a mass vaccination at Bushey. All the children of Mrs. Jordan (the duke's mistress, who was at the Spa as usual during the season), together with the entire household of the duke, were thus the first blood members of the royal family to be vaccinated.[8] This gesture of the duke's was perhaps the most historic event of the publication year. One might well say that with it vaccination was established, and Knight was immortalized as the first practitioner of vaccination in the British royal family. His name frequently appears in Mrs. Jordan's letters, and he vaccinated later children of the "alliance" as they were born.

Not quite in the class of a royal duke, perhaps, but a ruler in his own colony, another disciple was active far away in the Mediterranean. The gallant General O'Hara, who had been at Cheltenham with Mary Berry in 1795 and had promptly forgotten all about her when he was appointed Governor of Gibraltar a few weeks later, had not, however, forgotten all about Jenner. On the publication of the vaccination tract he became an active promoter of the movement in the colony. An hospitable if carefree character (though his devotion as a lover may have left something to be desired), he was always delighted to entertain any of his old friends of the Cheltenham days. Celia Lock and her husband arrived in Gibraltar late in the year and the general could not do enough for them.[9]

Only a few months previously poor Mary Berry had been faced
with what she anticipated to be a Cheltenham summer of loneliness and nostalgia as the guest of the first official endorsers of
vaccination—the Spencer family. "We go to Cheltenham to
meet the Douglasses and Lady Spencer," she wrote in her memo-
randum in August.[10] If any hostess could have made her forget
her sorrows it should have been the gay dowager Spencer.[11] Although well into middle age, this noblewoman was still a lion of
Cheltenham and London societies and had been one of the most
talked-of beauties of her day. Mary Berry was, indeed, a common denominator among the various scattered vaccination po-
tentials. From O'Hara onward, wherever she stepped a new patron
appeared—or so it seemed. Certainly prior to Mary Berry's visit
the summer of 1798, the Spencers were in no way concerned with
Jenner and his aspirations. At the soirees of Dowager Lady
Lavinia in Cheltenham, however, tongues wagged and interest
developed. Jenner's great hope was to have his practice adopted
by the armed forces of the country, and the Navy, as the Senior
Service, was the principle goal. Thanks to the Spencers his aim
was achieved, since Lord Spencer was the First Lord of the Admiralty among other things, and a most dynamic character—
part forceful naval strategist and part intellectual. It was he, who
after much soul-searching, sent Nelson to destroy the French fleet
at the Nile; and he was in great part responsible for the other
brilliant naval victories of the period. He was at the peak of his
prestige when Mary Berry visited his mother in Cheltenham, and
the town still was celebrating Nelson's great victory of August 1.
The other side of his character, however, was far removed from
wars and rumors of wars. He was a serious classical scholar and
antiquarian, and amassed one of the greatest private libraries of
his day at Althorp. At the time of his meeting with Jenner, there
was a certain coolness between Spencer and such local peers as
Berkeley, Sherborne, and Ducie, since he had deserted the extreme
Whig faction in the Lords to serve under Pitt. Despite his politics,
no one questioned his ability.

The accession of the Spencers to the vaccination cause represented the first great family bloc of peers to act. Lady Spencer's
father, Lord Lucan,[12] joined the crusade as did her daughter

Georgiana, Duchess of Devonshire, to whom, in particular, Jenner was eventually to owe so much. Georgiana's sister-in-law, the Duchess of Portland, was the mother of Jenner's future friend and benefactor, Lord William Bentinck. So was the web of influence woven in the highest places. Mary Berry was also in the middle of a similar web of connected bloodlines who were to support Jenner in the noble houses of Hardwick, Polwarth, and Egremont. It is strange to realize that this beautiful and talented woman, sought after by the cream of society, went to her grave a maid. O'Hara had, indeed, begged her to marry him before leaving for Gibraltar, but she had demurred. He then asked her to spend his last twenty-four hours in England with him and again she refused on the grounds of propriety. So, carefree and irresponsible to the last, he sailed out of her life forever. In Gibraltar he soon consoled himself with two new mistresses, both of whom bore him children. Mary seems to have felt no animosity, simply deep and lasting regret. She had bade a tearful goodbye to her friend Mrs. Damer before she left for the Spa. This good woman who had been in favor of the O'Hara match seems to have suffered almost as much as her jilted friend. Farington observed: "The 'extasis' on meeting and tender leave on separating between Mrs. Damer and Miss Berry was whimsical. On Miss (Mary) Berry going to Cheltenham the servants described the separation between her and Mrs. Damer as if it has been a parting before death."[13] Nevertheless, once she had arrived in Cheltenham there was a certain pleasing nostalgia amid the scenes of her idyllic courtship that at least partly tempered her deep sorrow. "This place and everything about it recall, in the most lively manner, scenes and recollections to my mind, which, though melancholy, I cannot call unpleasing," she wrote to Mrs. Damer. "They are thank heaven, unembittered by reproach, and undisgraced by folly. My imagination seems to pass over everything that has happened since, and to bring me back to the calm but lively enjoyment of a society in which I delight."[14]

From the observation contained in a letter of the following year, however, Lady Spencer was not immediately impressed by the rather overly brilliant young woman but eventually got used to her: "Miss Berry improves upon knowing her more," she wrote to her daughter the Duchess of Devonshire on July 23. "I do not know that she is au fond, a little too much flattery and too much satire I doubt, but she has many good sentiments and so much good sense and such a talent for conversation that it has already made Georgiana despise some of her girlish acquaintance and dread the coming of those we expect."[15] The Georgiana here mentioned was the duchess's eldest daughter who seems to have had a liver condition and had been sent to Cheltenham by Sir Walter Farquhar for treatment.

Mrs. Damer herself was an interesting enough person.[16] A daughter of the late Lord Aylesbury—the one who preceded Henry Jenner's employer—she became a sculptor of some celebrity while still quite young and was a force in London and Cheltenham art circles. She was already a widow at the beginning of the vaccination era, and it appears that she had lost interest in men. She enjoyed wearing male attire, and her views seem to have been very advanced for her time. Her devotion to Mary Berry was not exclusive. Other young women at the Wells, including the Lock girls[17] and the Ogilvys, were equally Mrs. Damer's sincere, almost motherly concern.

There was a mild epidemic of smallpox in Cheltenham during the late summer, and it seems that the supply of vaccine ran out, leading to an incident that did the vaccination cause a great deal of harm. In later years certain doctors claimed that, initially, Jenner himself had no faith in the efficacy of vaccination when the safety of his own family was involved. Baron writes:

While the infant (Robert) was in Cheltenham, the late Mr. Cother of that place came into Jenner's house and took the child in his arms, saying that he had just left a family labouring under smallpox. Jenner immediately exclaimed, "Sir, you know not what you are doing. That child is not protected; he was vaccinated but the infection failed." Believing that the natural smallpox would follow, he was greatly distressed and alarmed. He had no vaccine matter. He resolved therefore to adopt the next best expedient and immediately had the child inoculated with smallpox virus.[18]

Fortunately the baby came through safely, but Jenner's detractors said nothing of the inability to obtain vaccine and merely pointed out that the father had inoculated his own son in preference to vaccinating him.

In Cheltenham at the time was William Woodville who had been a physician to the Smallpox and Inoculation Hospitals at St. Pancras, London, since 1791.[19] He obviously had vested interest in the survival of smallpox inoculation and must have heard about Robert's inoculation. Woodville was an aging man and vacillated a great deal in his attitude, manifestly confused by conflicting interests. He did meet the Jenners in a professional capacity, however, before he definitely decided to oppose vaccination.

It would seem that the cottage in Berkeley was still not available even after the return from London, for on Jenner's having to make a journey to his native place, he still left the family behind at Cheltenham. Undoubtedly Dr. Cother was not in favor after his careless behavior at Jenner's house, and Dr. Minster, who was certainly working close to the family, was also ignored when one of the children fell ill during the father's absence. "It happened that he was here [in Cheltenham] during an excursion I made from hence to Berkeley," wrote Jenner, "and in the interval attended one of my children who had been seized with a violent fit of illness. On my return I found the child recovering and felt only too pleased with the manner in which Woodville had treated him."[20]

While Jenner had hoped to set up a practice in London for at least part of the year once the vaccination tract was published, its poor reception and his precipitate retreat made him reluctant to leave Cheltenham again once he had returned home. Indeed the Spa remained the only place in the length and breadth of England where he found any comfort or encouragement. Far from the publication of the *Inquiry* having any chastening effect upon the inhabitants of his native Berkeley, the opposite seems to have been the case. The hundreds of villagers who had flocked to be inoculated with smallpox three years before were not by any means ready to admit their error, notwithstanding the pro-vaccination policy at the castle. To be sure, Jenner's nephews George and Henry immediately conformed, and the former in particular became a dedicated practitioner of the new system; but the general population still stubbornly inclined toward Dr. Fewster's anti-vaccination ideas. Nor was this attitude confined to the illiterate ranks of the lower peasantry; the prosperous yeoman elements that should have known better were the most vociferous and even went to the extreme length of telling poor Jenner to his face how little they appreciated his activities.

One lady of no mean influence among them, met him soon after the publication of his *Inquiry*. She accosted him in this form and said in true Gloucestershire dialect, "Well! I can tell you there beant a copy sold in our town; nor shant be neither if I can help it!" On another occasion the same notable dame having heard about rumours of failures in vaccination came up to the doctor with great eagerness and said, "Shant we have a general inoculation now?"[21]

This was rather a cruel barb since the last general inoculation had been carried out by his nephews when he was a very sick man in Cheltenham. But passions were to run very high in the vaccination controversy. This was only the beginning.

Actually the reception he received in his native village was not a great deal different from that of the country at large, and some of his friends felt that he had given up the London idea too easily. Men like Cline, Baillie, and Farquhar[22] realized the tremendous magnitude of his discovery and felt that such a revolution in medicine could only operate from the capital. In addition, Jenner could, if he wished to protect his discovery, at long last live in style at Grosvenor Square with his ten thousand a year. (Prosperous doctors at that time earned about £300 per annum.) Jenner, however, with reasonable financial security, as he thought, on the horizon and the freedom to visit London whenever he cared, was more than content in the security and friendships of his Cheltenham circle. He made his position very clear in a letter to Farquhar at the end of that epoch-making summer.

Cheltenham, September 29th, 1798.

It is very clear from your representation that there is now an opening in town for any physician whose reputation stood fair in the public eye. But here, my dear friend, here is the rub. Shall I, who even in the morning of my days sought the lowly and the sequestered paths of life, the valley and not the mountain; shall I, now my evening is fast approaching hold myself up as an object for fortune and for fame? Admitting as a certainty that I attain both, what stock should I add to my little fund of happiness?

My fortune with what flows from my profession, is sufficient to gratify my wishes, indeed so limited is my ambition and that of my nearest connections that were I precluded from future practice I should be able to attain all I want. And as for fame, what is it? a gilded butt forever pierced with the arrows of malignity. The name of John Hunter stamps this observation with the signature of truth. However, this I promise you, *that as soon* as my engagements here cease, you shall see me in town.[23]

Jenner's engagements, though, kept him very busy indeed for the rest of the year. As soon as the autumn was past and his wealthy patients had departed, he resumed his experiments and before the winter was out had sufficient new case histories to fill a new book almost as long as the *Inquiry*. His friends did not see him in London, but since he included material from Cline, Woodville, and Pearson, it is possible that they visited him in the course of his work. At this point the two latter were still apparently enthusiastic about the new system.

Another doctor who was initially impressed by vaccination was Thomas Jameson of the Finsbury Dispensary.[24] He was among the first to practice the operation in London and in the course of 1798 actually settled in Cheltenham with his family; but once he was, as it were, on the very doorstep of the master, his enthusiasm evaporated, and he eventually attained a strange kind of celebrity as the only doctor in town who did not accept vaccination. Jameson was a Scot some four years Jenner's junior but already a member of the Royal Colleges of Physicians in both Edinburgh and London. With his wife, who also was named Catherine, he took rooms over a shop in the High Street near Minster as had Jenner. Though he had experimented with vaccination at Finsbury, he had not come to Cheltenham to promote that cause. His great interest was the mineral springs, and he began a program of research that led to the definitive work on the subject. Nevertheless, he was constantly thrown into contact with Jenner as both of them increasingly became a part of the local life. Fortunately Jameson's apathy—it could scarcely be called hostility—toward vaccination made no impact on the company at the Wells. He was apparently an indifferent general practitioner—much more at home with his research than with the stethescope—so that his influence on the public never became marked. A contemporary observed of him:

"His skill in the use of remedies was inferior to his knowledge of diseases; with this deficiency no learning can succeed in medicine."[25]

Lord Somerville, who had unexpectedly inherited the barony and estates from his uncle two years before, was one of the early few who were profoundly impressed by the *Inquiry*. Soon after its publication Somerville was appointed President of the Board of Agriculture, a post that made him an invaluable ally in cowpox research. Unfortunately Jenner's increasing support in the upper house was not matched in the Commons. Nor was all the "support" apparent in the medical profession just what it appeared to be on the surface. In a subtle way, one man at least was already wondering how he might turn the discovery to his own advantage. Dr. George Pearson of Jenner's own hospital, St. George's, immediately recognized the potential of the system on its publication, and before the year was out had published his own paper, *The History of Cowpox*.[26] In his innocence, Jenner saw this as a gesture of support and endorsed Pearson's researches to the extent of including examples in his own ensuing publication—a gesture he was to bitterly regret.

When the season was over the strain of making new but essential social contacts lessened, Jenner gladly returned to his country research. Despite the hostility of a large part of the medical world, the publication of the *Inquiry* had by now aroused sufficient interest to make vaccination a subject of discussion—written as well as oral. In fact from 1798 onward, Jenner was an active literary man. He had met enough prominent figures in his professional world to make possible continued debate and comparison of notes. Throughout the winter he not only compiled new case histories from his own operations but took examples from the work of such men as Cline, Pearson, and Woodville to produce the new volume entitled *Further Observations*, which appeared on April 5, 1799. Again Sampson Low was the printer and again the dedication was to Caleb Parry. It was in this work that smallpox inoculation was first condemned in print, the author quoting examples from the experience of his friends Trye and Tierney to prove his point. Whether by accident or design, a later translation of the *Inquiry* appeared on the very same day in Vienna, edited and translated by Aloysius Careno, incorporating the new material from *Further Observations;* and on August 19, Dr. G. F. Balhorn brought out a German version in Hanover. The word was spreading.

In Bristol, Dr. Thomas Beddoes[27]—who had established his Pneumatic Institute the year before—twice noticed Jenner's cowpox research mentioned in a comprehensive anthology of West of England Medical Contributions. Since both these contributions were anti-vaccination, however—one by a Gloucester apothecary named Charles Cooke and the other by a Stroud surgeon, Edward Thornton—Beddoes drew Jenner's attention to them before going to press and invited him to reply. This he did immediately, so that the anthology appeared with Jenner's more forceful rebuttal completely negating both doctors' observations. Beddoes's scrupulous fairness effectively neutralized what would have been a damaging piece of propaganda from the pioneer's own county.

A reaction to Jenner's discovery set in three long years after Phipps's vaccination; and for the first time Jenner, who had expressed his independence of London so forcefully in his famous letter to Farquhar, now found the capital's leading doctors seeking him out. Included in these was the brilliant and idealistic John Ring,[28] who apparently unaware of the Phipps case was impulsively moved by the humanitarian potential of vaccination when the *Inquiry* was published. Unhappily his initial reaction was short-lived. Ring succumbed to the pressure of the opposing forces, and his defection gave Jenner considerable distress. A friend of Woodville's, and a very conscientious if temporarily misinformed man, Ring eventually resumed his vaccination loyalty and became a lifelong friend of Jenner's. The two had a great deal more than medicine in common, both being interested in poetry and music.

By the middle of the summer a number of key figures in the history of vaccination appeared for the first time. Most of them came to Cheltenham to see the pioneer for personal discussion; others wrote him. The powerful influence of such figures from the capital as Lord Egremont, Lord Polwarth, and Dr. John Abernethy[29] lent weight to the growing movement that was steering the diffident doctor towards the Court of St. James and royal recognition. But from the provinces came two valuable recruits with

whom Jenner undoubtedly felt more at home. Dr. Darke of
Stroud, in the unsympathetic hinterland of Gloucestershire, eagerly offered his assistance and influence during an extended visit
to the town in August, and a Mr. William Fermor from Tusmore
in Oxfordshire probably appeared at the same time. The latter
gentleman was to become famous as the first lay friend of Jenner's
to write a work on vaccination. In a sense, Fermor was coming
home when he came to Cheltenham, since his family had been
established in the nearby parish of Deerhurst since the sixteenth
century and recently they had sold the impropriation of the
church to Powell Snell's father. It was probably Snell who introduced William Fermor to Jenner and a most valuable contact it
proved to be. The new recruit had everything that was so urgently
needed. He was wealthy, came of a noble family—the Pomfrets,
who had enormous influence in the county of Oxford, including
the university, had vast agricultural holdings, and most important,
were dedicated to the cause of vaccination. As a result of their
conversation, Jenner and Fermor decided to organize a research
campaign in Oxfordshire with vaccine supplied by Jenner, who
also agreed to send his nephew George to Tusmore to take charge.
Fortunately the cowpox was an occasional visitor to Fermor's area,
and he himself was already familiar with certain aspects of
the disease. Since there was ample money to spend, this venture
bid fair to be the most promising large-scale operation to date.
When his new friend left Cheltenham, Jenner promised that he
would visit him at Tusmore as soon as his immediate commitments
permitted. Back at his home, Fermor promptly entered the lists
in the battle against the anti-vaccinationists and proved a most
witty and potent ally. In one of his letters to Jenner he wrote, "I
told Dr. Moseley that in his assertions against it [vaccination] he
had acted the part of a devil's advocate at a saint's canonization,
who was to say all the hard he could against the saint in order
that his life might be thoroughly scrutinized, and his merits appear the more conspicuous."[30]

At the other end of the Cotswolds, in Bath, another key figure,
Dr. Thomas Creaser, was organizing the Bath Institution for gratuitous vaccination—the first in the country.[31] This brilliant and
fashionable medico who flourished towards the end of Bath's

golden age was not only the most uncompromising supporter of vaccination from its very beginning, but was the perfect example of the wealthy, intellectual doctor of the eighteenth century. His literary executor, the younger Fosbroke, writes:

As an operative and consulting surgeon at Bath he succeeded in the acquisition of the highest eminence and most extensive practice. The circle of his professional and private connections was most ample and select. . . . His scientific acquirements were many and valuable in their kind. With physiology and pathology he kept due pace with discovery and improvement from the day of Mr. Hunter to the time present. With most of the eminent characters, both of the metropolis and the country, who have existed during the last forty years, he had held some intercourse. For Doctors Parry and Jenner he entertained a permanent and enthusiastic esteem.[32]

The Bath field of operations in support of the cause was steadily expanding.

Everyone was not as prosperous as the fashionable doctors who were increasingly attracted to the vaccination fold, however, and with all the activity of his crusade swirling about him, Jenner was still concerned about his old friends. Thomas Fosbroke in his modest curacy at Horsley was bravely struggling along with his wife and two babies. At twenty-nine he had already embarked upon the antiquarian researches that were to make him famous, but he always seemed to be pressed for money. *The Economy of Monastic Life,* written, extraordinarily enough, in verse, appeared in 1795 and paved the way for his monumental *British Monachism,* but he made virtually no profit from either. He had little money to buy books or even the current magazines and was far removed from a decent library or the community of scholars. "My literary pursuits in the way of science are at present wholly at a stand [still?] from the distance of a library," he wrote to a friend in 1796, "and I can no farther presume upon that of Gloucester . . . for which reason I have often wished though perhaps in vain, to have been in range of the British Museum."[33] Well, possibly it would not have been feasible to move the British Museum to Gloucestershire but perhaps had he been a member of one of the great learned societies the resources of many scholarly collections would have been at his disposal. As it happened Samuel

Lysons had recently been made Director of the Society of Antiquaries. He usually spent a great deal of time in Cheltenham when visiting brother Daniel at Hempsted, and Jenner spoke to him about Fosbroke. As a result the young curate with but one book to his credit was duly elected to the Society of Antiquaries in 1799.[34] His whole outlook changed and his researches accelerated to the extent that the first edition of *British Monachism* appeared in two volumes three years later. Long the standard work on the subject, it went through two further editions in his lifetime. Whether by chance or design, one of the earliest lay vaccinators, Rev. T. T. A. Reed of Leckhampstead,[35] Buckinghamshire, was to be instrumental in Fosbroke's acquiring his first independent parish many years later. By then Jenner knew Reed very well, of course, and may have had a hand in the business during its formative stages. Reed wrote a pamphlet on vaccination in 1806 and became incumbent of Welford, Herefordshire, soon after Fosbroke became curate-in-charge there in 1810.

About the time that poor Fosbroke was looking for library facilities, an older friend completed his researches on a work that enhanced Jenner's medical reputation considerably. Caleb Parry's *Symptoms and Causes of . . . Angina Pectoris*[36] was published in the summer, and he paid warm tribute to the great part Jenner had played in the researches that had gone into the book. Some of this pioneer work in cardiac medicine was, indeed, done by Jenner alone. The Parrys were the center of a literary circle that included Edmund Burke—who had been Member of Parliament for Bristol—Samuel Taylor Coleridge, and Anthony Fothergill, who in 1785 had written the first book on Cheltenham waters.[37]

Fortunately for Jenner, the logic of his investigations and the purely objective judgments that the British medical profession, as a whole, refused to recognize were readily accepted on the Continent. Wars and political prejudices had no effect on the fight against the common enemy, smallpox. In September Jenner received a letter from Dr. Jean De Carro of Vienna,[38] a graduate of Geneva, who stated that he had already vaccinated with dubious serum obtained from Dr. Pearson. Since the cowpox was not prevalent in the Austrian Empire, De Carro begged the English doctor to send some of his own vaccine through the British legation. This letter led to the rapid spread of vaccination throughout Eastern Europe[39] and into Asia as far as India. A few weeks later in November a similar letter arrived from Doctors George Balhorn and Christian Strohmeyer of Hamburg. Though written in Latin, it was not too difficult for Jenner to decipher. The end result was that vaccination was established all over Europe and at least in part of the Near East before it was really accepted in England. In the last weeks of 1799 the *Inquiry* was translated into Latin for distribution from Vienna, and into German for distribution from Hanover.[40]

At the very end of the year there is evidence that the family strain, which must have obtained after the smallpox inoculations at Berkeley during the spring of 1795, was finally eased. Henry and George Jenner were now sincerely committed to vaccination. It was the former, as the senior partner, who broke a long silence—three years after Phipps's vaccination—and published a nineteen-page pamphlet entitled *An Address to the Public on the advantages of Vaccine inoculation, with the objections to it refuted.* It is dated December 26, 1799, so presumably it came out in the new year from the printer William Bulgin of Wine Street, Bristol, who was thus the first to issue a vaccination tract from that city. Henry was a man past thirty by this time, and his comments were taken with sufficient seriousness for an abstract to be printed in the *Medical and Physical Journal*; the following year a German translation of his article appeared. Rather more than his uncle, Henry Jenner was concerned about the apathy to vaccination in Bristol—the largest city in Gloucestershire—and followed up the tract with another one addressed specifically to *The Inhabitants of Bristol* (1801).[41] George emulated his brother and broke into print soon afterwards with a letter relating to some of his own case histories, written from London. Of the two, George was probably the more serious scholar, but both of them were now thoroughly committed to their uncle's cause. They published supporting material sporadically for the rest of their lives. Unhappily, even at the height of his prestige the civil service remained coldly aloof from Jenner, and he was never able to secure a living for George, who remained a poor man throughout his life.

It says a great deal for the immense power of the medical profession at the end of the eighteenth century that Jenner's support by the highest families in the land—as well as abroad—was not sufficient to give his discovery a fair and easy passage. Putting aside personal or professional jealousy, there was a solid force of vested interest involved. The vaccination revolution would remove from the books a disease that was probably a main source of revenue for thousands of practitioners. It would mean the end of all the smallpox hospitals, and finally, the eradication of smallpox inoculation—an operation that had been an important part of the physician's work for half a century. In addition to all this there was a certain aspect of vaccination that readily lent itself to the exploitation of mob fear. The injection of animal tissue into a human being could all too easily be pictured as evil and against God's law. And so it was that certain well-trained but cynical doctors used the ignorance of the people to oppose a man who would save them from the horrors of a disfiguring and fatal disease. As a balance to this, the most important and prestigious of the anti-vaccinationists, Dr. Ingenhousz, died before the year was out, but his patron Lord Lansdowne remained.

One can to a certain extent understand the reluctance of men like Ingenhousz and Woodville to support the new system. Woodville had been appointed physician to the St. Pancras Smallpox Hospital and Inoculation Clinic at the age of thirty-eight, after a most distinguished career, and Ingenhousz was the most celebrated inoculator in all Europe. Both were probably very sincere, but the same might not be said for Moseley and Pearson, who showed themselves from the very beginning as calculating businessmen.

As the century neared its end, Jenner found his social connections soaring ever higher and his financial resources sinking ever lower, since his crusade activities left too little time for professional earnings. Patronage by the mighty would no doubt lead to official rewards eventually, but in the meantime he had to feed his family, and this was getting very hard. To be harassed by household bills in the evening and approached by members of ruling houses the following morning was something that was difficult of adjustment. The first foreign royalty to recognize Jenner's efforts was in the person of Princess Louisa of Prussia, and he was somewhat swept off his feet when she sent a request for serum just

before Christmas, 1799. Still having Henry's two doctor sons under his wing, so to speak, he offered to send George to show how
to administer it. This suggestion was politely refused, but the
serum was gratefully received and vaccination duly implemented
in Prussia. It is hard to see how Jenner could possibly have financed his nephew's expedition to that far country had the princess accepted his offer. But more of his native patrons were extending their contacts into the regions of the world where their
services might be at his disposal. The Elgins opened up a new
potential for the international spread of vaccination when the
young earl was made Ambassador to the Ottoman Empire.[42] Well
as he knew Lord Aylesbury, Jenner had never met the Elgin
cousins though later events suggest that Aylesbury may have written and told them of the new discovery of this Cheltenham doctor.

In the meantime the circle of influence at home continued to
widen. Captain John McMahon, private secretary to the Prince of
Wales and later Keeper of the Privy Purse, was a regular summer
resident of the Spa, and was the connecting link in the many
cliques and coteries.[43] He was the confidant not only of the royal
princes—Clarence, Sussex, and York, as well as of the heir himself
—but also of their mistresses and their circles. He was a sought-
after guest at every rout and ball. The Locks and the Berrys together with the nobility eagerly courted his patronage and his
advice. Perhaps an important aspect of his influence was the fact
that he was not merely a court official. He circulated in art circles
and was a great enthusiast of the stage. In fact, his compassionate
relationship with such royal mistresses as Mrs. Jordan and Mrs.
Robinson[44] clearly shows his respect for their art far beyond his
concern over their associations with his royal employer. It must be
remembered that the household and world of the Prince of Wales
with its permissiveness was totally different and totally separate
from that of the King's. Members of each frequented the walks
in Cheltenham. Both worlds were essential to Jenner's interest,
and at first it even seemed that he would meet the Prince before
the Sovereign. While Lord Elgin was promoting vaccination in
the Middle East, his family had assumed a very vital position
on the birth of a daughter to the Princess of Wales. The infant—
who, had she lived, would have been Queen of England—was

placed in charge of the Dowager Lady Elgin. As Farington observes with great surprise: "The Princess of Wales only has the young Princess brought to her twice a week. Lady Elgin has the entire care of her. The child already has a sense of its situation in life and deports herself with a consciousness of it.—It is quite remarkable that she calls the King Grandpappa—but the Queen always *Your Majesty*."[45] This same young princess fell even deeper into the hands of the vaccination camp a few years later when a powerful Jenner supporter, Dr. Richard Croft, was assigned her medical care.[46] Croft was Matthew Baillie's brother-in-law.

While on the subject of influence in high places, it might be well to notice what was happening at Leckhampton Court, where Dr. Trye with his newly acquired wealth was expanding the estate and at the same time enthusiastically promoting vaccination. He had two spheres of influence: the world of the Gloucester Infirmary (to which he stayed in harness to the day of his death) and the vast freemasonry of the local families. Undoubtedly this close network was of the utmost value in the coordination of pressures on official circles. The estates of important society surrounded the town like a vast spider's web. The Hicks at Whitcomb, the Hardwicks at Arle, the Sherbornes at Northleach, the Ducies at Woodchester, the Snells at Guiting, the Russells at Charton Kings, the Coopers at Dursley, and perhaps a dozen others were the centers of great-house hospitality that catered to even larger gatherings than the salons of the town itself. Astley Cooper, incidentally, bid fair to amass greater riches than his brother Bransby had acquired through his heiress. Already in 1800 when he was elected to the Royal College of Surgeons, his professional earnings were among the highest in London. Henry Cline, who had taken Cooper under his wing after he had left Hunter, saw his own fame eventually challenged and surpassed by his pupil. Cline, now the most vigorous proponent of vaccination in London, was thus equally involved in the rise of the country's greatest surgeon. But wealthy landowners among the nobility and perhaps wealthier society doctors were still poorer than bankers. Amelia, the most beautiful of the Lock girls, was instrumental in bringing the millionaire banker John Julius Angerstein to Cheltenham.[47] If Sarah Siddons had brought the impressive Moore clan, it was this magnificent twenty-two-year-old who netted the richest vaccination fish of them all. Old Angerstein was even then a legend. The directing force behind Lloyds and a man of inestimable wealth, his origins were veiled in mystery; some called him German, some Russian. In his early banking career he had struck up a friendship with William Lock of Norbury—a financier of much more modest scale —and the two families drew very close with the passage of years. Amelia Lock, the youngest daughter, was born in 1777 and grew up to be one of the toasts of society. Sir Thomas Lawrence, the painter, who was a family friend, was one of her many admirers and most of the fashionables followed him. "We hear of Lord William Gordon dying of love for her, and a Mr. Hammenday being quite in despair at her refusing him." It was the son of John Julius Angerstein whom she married, however, on September 28, 1799, and as of then the great man himself became a summer resident of Cheltenham, a friend of Jenner's, and eventually one of the leading organizers of the vaccination campaign in Britain. Like most bankers he was a possessive man and he no doubt looked upon the girl as he did his many priceless works of art. "Her father-in-law," it was said, "became extremely fond of her and no doubt ruled her as he did all his family, with the authority tinged with arrogance which extreme wealth usually develops." Angerstein was also a close and sympathetic friend of that somewhat unusual young woman, the Princess of Wales, and it was probably he who introduced Jenner to her. (Whether or not the association with Her Royal Highness was an asset in the long run, however, is another matter.)

Shrewd man of finance that he was, Angerstein was not interested in profiting by his support of Jenner. He never saw vaccination as a commercial possibility, though there were many who did. Despite the adverse impact of the movement on the large element in the medical profession who prospered in the field of smallpox treatment, it was inevitable that sooner or later the financial potential of the discovery would have to be noticed. It was clear from Jenner's behavior since the vaccination of Phipps and even more so after the publication of the *Inquiry* that he was not interested in protecting his system or even making a reasonable profit. He was solely concerned with its social effect. Consequently George

Pearson, who had marked attentively the gradual spread of interest through 1799, decided that there was considerable profit available for a man of keen business propensities. Jenner was an idealistic provincial from whom it would not have been difficult to take over control. Pearson lived in London where all medical development centered, and he could promote his own campaign while Jenner was dreaming and hoping in faraway Cheltenham. Pearson, indeed, had benefitted considerably by the attention he had received from the pioneer, and the fact that some of his own operations had been included in the 1799 book enhanced his reputation as a vaccinationist significantly. A much more aggressive, not to say ruthless, man than Cline, Pearson set out to be the director of the campaign in the capital. He proclaimed himself the authority on the subject, and by way of a series of public lectures, he inaugurated an independent program of vaccination entirely on his own. His early recognition by Jenner apparently made many simple people believe that the master was content to leave the organization of affairs to this younger and more dynamic London doctor.

It was Pearson's growing confidence in his own ability that led to what Le Fanu calls "the controversy that cost Jenner most grief and trouble."[48] For the first few years of vaccination only virus carefully selected by Jenner himself was the basis of serum used anywhere in the world, and the virtually perfect record of this practice inclined the ambitious Pearson to develop supplies of his own rather than be delayed by the limitations of Jenner's pedestrian pace. As a result he and Woodville, impatiently pressing their London operations, contaminated some cowpox matter with smallpox matter. That moment of carelessness brought about a wave of smallpox infection. Inevitably, the cry went around that vaccination was actually *giving* people smallpox, and Woodville, at least, believed this to be so. It was obvious, he decided, that there was no essential difference between cowpox matter and smallpox matter. To John Ring, also, this seemed apparent. These two latter were honest men who simply felt that the great vaccination hope had proved illusory; they had no venom or resentment against Jenner. Pearson, however, was another matter altogether. He had been, as he thought, on the crest of the wave when the disaster came and had much farther to fall. Indeed, he had so far impressed the most influential vaccination patrons in the capital, that, in the absence of any apparent objection from the quiet doctor in Cheltenham, he inaugurated a national vaccine institute with no less a person than the Duke of York as its patron. Not content with this, Pearson next had the unwise effrontery to offer Jenner a subordinate role in the organization—a position immediately under himself. Needless to say the offer was treated with the contempt its impudence merited, and Jenner belatedly awoke to his erstwhile ally's treachery. The incident of the contaminated matter followed soon afterwards, in January 1800.

Pearson conceded no possibility of his own carelessness. The die for him was cast, and he had to nail his colors to the anti-vaccination mast. Inevitably, he got into print first while the shock of the post-vaccination smallpox fatalities was still widespread. He immediately wrote to the *Medical and Physical Journal,* and the January issue announced his "discovery" of something resembling smallpox pustules resulting from vaccine inoculation.[49] Since this periodical was a monthly, Jenner's reply only came out in the February issue after a great deal of damage had already been done. Nevertheless, Jenner pointed out bluntly that he suspected "that where various postules have appeared, variolus matter had occasioned them," since no such phenomenon had occurred after the launching of vaccination. Nonetheless, January was a period of great anxiety for Jenner, and while no really exalted public figures were deflected from the cause, a vast number of lesser lights and, in particular, disgruntled doctors were encouraged to unite against Jenner. Perhaps the vaccination myth had been exploded. Unfortunately, also, throughout the controversy that persisted all through the spring, Ring and Woodville stubbornly supported the position of Pearson, even when that gentleman's case had been finally discredited.

Among the places to which Pearson sent his impure matter was the village of Petworth in Sussex where Lord Egremont's[50] surgeon, Mr. Andre, innocently vaccinated fourteen people with it. All of them became dangerously ill. As it happened, an old Gloucestershire friend of Jenner's, the Reverend Mr. Ferryman who was in Petworth at the time, was permitted to view the patients, and was horrified to see that they were suffering from small-

pox rather than cowpox. Fortunately Lord Egremont acted swiftly
to prevent the disease from spreading, and he had the patients removed from the village to his own mansion, where later one of
them died.

Undoubtedly, Egremont's prompt action prevented a serious
epidemic, but a side effect was a correspondence between his lordship and Jenner, which was of inestimable value to the doctor at
this critical time. The peer was open-minded enough to write a
description of the incidents, requesting the doctor's comments,
rather than taking the more simple course of joining the opposition. Ferryman also wrote to his friend adding his detailed account of the tragedy. Jenner replied with great fervor and at
great length, while enclosing a supply of healthy serum. "The
included virus is secured in a way that I imagine cannot fail to
infect, if Mr. Andre will reduce it to a fluid state by moistening
with water on the point of his lancet previous to its insertion."[51]
No sooner had his letter been dispatched, however, than the doctor sent a further one offering the services of his nephew George
at Petworth to make sure the correct procedure was followed. Jenner had just heard that a servant in the household of a Lady
C—— had received smallpox by being injected with the same
matter that had caused the Petworth disaster. The result of all
this was to make Lord Egremont a staunch promoter of the cowpox inoculation. "From Lord Egremont," Jenner was able to
write to Gardner:

I have also had a pleasant account. The matter I sent to his lordship
has dissipated all doubts and prejudices, he says, from the minds of the
people around him. Forty have been inoculated and all have had the
disease as I have described it. You must observe that fourteen had
previously been inoculated with matter from Pearson and *all* had
variolus-like eruptions . . . I think the surgeon at Petworth who inoculated both sets of patients, mine, if I may call them so, and Pearson's,
should publish immediately the result of the two inoculations.[52]

By now very impressed, Lord Egremont suggested meeting the
doctor in London for the purpose of planning the establishment
of a new vaccine institution. Jenner, however, begged to be allowed to meet him in Petworth instead, and, his host agreeing, he
arrived there with Catherine's brother-in-law, Mr. Ladbroke, on

February 15, 1800. While Jenner had been in correspondence with Egremont since the previous autumn, it is uncertain whether they had actually met before, though they had many common acquaintances. The peer, who was an eccentric in an age of eccentrics, was a great patron of the arts and held permanent court at Petworth. He usually had several painters in residence and left them to their own devices.

Jenner spent an interesting nine days at the mansion and was entertained in regal style. Egremont was completely dedicated to helping in any way that he could, and a series of treatments was completed that thoroughly vindicated the vaccination case. To be sure, the doctor worked extremely hard and performed some two hundred vaccinations before he left, "without one deviation from the ordinary course having taken place," and thereby summarily triumphing over the machinations of Pearson and his colleagues. The visit had certainly cemented his friendship with Lord Egremont and probably gave him the opportunity of meeting the poet William Hayley, with whom he was sporadically associated for many years after.[53] But of more importance was the effect of his efficient rescue operation upon the more exalted supporters of vaccination. Immediately after his work at Petworth was concluded, Jenner received a summons from the Duke of York, the discomfited patron of Pearson's vaccination institute. He waited on his royal highness a few days later on March 1, and after a prolonged conversation and some correspondence between members of both factions, a halfhearted attempt to heal the breach between the opposing forces was discarded. On March 17 Jenner was informed by Lord Egremont that both the Duke of York and he had decided to withdraw from the institute altogether. It was a major victory for the harassed and nigh penniless pioneer, who had been challenged by vested interests that may well have daunted a lesser man. This victory made his reception at the Court of St. James almost inevitable.

The path to the royal presence from Petworth was not a long one. Where Pearson had stepped down Jenner would step up. He had been gathering new material since the publication of the *Further Observations* and combined everything in a splendid second edition of the *Inquiry* that ran to some one hundred and eighty-two pages—about three times the bulk of the initial work. "The foregoing pages," he wrote, "contain the whole of my first treatise on the variolae vaccinae published in June, 1798. . . . I was induced to offer to the world *Further Observations . . .* published in the beginning of the year 1799. These treatises I have here combined, together with some additions." He dedicated it to H.M. the King. It was a heartening end to the pilgrimage that he had started so anxiously nearly five months before. His friend Fermor expressed his conclusions in a forty-seven-page pamphlet, *Reflexions on the Cowpox as a Security against the Smallpox,* which was published in Oxford on May 2.[54]

After a visit to Tusmore, Jenner spent a few more weeks in London trying to capitalize on the gains of the first half-year of vaccination, though it is likely that he had other interests in the town. Matthew Baillie's sister Joanna presented her "psychological" play, *De Montford,* which opened at Drury Lane on April 29, and a real gathering of the Cheltenham clans it turned out to be. Mr. Kemble produced it and played the male lead, Mrs. Siddons played the female lead, the Duchess of Devonshire wrote the epilogue, and Michael Kelly wrote the music! These massed talents notwithstanding, the play was a failure. Neither literature nor science, it miserably fell between the two stools. As the critics wrote, "The acting of Mr. Kemble was amazingly powerful" and "Mrs. Siddons exerted herself powerfully"; nevertheless it only ran for twelve nights and the final curtain came down on May 13.

Of somewhat more interest was the industry of another Gloucestershire expatriate, Thomas Paytherus. Despite Jenner's vindication at Petworth, the subject of the impure vaccine and slipshod practice was still very much in the public mind. Paytherus compiled a record of the evidence of Woodville—the most expert of the anti-cowpox faction—as opposed to the concrete achievements of Jenner and had it printed anonymously by the doctor's own publisher, Sampson Low. It was issued in the identical format of the *Inquiry* and entitled: *A Comparative Statement of the Facts and Observations Relative to the Cowpox; Published by Doctors Jenner and Woodville.*[55] The obvious intention was to give the impression that the work was *written* by the two men, and also to show Jenner in the strongest possible light. Why the writer should have done this is not clear, unless he felt that Jenner would be more readily noticed than himself. Be that as it may, it was an incisive, logical document and struck a welcome blow at the by-no-means-chastened opposition.

By July, however, London fashion had departed to the various resorts chosen for the hot weather, and there were no people of importance to proselytize. Jenner returned to Cheltenham alone on July 10, when the season at the Wells was in full swing. Perhaps he was called by some sudden pressing business and could not wait for the rather more sedate travel arrangements necessary for Catherine and the children. Certainly after such a long absence his affairs at St. George's Place would have been accumulating steadily. On the other hand, Catherine's health must have been in a very satisfactory state for him to be willing for her to remain in the capital alone with the children at that humid time of the year. It is possible that by the summer he had simply run out of money and had to pick up as much of the seasonal trade at the Wells as he could. All the encouragement and personal vindication he had received in London in no way compensated for the half-year he had spent away from any kind of lucrative employment. Nevertheless he seemed to be in a happy enough frame of mind when he returned home. "I am just now got to Cheltenham," he wrote to John Clinch on July 15, 1800, "after having spent near six months in London." Then he immediately turned to the urgent business of vaccination in far-off Newfoundland. "Lest the thread sent to you by George should not take effect I have enclosed a little bit more newly impregnated by the cowpox virus; use it like a smallpox thread; but small as it is, divide into portions that you may multiply your chance of infecting. Wet it before insertion; or rather moisten it."[56]

Since this letter was written on Jenner's arrival in Cheltenham direct from London, it would seem that he at last had a local source of cowpox vaccine available without having to go to Berkeley for it. John Goding mentions a summer house on Cleeve Hill where Jenner obtained his supplies but does not mention when.[57] What was more serious in several ways was the free and easy manner in which the less responsible Cheltenham folk were indulging in amateur vaccination practice, both to the danger of

their health and the detriment of poor Jenner's livelihood. As
Powell Snell observed, "The housewife scratched with her needle,
the cobbler with his awl, and even shepherd boys each other with
their pocket knives."[58] Nor was this wide application of Jenner's
system of the slightest help to him financially. Since he repudi-
ated any thought of protecting his discovery, its wide practice in
the West of England brought no reward but prestige. Again quoting Snell: "Every village surgeon adopts it"[59]—and one might
have added every town surgeon in Cheltenham, Gloucester, Bath,
and Bristol. Jenner's friends began discussing plans for the promotion of a parliamentary grant as soon as possible. Everyone
seemed to be benefitting except the great pioneer himself. Now
recognized in the highest possible official circles, he was yet left
with no tangible assistance to aid him in his work—or, indeed,
compensate him for loss of revenue stemming from weeks and
months taken away from his practice.

Jenner's return to Cheltenham was timely. The season still had
several months to go, and the reception he had received from the
royal family in London greatly increased his prestige in the local
society. Nor was his fame confined to vaccination alone. The nobility led by the Aylesburys and the Spencers turned some very
lucrative general practice his way. He was also consulted by many
of them professionally and was likewise employed in vaccinating
their children. In this manner he might make a sufficient amount
in the second half of the season to support the family through the
lean months of the winter. Lord Ellenborough was among those
who had his large brood of children vaccinated at this time, and
the ensuing ones (for a total of nine) as they appeared.

But the children of the rich were only a portion of those in need
of vaccination. During the latter part of his stay in London Jenner had been impatient to get home so that he could resume his
campaign to ensure that all the poor of the town were vaccinated.
He was eager to proceed with the smoothness and lack of opposition that he could expect nowhere else. "He offered gratuitous
inoculation to all the poor who thought fit to apply at stated
periods," wrote Baron. "These benevolent invitations were, in the
main very generally accepted, parents bringing their children
in great numbers both from the town and adjoining parishes."

But the stubborn Gloucestershire peasants were still not convinced, all too many remaining under the influence of their Berkeley brethren and variola inoculation. This phenomenon continued despite the serious mortality rate outside of Cheltenham during the epidemic of 1798–99. There was one village in particular that had suffered extremely by its dogged resistance, but soon after Jenner's return home he was greeted with the news that it had decided to cooperate. He was very gratified until he learned of the actual reason for the change of heart, and a very macabre reason it was: It appeared that the churchwardens were so upset by the cost of coffins to bury the smallpox victims that they peremptorily ordered the villagers to go into Cheltenham and "avail themselves of Dr. Jenner's offer."[60]

With it all, however, life was very tranquil after the harassing pace of London. Catherine arrived on July 29 with the children apparently none the worse for their long hot sojourn in the capital. But the Cheltenham respite was actually precious time stolen from the essential campaign Jenner and his patrons would have to continue to pursue at the center of the medical world. He would have to return to London in November, but at least, as Baron put it, "during his stay in Cheltenham he had some little relaxation from the incessant efforts we have seen him compelled to make."

But when sufficiently stirred, Jenner could still respond swiftly. A little over a week after Catherine's return the outside world intruded in a most welcome manner. He received a letter from Monsieur Le Compte de Laroque of Lyons who had completed the first French translation of the *Inquiry* in February. It had been posted in France on August 5 and addressed to Jenner in London, whence it had been forwarded to him in Gloucestershire. His reply, which was reprinted in a later edition of the translation, was dispatched on August 8 (*Response Du Docteur Jenner, Cheltenham, compte de Gloucester, 8, aout.1800*).[61] This suggests that he answered the letter within hours of his receiving it. Three days transit for the mails from Lyons to Cheltenham via London in time of war was phenomenally fast, and Jenner's reaction was untypically swift, undoubtedly moved by the vast new world a translation into the French language opened up. (An Italian translation appeared in Pavia soon afterwards.) Laroque wrote again on

August 21, to which Jenner also promptly replied, but after that there seems to have been a cessation of the correspondence. Perhaps all the points of interest had been settled, however, since Laroque proceeded to translate with the doctor's full authority Jenner's ensuing tracts as they appeared. The Frenchman actually lived at Privas, some eighty miles south of Lyons, and eventually made the not inconsiderable journey to London where he met Jenner in 1803. Even though the first draft of the French translation was published apparently without the writer's authority, with its appearance and that of the Italian version, *The Inquiry* was disseminated over the mainland of Europe within two years of its original publication in London. This, of course, was in addition to the circulation of the English edition in North America. Perhaps it is understandable that the pioneer felt he was entitled to relax for a month or two to nurture his own people in Cheltenham.

In July recognition came to Jenner's young disciple, Dr. J. H. Marshall of Stonehouse, who, with another vaccinationist, Dr. John Walker, was delegated by the government to make a tour of the Mediterranean colonies and adjacent lands in order to carry vaccination to the whole region; Gibraltar and Malta were to be the bases of operation. As previously mentioned, General O'Hara was already an enthusiastic supporter of the movement, and he was delighted when the government officially supported his position. All this was delineated in a letter that covered the events of the summer and reached Cheltenham at the end of October. Marshall wrote from H.M.S. *Foudroyant* on October 19, 1800:

My Dear Sir,

Since my last letter to you from hence the progress of the cowpox inoculation has been rapid, and is now generally adopted, I may say without exception in this island; the Governor has also patronised an institution for the cowpox or Jennerian inoculation, the rules of which I shall transcribe and send you with this. At Gibraltar, where we were received with the greatest attention by the Governor, General O'Hara, we were grateful by observing the cowpox proceed in the usual mild and easy progress to its termination as in England; nor did we perceive that the unusual heat of the climate (in the month of August) in the smallest degree aggravated the symptoms, though the soldiers of the garrison continued their fatiguing duties as customary previous to their inoculation, nor was any alteration made either in their diet or allowance of wine. The children of the inhabitants also experienced its mild and gentle progress, nor in any one instance were its symptoms in the least aggravated.[62]

Marshall continued to send back similar reports of his travels to Jenner for the next two years until his return to England in the summer of 1802, very much like a junior official reporting to headquarters. The master did, indeed, have his emissaries in an ever-increasing complex of overseas bases. But there was at least one local friend who was not entirely happy at the pace of the movement in England despite all the acclaim from abroad. In this, the first year of the new century, the bluff, nonintellectual Powell Snell was shrewd enough to see the barriers that were being raised, not only against vaccination, but—more important—against Jenner himself. To be sure, in the insulated world around the Wells all seemed secure; but Cheltenham was not England and the gregarious poetaster who travelled a great deal about the country heard much of what was being said. He also noted how smallpox inoculation continued to flourish despite the availability of cowpox serum. Undoubtedly he was the first of Jenner's lay friends to see the danger of this and cry out against it. Little good came of a situation where for every ten people saved from the disease by vaccination, ten more were deliberately infected by the variola injection. Almost within earshot of the great Marquess of Bute, who was still in residence, Snell wrote thus of the peer's grandmother on August 1: "Alas fair Montague, thy reign is o'er." Belatedly and with profound charity under the circumstances he proceeded to compose his own poem to Jenner long after the doctor and Thomas Fosbroke had lampooned him in verse. It not only reveals the warm feeling the Squire of Guiting held for the doctor after their five years as neighbors but expresses a confident finality that the smallpox problem had been solved.

> . . . Lo, hence no more the pest innate shall spread
> Its venomed fire and plume its purple head
> The subtle antidote of Jenner's skill,
> Shall check the birth and latent seeds of ill.[63]

The work itself is negligible as poetry but contains a great deal of information about the relationship of the two men and Snell's concern that his friend was not always appreciated as he should be. He specifically comments upon the lukewarm attitude of the Royal Society and urges them to recompense the doctor (who was indeed one of their number), "whose envied lore adds such a treasure to their chosen store." Entitling his work "My Learned Friend Edward Jenner," Snell extolls the doctor's role as husband, father, and friend; but he might also have referred to the many things they had in common. At the age of sixty the dashing squire, while still very much the lady's man, was increasingly concerned with the deeper matters that were also close to Jenner's heart. Their interests in the realm of natural history were almost identical, and Snell was fascinated by the still mysterious and disreputable nesting habits of the cuckoo. The migration of birds was also a common interest and the squire's plantations at Guiting Power undoubtedly provided valued observation posts for the doctor when he first came to Cheltenham. The similarity of the two men's approach to life, however, is probably most strongly brought out by their interest in animals. They both versified copiously on animals—domestic pets in particular. Snell immortalized in rhyme a good proportion of the Cheltenham dogs and cats of his day (an interesting and artless balance to some of the very sophisticated verses he composed to the various nymphs at the Wells), and his lines are remarkably similar to Jenner's in the same field. Though the doctor's style comes nearer to genuine poetry, it is difficult to determine whose influenced whose.

What little that has been written on Powell Snell suggests a man of scatterbrained if harmless character—the typical eighteenth-century country gentleman; but further investigation reveals unmistakably the qualities that made him a friend of Jenner's. His early awareness of the futility of smallpox inoculation was not the only indication of his forward thinking. His concern for children and their exploitation among the lower orders was half a century ahead of his time. He bitterly opposed the system of climbing boys—child chimney sweeps—and preached against it more than a generation before it became a national concern. Only three weeks prior to his poem to Jenner, Snell declaimed in defense of these hapless urchins:

. . . poor sable tinted tribe,
Half of whose days in loathsome flues is spent
With hunger, thirst and penury opprest
Of tyrants merciless the tattered slaves.
Whose harpy talons often seize the mite
The 'date obulum' of pity's hand.[64]

Behind Snell's frivolous facade, there was manifestly a humanitarian compassion that even Catherine had to acknowledge, even while she must have raised disapproving eyebrows at some of this aging gallant's escapades. He was as likely to pen lines to a scornful eighteen-year-old maiden as to some serious social evil. In fact, at the very time that Snell was concerned about exploited child labor and vaccination, he was also eating his heart out over Miss Kate Thompson, a nymph young enough to be his granddaughter. He might be thought a strange companion, even for the catholic taste of Jenner, but Snell was the prototype Georgian buck. Cheltenham, Bath, and Clifton swarmed with these lusty sorts, and the good doctor was completely at home with them. They too were a part of his very full world. All this fringe of frivolity—though there is a great deal of the tragic in Snell—was the stuff of Cheltenham. Nor were all the versifiers who strolled the groves older men. Young William Drayton appeared about this time and became a most devoted follower of Jenner. John Worgan, also, was writing poetry in Bristol, though he had not yet invaded the local scene. In a few years they all gravitated to St. George's Place in the train of the great doctors (most of whom were also writers).

The day would come when one of the main pleasures of Jenner's life would be patronizing these young intellectuals, but during 1800 there were many problems of a much more urgent nature to be faced. Jenner was not an energetic man by nature and he had all the weaknesses of the artist despite his brilliance as a medical man. He loved the distractions of the Cheltenham scene even while he was aware of the urgent load of correspondence facing him when he came home that penniless summer. The younger Fosbroke, who perhaps knew him more intimately than anyone else, writes:

Seated to execute something half-finished, now applying to, now receding from his task, showing dread of interruption yet pleased to be interrupted, the dislike of confinement of any requisite undertaking till it could be no longer postponed, and delay favoured with smiles, till it became needful to thrust it off with a violent impulse, showed rather the want of discipline and regularity in earlier days, than any natural inaptitude for more sustained and severe study.[65]

More than any man he needed a very efficient and devoted private secretary—a luxury he was not fated to have for several more years.

By the end of the century, however, when two-thirds of his life was past, Jenner could gain satisfaction from the fact that vaccination was definitely established. His *Inquiry* was read in the major European tongues, the practice had reached four continents, and smallpox deaths had been decimated. Whatever worries Jenner might have had over his personal finances, he must have felt that his discovery would now spread unimpeded over the earth as the new century dawned.

∽ IV ∽
Poverty and the Patronage of Princes
1800-1803

Unhappily the idyllic domestic life at St. George's Place was exchanged much too soon for the slavery of London. Jenner had obviously not rested sufficiently when he returned to town in November, and he paid bitterly for it. His old enemy, typhoid, struck him down just before Christmas and confined him to bed for several days. Since his narrow escape from death in 1794, he had always been fearful of this disease, particularly when in an overworked or run-down condition. But Jenner had more friends in the capital now and everything to get well for, so he resisted the temptation to return home and was eagerly back in the fray by the New Year. "His vaccinations among the higher ranks were very numerous; and many of the nobility were desirous of having from his own mouth information on the great question which then engrossed so much of the public attention."[1] And the tentacles of support were reaching out from Well Walk to Belgravia. This was emphasized very clearly when his new friend Lord Spencer, whose mother was such an important figure in Cheltenham society, gave a kind of vaccination soiree at his town house for Jenner to expatiate on his theories. Lords Lucas, Campden,[2] and Macartney were present, as well as Mr. Greville and a host of other celebrities. On the lighter side, Jenner went on sightseeing trips around the capital with his children and took them to see the illuminations in honor of the Queen's birthday. Being now almost desperately dedicated to obtaining some kind of financial grant from the government, Jenner reconciled himself to a much-extended period in London on this occasion and even entered his son Edward at Mr. Evan's school in Islington on January 21, 1801.

While the circle of his acquaintances among the mighty was certainly extending, real security could never come if he had to permanently subordinate his bread-and-butter practice to his crusading spirit. From 1798 Jenner had been required to spend a large part of each year in London and would have to do so until Parliament acted. These months represented periods of continual lobbying and visiting with little time for remunerative work. The weeks had sped by after the doctor's cordial reception by the royal family, but since no signs of gainful rewards had appeared Jenner had written to Sherborne asking his help in the matter. Acclaim was not edible, and Cheltenham's Lord of the Manor, Sherborne, was very forceable in his attitude to public compensation. When Jenner was being wined and dined in the most elaborate manner in town, he received the following letter from the peer.

My dear Doctor. Many thanks for your circumstantial letter; I am sorry to say I do not know Mr. Addington even by sight; they tell me that the King is recovering very fast and we may expect a drawing-room very soon which I will attend and I will then speak to Mr. Pitt. If patriot Grattan gets £50,000 for his patriotism, then true patriot Jenner deserves much more: I am sure not less; and less would be perfectly shabby to think of. I perfectly recollect Grattan's business —it was settled among his friends to propose £100,000 for him; determining to ask enough, and fearing that the sum should not be granted, one of his most particular friends was to get up afterwards and ask for £50,000 which was immediately granted, and he took £47,500 for prompt payment.[3]

It was a pity that the wily peer's advice was never taken by Jenner's friends, because, as we shall see, when a grant was forthcoming it was ridiculously low. The praise continually came pouring in to Jenner from all quarters of the success of his system that was enriching mankind but not bringing him a penny piece. Dr. Davids of Amsterdam wrote, addressing him: "The benefactor of Mankind, Dr. Jenner—I am happy to introduce the cowpox through the whole country [Netherlands]. The name of Jenner is adored." Nevertheless, this patient man once more returned home heavy with new laurels, and light from empty pockets.

The only tangible or negotiable thing he brought back to Cheltenham was a splendid service of plate from the "Nobility and Gentry of Gloucestershire," through the loyal exertions of the Countess of Berkeley and the Reverend Mr. Pruen. In a crisis, he could always realize money on it. There was the usual correspondence to attend to when he got home, in particular a most important letter from Dr. Benjamin Waterhouse at Harvard that must have arrived in London just before he boarded the coach.

The increase in the number of celebrities—both fashionable and intellectual—frequenting the Wells in the summer of 1801 was very marked. The Jenners arrived when the season was in full swing, and one of the principal topics of conversation was the parliamentary grant. St. George's Place became a kind of Harley Street or medical center when Dr. Minster leased the whole terrace where Jenner lived from the livery stable proprietor, Mr. Lambert.[4] Since the houses on either end were let to Newell and Jenner, respectively, and number six—Athelney House—was probably already occupied by Dr. Fowler,[5] Minster himself would appear to have occupied the remaining one—number seven. In Manchester Walk, a lane off St. George's Place, Dr. Pope lived and, as we have seen, Dr. Hooper was ensconced at the Great House. The back of the terrace looked directly on to the churchyard, which in those days was just a quiet tree-embowered oasis that Moreau described as "one of the most beautiful in England."[6] Perhaps a house backing onto a churchyard had another advantage for the eighteenth-century doctors. There was a long tradition that a vault in the garden of number six—since filled in, alas—was a place where Jenner and his friends performed their anatomical dissections.[7] What is more concrete, however, is the fact that Jenner's tardiness in getting home this summer left him out of a very interesting development that had arisen when the Enclosures Act was being implemented. The skeleton of a murderer named Armstrong was discovered in a Cheltenham field where a fence was being erected. Minster and Newell promptly made a bid to the vestry for the purchase of the remains, and they returned to their respective homes with the spoils—Minster had the head and Newell the rest of the body. Corpses for dissection were hard to come by in those days. On the death of Newell, the murderer's skeleton was sent to the Royal College of Surgeons.[8]

Dr. Darke was still in Cheltenham when the Jenners got back, and he spoke with a reassuring enthusiasm Jenner direly needed when faced with the unpalatable task of appealing to the government for funds. Jenner wrote to Hicks at Eastington:

Darke . . . mentioned some strange cases of the preventive power of cowpox. He can also favour me with the cases of those who have resisted variolous inoculation because they have undergone the cowpox at some distant part of their lives. Evidence of this kind I cannot obtain too abundantly as it is at this point that the public mind makes a pause, from the early impression that was made of its proving a temporary preventive only.

By and large, most of Jenner's disparagers seem to have kept away from Cheltenham, and I can find no record of Ingenhousz, Pearson, or Moseley on the visitor lists. Woodville is, of course, the exception, but he was at that time about to change his allegiance and support the new movement. All in all, Jenner's spirits always seemed to rise when he returned home; familiar places and familiar faces meant a great deal to this sentimental man and a splendid company was certainly awaiting him.

Charles James Fox,[9] who was Moseley's patient, had yet to be converted, and it was at Jenner's house that the event took place. Fox had never been acrimonious; he had merely professed a certain lofty amusement at people who had deliberately encouraged the injection of a very dirty disease into the system of a completely healthy person on the assumption that it might cure an even dirtier one. Dr. Jameson had pretty much the same attitude. It was incredulous rather than hostile. "In his usual playful and engaging manner Fox said one day to Jenner, 'Pray, Dr. Jenner, tell me of this cowpox that we have heard so much about:—what is it like?' 'Why, it is exactly like the section of a pearl on a rose leaf.' This comparison which is not less remarkable for its accuracy than for its poetic beauty, struck Mr. Fox very forcibly. He laughed heartily and praised the simile."[10] Nevertheless on his stroll back to Vernon House that summer evening, Fox thought in a less frivolous manner and became one of vaccination's strongest supporters—and he was a very powerful man.

With the Foxes in Cheltenham was Lucy Fitzgerald, who had

been there with Celia Lock and Lord Edward in 1798. After the latter's death in the Irish rising, all his estates and possessions had been seized by the Crown by bill of attainder, and his wife was left in abject poverty. Fox with characteristic courage and generosity supported a fund to provide two hundred pounds per annum for Lord Edward's widow, Pamela. When one realizes the opprobrium under which the rebel cause stood, Fox's was a gesture of the greatest significance in a man in so high an official position. The Duchess of Leinster, Fitzgerald's mother, continued a regular patron of the Wells, though she was not present this summer. From her home in Wimbledon she was hoping and praying that poor Lucy Fitzgerald would find herself a husband. She wrote:

> You must not think of coming to me, so far from being of use to me, Angel, I should only fret: no, no, you cannot be better than where you are, taking the Cheltenham Waters. . . . I hope that your success at Cheltenham will have put you a little in conceit with your dear self, I hope too, that it will, in the end, produce something good in the marrying way, to see you happily settled, sweet girl, is the first wish of my heart.[11]

As a matter of fact the worthy duchess need not have worried about Lucy in the least. She was well able to take care of herself. An unashamed rebel, she thoroughly enjoyed her rather hectic life. She married of all people an admiral in the Royal Navy, Sir William Foley, in 1803, though she proclaimed her loyalty to the cause of Irish independence for the rest of her life. At the end of the wars, incidentally, Foley sat beside Jenner on the magistrate's bench in Cheltenham.

Fox's house in Cheltenham was near the little lane that leads from the banks of the Chelt at Barratt's Mill to the High Street. It backs onto the rear of 450, High Street, where Lord Byron lived in 1812, and where the lesser poet Thomas Haynes Bayly[12] died in 1839. The Duchess of Devonshire and the Jerseys already had seasonal residences near here, and after a visit to Matthew Baillie in London for treatment of his club foot, the thirteen-year-old Byron was brought to Cheltenham by his mother to visit friends and take the waters. The family had connections in the neighborhood and the poet's young cousin John Byron eventually became rector of Elmstone Hardwick. In Cheltenham the wife of the miniature painter, Millet, seems to have seen a great deal of the Byrons; she was also a close friend of Mary Anne Chaworth's,[13] whom the poet Moore met in the town some years later.

Still on the subject of the Romantic poets, it is interesting to note that Charles Parry had given Jenner's 1798 book to Dr. Johann Blumenbach under whom he was studying medicine at Gottingen.[14] Parry spent the summer vacation that year touring the Continent with the poet Coleridge. Parry himself when he settled in Cheltenham wrote a certain amount of verse. Since the younger Fosbroke reveals that Jenner and Coleridge eventually became friends, they probably met through Parry. Blumenbach soon afterwards started his correspondence with Jenner, and once again there was the mutual interest in natural history as well as vaccination—a common phenomenon with most of these men.

It is always hard to tell the exact sequence of the letters Jenner was receiving from all over the world by this time, since the Cheltenham postal service was very unreliable. Indeed, until 1800 there had been no post office as such in this fashionable resort. Letters had been dropped off by the mail coach at the cottage of whomever was the local postmistress-cum-town crier, and she delivered them when she had time. Consequently, the date the letter was written was not always a clear indication of when it was received. In 1800, a Mr. Smith did open a post office at 127, High Street (on the corner of North Street), but he had no postman or system of delivery. Letters from America probably required a six- or seven-week transit time, so that several letters (from Waterhouse) posted from Boston in the spring might have been awaiting Jenner when he arrived home. As it was, he soon had a great deal of international correspondence on his hands within a few weeks of his arriving home. There were letters from Doctors Curier, Coloumb, and DeLambre at the French Institute, two from Blumenbach, and two from Louis Sacco, an Italian vaccinationist.[15] In addition, of course, there was a daily arrival of the domestic post, which was always heavy.

All through the autumn news came of the steady spread of vaccination on the Continent. Jenner had given some cowpox matter to London doctor Alexander Marcet[16] to send to Copenhagen, and it proved so beneficial that the King of Denmark appointed a committee to arrange the spread of the system throughout his dominions. At the same time the Cisalpine Republic gave official sanction to the practice and Dr. Sacco was placed in charge. On October 16, he wrote an enthusiastic letter to Cheltenham announcing his promotion and also the fact that he had found an indigenous cowpox virus in Lombardy. He addressed Jenner in the most glowing terms: "It is to the Genius of Medicine, and the favourite child of nature that I have the honour to write. The name of Jenner will always be beloved by all posterity." He concluded: "May you live, my dear sir, a long while for the good of humanity and for the sake of all those who love you."[17] Similar tidings came from the courts of Prussia, Poland, and Sweden, keeping Jenner busy both acknowledging letters and dispatching his own serum whenever he could. He glowed in the recognition he received abroad and realized with a certain wry satisfaction that he was probably the most poverty-stricken great man in Europe. Reading his own praises from all over the globe was a delightful distraction—like conversation—that did not cost any money. These delightful distractions continued, despite the financial crisis, and though Jenner did not dispose of his magnificent set of plate, it is said that he was forced to sell his carriage horses. Nonetheless, he permitted himself a moiety of social spending; on September 4, Jenner and his friend Hicks attended a performance at the Theatre Royal in honor of the Prince of Wales, who began to take interest in the town where his secretary spent so much time.

One of the first tasks Jenner assigned himself when he had disposed of his more pressing correspondence was a short pamphlet for William Fermor of instructions for securing successful vaccination. He sent it off to his friend on September 7, and Fermor had it printed in the October issue of the *Medical and Physical Journal* under the title, "Dr. Jenner in Reply to Mr. Fermor." In the letter to Fermor, Jenner mentioned that incessant interruptions had prevented him from writing "a fourth paper" describing the best mode of inoculation. He appears to have applied himself to the task as soon as he was able, however, and he had it finished by the end of the year. Despite his fortnight in Berkeley at the beginning of December and his departure from there to London on the ninth, the fourth pamphlet was published, according to the conjecture of Le Fanu, by February. It was not always his own writings that Jenner distributed to applicants for assistance. In response to a request, he sent one of Creaser's excellent instruction sheets, and to Lyman Spalding on November 10, he sent "a little paper which will perhaps furnish you with valuable intelligence. Tho' it does not come from me it has my sanction."[18]

In Jenner's house there was a pleasant sitting room at the back of the ground floor overlooking the churchyard, and here one might write or daydream without any of the distractions of the center of the town. Also one might hear all the muted sounds of activity in the other three houses of the terrace, but not loudly enough to be disturbed. The occasional carriage going back and forth to Lord Fauconberg's at Bayshill Lodge[19] or wealthy patients waiting on Dr. Hooper at the Great House, would be the only traffic sounds to disturb Jenner's reverie.

That emancipated lady, the Countess of Berkeley, now completely recovered from her illness of 1797, was increasingly interested in Jenner's activities in Cheltenham. He was a dependable, valued ally in her complicated social problems and knew more famous people than she did. Despite her coronet, she experienced the snubs and coldness of the many who disputed her right to the noble state. A seasonal resident of the town was the gay if elderly Sir Isaac Heard, Garter King of Arms, who, though in his seventieth year, was active and much sought after as the ultimate authority on lineage and precedence. He would be a great comfort to Lady Berkeley if he could be persuaded to form an acquaintanceship, so she wrote to Jenner on November 13, 1799, begging him to invite Sir Isaac and his wife to Berkeley Castle. "You can inform him," she said, "that the Castle beds are well-aired."[20] Unfortunately we do not know whether the invitation was accepted, but years later, when the Berkeley's "took-over" Cheltenham, Sir Isaac became one of their circle, together with the young Lord Byron, to whom the elderly man became very attached.

Another and perhaps the most interesting lady of the Berkeley household who supported Jenner was Elizabeth,[21] the daughter of the fourth earl. She had married Lord Craven in 1767, when she was seventeen, but found him extremely dull and left him for the Margrave of Anspach. In 1791 when her lord died, Elizabeth married the margrave. She was a wide traveller, an industrious, talented writer, and a dramatist of some distinction. She was one of the first to write to Jenner after his vaccination of Phipps, and even after she had moved from the Berkeley family circle she always remembered him. It is interesting that Jenner, a man on the wrong side of fifty and of unspotted reputation, continued to be revered by so many of the gayest and most notorious ladies of the age. I suppose a man who, besides being a distinguished doctor, could talk on most subjects and had the enthusiasm of the idealist, would have been popular in all the salons. The fact that poor Catherine never accompanied him made his range of visitations quite unrestrained by what she would have considered proper.

The margravine was perhaps the least conventional of all the splendid beauties to be encountered among Jenner's wide range of acquaintances. She defied the edicts of society, and challenged the royal family itself by demanding recognition as a princess after she had regularized her liaison with the margrave, with whom she had been living for five years. Unlike her brother, the fourth Earl of Berkeley, she had no children by her paramour before or after her marriage to the margrave. She was, however, forty-one years old when she became Margravine of Anspach. Nevertheless, brother and sister seem to have had the same advanced ideas about their private lives, the earl living as openly with Mary Cole as Elizabeth did with the margrave. This latter gentleman, unlike his wife, does not seem to have been a particularly generous patron of the arts. "The Margrave of Anspach [Queen Caroline's nephew] calls upon Loutherburgh very frequently," observed Farington, "and professes great regard for him, but Mrs. Loutherburgh remarked that he never employed Mr. L. to paint a single picture. Liberality does not seem to be one of his qualities. Though he occasions a great deal of trouble by calling often, he never gave anything to any servant of theirs." Perhaps the sour disposition that Jenner had noted in the artist many years before had something to do with it.

A renowned beauty in her day, Elizabeth retained her looks well into middle age. She sat for George Romney in 1796 when she was

forty-six years old. She was reputedly a vain woman and not above
the occasional catty remark. A few weeks after she posed for Romney, we have a further report from Farington. "Humphrey was a
considerable time with the Margravine of Anspach (Lady Craven)
yesterday at Brandenburgh House,—she spoke of Lady Jersey, and
allowed her beauty, but said she had thick legs."[22] There might
have been an element of spite, for Lady Jersey was received at
court despite her wild life—she eventually became the Prince of
Wales's mistress—whereas the margravine, though married to the
Dowager Queen's nephew, was not. But this fascinating woman
has a particular interest for us in that she was perhaps the first
really exalted personage to recognize Jenner's ability as a medical
man (as opposed to a naturalist). She had four children by Lord
Craven and before she left him came very near death when
brought to bed with her youngest son, Henry Augustus, born on
December 21, 1776. "Lady Craven, sister of Lord Berkeley confessed she owed her life to Jenner. Attacked after the birth of her
youngest son with fits, which rendered her totally speechless, and
in the opinion of six physicians dangerously near death." From
her own description of the incident, Jenner had not come in a professional capacity, but merely "to pay his respects." He was therefore committing a serious breach of medical ethics by becoming
involved in her treatment, but since her language manifestly indicates a social relationship between them, he undoubtedly felt justified. He immediately realized that his visit to the room of his dying
friend did not have to be that at all. She wrote:

He came to pay his respects to one he imagined at the point of death
and for whom he had the sincerest regard. He had the courage to inform Lord Craven that my case was totally mistaken and it was owing
to such a mistake that all the singular disorders that I had, had followed . . . the complications of complaints which had come upon me
arose from milk having become fixed about the region of the stomach
and lungs. He ordered me to be sent to Barham, where he came himself and attended me, till by his proper management I was in a fair
way of recovering.[23]

At the time Jenner was twenty-seven years old and his patient a
year younger. We have no record of what the six learned physicians had to say at his cavalier dismissal of their diagnoses, but

since it saved the life of the Countess of Craven, their comments no doubt would have been in private. The baby involved also survived and ultimately became General Craven. Of more interest, however, the eldest son, later Lord Craven, became prominent in Cheltenham society after Jenner took up residence and actually met his future wife there.

The introduction of vaccination into the armed forces this year (1803) was yet another milestone passed with the aid of these noble patrons. Although the actual decision was due to the edicts of the Duke of York and Lord Spencer, another interesting figure emerged in the person of Thomas Trotter.[24] This man first corresponded with Jenner in February, and it was he who implemented the decision of the First Lord of the Admiralty to make vaccination compulsory in the Royal Navy. Trotter moved in very exalted circles and his ability as a medical man was equalled by his facility as a writer and—in rather a minor key—poet. His enthusiasm for vaccination was, perhaps, exceeded only by his personal esteem for Jenner. In the course of the spring he arranged for a medal to be struck in honor of vaccination and presented to Jenner by the surgeons of the Royal Navy. As First Lord of the Admiralty, it is Spencer's name that appears on the medal, but the whole idea was Trotter's. He and Jenner maintained a sporadic correspondence for the next few years and, in 1803, Trotter dedicated his *Essay on Drunkenness* to the doctor. What was especially interesting in the story, however, was the role of the distaff side, circumstantial evidence though it be. Trotter had a beautiful daughter named Elizabeth, who married the heir of the Marquess of Thomond in 1799. As a result she found herself the sister-in-law of the gallant Admiral (then Commander) O'Brien. Yet another gracious lady to come under Jenner's spell, she, with her husband, became an enthusiastic supporter of vaccination; particularly when she became Lady Thomond in 1808. Since the medal from the naval surgeons was also the first official award of any kind that Jenner received for his services to mankind, the sailor Trotter, and perhaps his daughter, should surely have a modest place in medical history.

These worthy pioneers who sailed the seas recognized the great benefactor before their brethren on land, and they were enthusiastically emulated by those who dwelt far beyond the seas. Benjamin Waterhouse was without question the main vaccination pioneer in North America, and it may be well to consider the events that led up to the general acceptance of the system on that continent. Actually, the first cowpox inoculation was performed by John Clinch in Newfoundland, if one wishes to be technical, since Jenner had sent him serum in 1798 right after the publication of the *Inquiry*. The two friends were in continual correspondence, and it was likely an automatic gesture for Jenner to pass on the discovery as soon as it was announced to the world. Nor were there any complications: the governor of the colony was only too eager to cooperate since the Indian population had suffered from decimating epidemics of smallpox for centuries. But Newfoundland was a remote and thinly populated island. It was in New England, some four hundred miles south, that the new practice made its real impact, and from there it spread all over North America.

As early as 1799, when Jenner was fighting the first opposition in England, old Dr. William Aspinwall of Brookline, Massachusetts, and a Harvard graduate of colonial times, closed down his flourishing Smallpox Inoculation Hospital after reading the *Inquiry*. It was a gesture of medical integrity that still stands out in the history of vaccination. "This inoculation is no sham," he wrote, "as a man of humanity I rejoice in it, though it will take from me a handsome income."[25] He spoke truly: his hospital had been established in 1783 and was a lucrative and highly respected institution. Its demise was a triumph of God over Mammon that tragically had no counterpart on the English scene.

Doctors Aspinwall and Waterhouse were not the only links between Harvard and Jenner in the period immediately following the *Inquiry*. At least one young man might well have been in Cheltenham itself. John Collins Warren graduated from Harvard in 1799 and spent the next three years making a grand educational tour of England and Scotland with a period in France. In London he studied under Astley Cooper[26] at Guy's Hospital and was probably there when Jenner was made a Fellow of the Physical Society of that institution. The diploma was signed by Cooper with the date February 20, 1802, and Warren returned to Boston the following December. It is interesting to note, however, that on May 25, long before the young American doctor left England, Jenner was awarded the Diploma of Fellow of the American Society of Arts and Sciences in Massachusetts, signed by Dr. Joseph Willard, president of Harvard. One does not suggest, of course, that there was any connection between a mere travelling medical student and the actions of so austere a figure as Dr. Willard, but it does indicate the topical concern with Jenner at Harvard at that time. It would be reasonable to assume that Cooper may have introduced an enthusiastic American student to Jenner when visiting Bransby in Cheltenham. Another Harvard graduate Jenner would meet in due course was Sir Thomas Bernard, son of the penultimate colonial governor of Massachusetts.

In the meantime, when the first flush of the novelty of vaccination had worn off in Boston, Waterhouse found himself facing the first murmurs of hostility. It was nothing compared with the animosities in England, but nonetheless discouraging after the promising beginnings. Like Jenner, Waterhouse would have appreciated having more active allies instead of mere well-wishers. In a letter to his English friend, from Cambridge, Massachusetts, on November 5, 1801, he wrote:

The characters in America most distinguished for wisdom and goodness are firm believers in *your* doctrine. They are not, however, overforward in assisting me against this new irruption of the Goths. I do not wish them to do more than make the cartridges, or at least hand them. At present they leave me too much alone, and it is probable will only come openly to my assistance when I do not *want* them. Had I not a kind of apostolic zeal I should at times feel a little discouraged. The natives of America are skilled in bush fighting.[27]

What Waterhouse did not know was that the tide was about to turn very decisively before the year was out. In December an embassy of a number of Indian tribes came to Washington under the leadership of a chief named Little Turtle. President Jefferson told this man all about Jenner's discovery, and its value in conquering the fearsome disease of smallpox. When the interpreter imparted the information the chief begged to be the first one treated. "On their departure," wrote Waterhouse, "the President caused them to be supplied with the virus; and the interpreter (a white man) took a copy of the directions for conducting the process I had transmitted to the President."[28] Undoubtedly, President Jefferson was the first head of state in history to preside over a mass vaccination. Indeed, his vital interest and activity in the eliminating of smallpox was a long-overdue example to a dilatory British government. In a letter to Dr. Ring on December 18, Dr. De Carro, the Austrian pioneer from Vienna, wrote: "Remember me to Dr. Jenner . . . his fame increases daily; but I blush for all the governments, that have not hitherto bestowed any public mark of their gratitude on that immortal benefactor of mankind."

This very fame, indeed, wreaked a heavy toll on the energy and resources of said immortal benefactor. He was constantly called upon from abroad to supply reliable vaccine. There was no serum in London, so when he returned to Cheltenham he always had to fulfill his many commitments in this department before he could rest. A tired man, well past fifty, Jenner would travel the slopes of Cleeve Hill in the summer heat to personally extract the precious matter from his local supply herds; and this year was a busy one. He sent serum to the Barbados by a Mr. Holder, who "inoculated several sailors with it on the voyage, so that he was enabled to make use of recent virus on his arrival. The success was complete; and the inhabitants received the preservative with much thankfulness." Upon receiving serum from Jenner, Clinch wrote from Newfoundland: "The matter sent me by your nephew produced the effect completely, although from the date it was kept four months."[29] And Waterhouse, of course, was still using the matter from the Cheltenham meadows that had been sent some time before. "I began with the matter your doctors Lettsom, Woodville, Pearson and Creaser sent me on the twenty-fourth of March, and have inoculated not quite a hundred, and have not had one dubious case among them all. I have given the virus to most of the leading physicians in Boston and its vicinity."[30]

Unfortunately for Jenner, the constant demands were never accompanied by a remittance and yet he somehow contrived to struggle along. Nevertheless, it was obvious that action on Jenner's behalf could not be delayed much longer, and eventually an advertisement was placed in the Gloucester newspapers—there was as yet no Cheltenham paper—setting out the situation and announcing that a petition to obtain a grant for Jenner was to be brought before the House of Commons. In due course it was decided that the claim for a grant should be brought before Parliament during the next session.

It might be noted here that the only sign of any reciprocal gesture during these hard times came from Dr. Sacco on October 16, when he sent, by way of Woodville, some vaccine from the plains of Lombardy to Jenner in Cheltenham. Sacco, of course, requested that Jenner send him some in return. This left the English doctor a little worse off financially as a result of the transaction, but he was profoundly grateful for the small crumb of kindness. "I am extremely gratified by your goodness in sending me your pamphlet on Vaccine Inoculations . . . and above all, the virus from the plains of Lombardy."[31]

At Brunn in Moravia, the young Count Francis Hugh de Salm spent huge sums of money to pay for vaccination on a large scale, though ironically not a penny seeped back to Jenner. It was the native doctors who benefitted financially. "This truly philanthropic nobleman having obtained genuine vaccine virus with appropriate directions for its employment called in to his assistance two physicians and sent a third to be fully instructed in the practice. He likewise held out rewards to the physician who should vaccinate the greatest number in that country." This wealthy young man came to England to meet Jenner during the summer with a letter of introduction from De Carro who stated: "The propagation of your discovery in the Austrian Monarchy has been more forwarded by him than by all the imperial faculties of medicine."[32] It was yet another sop to Jenner's ego before he devoted the remaining months of the year to preparing his parliamentary appeal and ranging his Cheltenham allies for the struggle. The local peers, of course, were already laying the groundwork among their friends in London. Lord Sherborne, the most vociferous, and the Berkeleys, who contrived to have Admiral Berkeley as chairman of the committee that was ultimately formed, organized the pro-vaccination doctors into a far more powerful lobby than the less organized but more numerous opposition.

Jenner left Cheltenham on November 6 and spent a month at Berkeley to collect his thoughts and see a few old friends. He then proceeded to London, where he arrived on December 9 with a few weeks left to prepare his campaign before Parliament returned in the new year.

As soon as the Christmas festivities were over, a petition was drawn up and presented on January 12 to the House of Commons by—among others—Lords Sherborne, Rous, Egremont, and Wilberforce, and Sir Henry Mildmay.[33] On March 17, the petition was referred to the committee under the chairmanship of Admiral Berkeley. The appeal for a grant was based jointly upon the reward due to such an important discovery for the betterment of mankind, and the pecuniary loss Jenner had suffered by devoting all his time to the vaccination research. Also to be considered, of course, was whether Jenner was the real discoverer of vaccination. The committee sat for precisely five weeks—from March 22 to April 26—and practically every doctor of importance testified.[34] The quality of the evidence was very definitely in Jenner's favor. Even the King strongly recommended a substantial award. Lord Rous used prima facie evidence of the most intimate nature. His own son had been vaccinated a year before at the age of three and had been perfectly protected from the dread disease. But it was the great doctors who used the superlatives. "In my opinion," said Matthew Baillie, "it is the most important discovery ever made in medicine." He then added: "If Dr. Jenner had not chosed open and honourably to explain to the public all he knew upon the subject he might have acquired a considerable fortune." This was, of course, a profound understatement. Not only had his idealism caused Jenner to miss the opportunity for riches—it had reduced him to penury. The enthusiasm with which Jenner had written his friend Clinch in 1795 about his new residential arrangements had not foreseen the need to spend so much of his time in London. Cheltenham with its wealthy patients had seemed to be the solution for financing his research, but he had reckoned without the bitter opposition that consumed so much of the time he should have dedicated to remunerative practice. By leaving Berkeley to promote his discovery in a wider world he had given up a security of many years' standing. Baron succinctly describes Jenner's plea to the committee.

He then goes on to state that by leaving his place of residence in the country where he had been established many years in a pleasant and lucrative profession, which, after so long an absence it was not probable that he should ever regain, he sustains another serious evil. The minor expenses such as postage etc., etc., he forebore to mention.

Sir James Erskine Sinclair supported Jenner's case with very logical statistics. "He noticed the *actual expense* which Dr. Jenner had incurred in presenting his enquiries, at the least £6000; if then £20,000 was objected to as too large, he would propose £15,000 as in some measure remunerating." Along somewhat more ingenious lines of reasoning, Mr. John Courtenay[35] pointed out that, "it appeared in evidence that 40,000 men were annually preserved to the state by Dr. Jenner's discovery—by this number £200,000 was annually brought into the Exchequer; and certainly, Dr. Jenner, the efficient cause, was well entitled to £20,000." Another member of Parliament, Mr. Fuller, observed, in justice, that the larger sum (£20,000) was due to the doctor for the simple reason that he had not protected his discovery. "He could look to no remuneration by patent." Others made simpler but perhaps more direct comments on the discovery. To Cline it was simply "the greatest discovery ever made in the practice of medicine." Ring stated more strongly, "It was beyond all comparison the most important and valuable [contribution] ever made by man." The untold wealth that Jenner might have amassed was not overlooked. Many doctors, including Farquhar and Bradley,[36] maintained that he could easily have made his ten thousand pounds a year. The latter, pointing out that two million people had already been vaccinated in the world without a single fatality from smallpox, estimated that in five years this income could have easily risen to twenty thousand. It was left, however, to the learned James Sims, President of the Medical Society of London, to touch the peak in superlatives. He not only agreed that it was the "greatest and most useful discovery ever made in medicine," but added that, "Dr. Jenner, had he kept it a secret might have died the richest man in these dominions."[37] The humanitarian William Wilberforce simply reminded the House that Jenner had devoted twenty years of his life to the research that led to the discovery. Creaser and Beddoes pointed to the abuse and vindictiveness to

which Jenner had been submitted, particularly through the ignorance and willfulness of Pearson. Fortunately the admission of
testimony from nonmedical and nonscientific witnesses gave Jenner's many influential friends the opportunity not only to express
their support but to cite the instances *in their own families* of
the efficiency of his discovery.

As to the question of whether Jenner was really the discoverer
of cowpox inoculation—a question raised mainly by Pearson—
there was strangely little fight. Pearson himself conceded that he
had first heard about it from Jenner, but maintained that he had
heard it independently from other sources also. The whole case
actually rested upon evidence collected by a Reverend Herman
Drew from certain farmers and others in Dorsetshire and Wiltshire who claimed to have, at one time or another, experimented
with cowpox serum. Since the disease was well known in the
West Country, there was undoubtedly some truth in the materials,
but nothing like a systematic pattern of research had been followed. No one had actually tried to develop a cure for smallpox
out of all the years of folk knowledge that had existed. It remained
for Sir George Baker, the royal physician, to dispose of these
claims. A spry man of eighty, and, incidentally, a great admirer
of Mrs. Jordan's, he made his second impact on Jenner's life in
the most decisive manner. It was to Baker that Drew sent his
evidences of the rival claims. To Sir George they seemed sufficiently trivial to be ignored. "It is impossible to ascertain the precise contents of these documents," observed Baron. "It is, however, certain that they were not deemed of sufficient importance
by that eminent and enlightened physician either to be given to
the public or to render him very anxious for their preservation,
as they remained unheeded and have been allowed to perish."
Baker gave evidence to this effect and, of course, had a profound
influence on the ensuing debate. His attitude was particularly
noted by the royal family. It is worth noting that the year 1788,
the one in which Sir George showed his first interest in Cheltenham, was the year that Jenner took his drawing of the cowpox
pustule to John Hunter in London. Hunter showed it to a close
friend of Baker's, Everard Home, who inoculated one of his
own children with the serum, as he revealed in his testimony.

Jenner's opposition on the whole was weak and unconvincing, so that the main debate became a question of how much the grant should be rather than whether there should be one. The Chancellor of the Exchequer, Spencer Perceval—who soon afterwards took a house in Cheltenham—observed that "no money value could be put on the discovery as it was beyond all calculation." The debate upon the amount took place in June, and Jenner was finally awarded ten thousand pounds. Not only was this sum a paltry amount, Jenner would wait two years to receive the funds.

In considering the paltriness, as well as the tardiness, in payment of Jenner's grant, however, it might be well to comment on another aspect of the grant debate. The proceedings brought out in sharp relief the mass of support Jenner had in the more responsible medical circles against a background of vested interest and fashionable jealousy. In addition to the distinguished names I have already mentioned, the leading figures among the "elder statesmen" of medicine testified on his behalf. In a bare four years since the publication of his book, most of the established senior men of the profession had been converted so completely to vaccination that they were willing to appear before the bar of the House of Commons to plead their belief in its efficacy. Old Thomas Dale,[38] in his seventy-fourth year, could have been Jenner's father, and was outstripped in seniority by Sir George Baker alone. Thomas Keate,[39] surgeon of Jenner's old hospital, St. George's, William Saunders[40] from Guy's Hospital and the old faithfuls, Farquhar and Lettsom[41] were all equally eager to support their younger colleague.

An earlier graduate of St. George's Hospital, Thomas Denman,[42] the most celebrated accoucheur in the country at the time of the grant debate, had two daughters: Sophia, who married Matthew Baillie, and Margaret, who married Dr. Richard Croft. All three, the father and the two sons-in-law, were among those who duly appeared to plead Jenner's cause. Croft, who was a year younger than Baillie, had a most brilliant career as accoucheur to the Duchess of Devonshire and physician to George III while still a relatively young man. He was impulsive, volatile, and often erratic in his social relationships, but still sought after for his undoubted ability. After the death of his brother, Sir Herbert Croft, in 1816, he succeeded to the baronetcy, but thereafter his life took a most tragic turn as we shall see.

The youngest but perhaps the most learned of this impressive array was Dr. Robert Thornton who,[43] in 1797, at the age of twenty-nine, had commenced his great *New Illustrations of the Sexual System of Linnaeus* (which he finished in 1807) and was already recognized as one of the most learned men in the field of biology. He took a major part in the debate and made an exhaustive, 318-page report on the impact of cowpox entitled *Facts Decisive in Favour of the Cow Pock* (London, 1803). Thornton dedicated the book to Jenner and, in 1806, reprinted an article of Jenner's (that had appeared in the *Medical and Physical Journal* in 1804) in *Vaccinae Vindicia*. That seems to have been the extent of their relationship. I can find no record of any meeting or correspondence. Le Fanu records nothing in print relative to Thornton and vaccination after 1806.

All in all, some thirty-one doctors had testified—some of whom travelled great distances to do so. With the opposition lobby so vociferous, this rallying of the clans must have been a blessed compensation for the impoverished Jenner. The debate had brought together this formidable cross-section of the medical world and represented every facet of experience. If he took nothing back to Cheltenham with him, Jenner certainly arrived home secure in the knowledge that his discovery was widely accepted if not officially established. It was quite apparent, however, that the unreasoning, illogical opposition to vaccination was also firmly entrenched and if it could not stop, it did, indeed, hamper the fight against smallpox as long as Jenner lived. He was always required to look over his shoulder and spring into action where it was needed. Nor was the enemy always the vindictive rival; sometimes it was plain ignorance. In the middle of the long hearing Jenner was still vitally aware of the menace of careless, inexpert cowpox inoculation.

On one of his rare visits to Bristol (probably to consult with Beddoes), he was staying at 26, College Green on May 15 when he wrote to *Felix Farley's Journal* that "so many accidents have happened in vaccine inoculation within the city of Bristol, which have been mentioned by way of reproach, Mr. Jenner thinks it justice to himself and the cause to assert that such accidents attach only to the improper management of the inoculation, etc."[44] The tenor of the comment is defensive and manifestly reflects continuing criticism of his work in South Gloucestershire.

Almost unnoticed in all the excitement of the debate, vaccination had lost a valuable friend and Cheltenham a popular, familiar face earlier in the year. General O'Hara died suddenly in February at his post in Gibraltar. He had been the heart of society at the Spa in his day, being so close to the Berrys, the Locks, and the Leinsters in an association that went back far beyond Jenner's time.

With the Treaty of Amiens the English watering places were more or less left to the natives, who celebrated the new era in their own provincial circle. There would not be the usual brilliant cosmopolitan gatherings, so on his return from the capital Jenner spent a few quiet weeks in Berkeley. While there he was visited by Dr. Joseph Franck, of Vienna, who bore a letter of introduction from Dr. Babington of London. "Dr. Franck has too much good sense and politeness to wish to trespass upon your valuable time. He merely desires the honour of being acknowledged as an acquaintance, which I flatter myself when you come to know him, you will not repent having granted." Characteristically, Baron gives no information about the two men meeting.[45]

When he did get back from Berkeley, there was quite sensational news awaiting Jenner from a completely different quarter; though it must have been dampened by the worries of his increasing penury as he waited for the grant money to be paid. A report from one of the many places where Jenner had sent help or serum bounded into the public eye. In what must have been record time, smallpox had been completely eradicated from the primitive country of Ceylon. Young Thomas Christie, medical officer to the government of Ceylon, had been one of the first converts to vaccination. At the beginning of 1802 he inaugurated a campaign to clear the island of smallpox in the quickest possible time. This ancient land had suffered from the scourge more, perhaps, than any country in Asia. Whole communities were frequently devastated, with weakened survivors of the disease often devoured by wild animals to complete the pattern of extinction. Christie, who was only twenty-nine when he engaged upon this task, corresponded with Jenner, who went to great pains—unsuccessful as it turned out—to send him the vital vaccine and gave him all the necessary advice. The Ceylon campaign was as effective as it was swift, and smallpox was totally eliminated. Christie himself was so moved that he resolved to settle in Cheltenham when his turn of duty with the East India Company terminated in 1810, in order to live and practice near the great vaccinator. Jenner, however, would be overshadowed by purveyors of the vaccine to the distant parts of the globe who all too often received the honors that should have gone to its discoverer.

Christie was not obliged to struggle with the obstruction and jealousy that bedevilled Jenner in England and he received the wholehearted support of the colonial government. He was one of the first—as well as Aspinwall of Brookline—to see the evil of smallpox inoculation, when a perfect vaccine was available of an almost innocuous form of the same disease. Christie wrote:

At the time of the first establishment of the Small-Pox Hospital in Ceylon, no authentic account of the success of Dr. Jenner's discovery had reached us, but soon afterwards we received his own original publication, that of Dr. Aikin and the greater part of Mr. Ring's work on that subject. . . . Several packets of matter were received from England by various surgeons; all of which were tried but the length of the voyage had made them effete.[46]

Undaunted, however, the Ceylon authorities attempted to obtain cowpox serum from the local cattle, but this also was unsuccessful, as was Jenner's personal effort.

Dr. Jenner and others were strenuous and persevering in their efforts to transmit the vaccine to India by sea. The first attempt of the kind, it is believed, was made by Dr. Jenner himself who sent out packets of matter with ample instructions by the *Queen,* Indiaman, which was unfortunately burnt on the coast of South America in 1800. A plan was also concerted by Dr. Jenner, under the auspices of the British government, to send out the vaccine to India, with a detachment of royal artillery which sailed in the *Wyndham* and *Walpole* from England in February, 1803, destined for Ceylon.[47]

As it happened, by the time Jenner's vaccine arrived, the island had already been purged of smallpox with serum forwarded by

Lord Elgin from Constantinople via Basra and Bombay. Using every conceivable means of obtaining the precious remedy, Christie had been in correspondence with the peer, as well as with Jenner, and Elgin had presumably made earlier efforts to get supplies through.

The attitude of the native population facilitated this rather sophisticated operation. They were certainly more enthusiastic than the peasants around Berkeley. Christie continued:

At the first introduction of the vaccine virus into Ceylon, a regular establishment existed for the promotion of Small-Pox Inoculation, to which the natives were in a great degree familiarized, and it was only necessary to transfer the services of the individuals composing this establishment to the preservation and diffusion of Cow-Pox, which the natives in the first instance, seemed to consider a milder species of the same disease; and it is to the decisive measure of the Government, in immediately adopting this plan, and the steady and liberal support afforded to it, that we ought to attribute the more rapid extension of the practice on its first introduction into Ceylon, than in Bengal and some other parts of India.[48]

Christie went on to record how Jenner's friend, Lord William Bentinck, had, when appointed Governor of Madras at the age of twenty-nine in 1803, cooperated in the Indian mission.

Dr. Jenner forwarded by Lord William Bentinck, Governor of Madras, a number of coloured drawings of the Vaccine postule with a variety of pamphlets on the subject which were distributed throughout the continent of India by the late highly respected Physician-General of Madras Dr. Anderson, than whom no person could be more assiduous in promoting vaccination.[49]

These apparent dandies of the Cheltenham Wells—the Elgins, the Bentincks, the Wellesleys, the O'Haras, the Abercrombys, the Hardwicks, and the Hutchinsons—were the men who helped Jenner spread vaccination over the face of the earth. While on the King's service beyond the seas, they carried the torch from St. George's Place, leaving the domestic crusade to the less adventurous but just as dedicated Aylesburys, Boringtons, Berkeleys, Sherbornes, and Bedfords.

Nor was Ceylon the only major overseas event of 1802. Much nearer home more powerful people were taking notice. Soon after the doctor arrived in Cheltenham he received the following letter from Lord St. Helens who was British ambassador to the Court of St. Petersburg. His Lordship had arrived in London on leave only to find that Jenner had already left the capital:

Sir,

Since writing my other letter to you of this date I have learned by the servant whom I sent with it that you are now in Cheltenham. I have to request, therefore, that if you do not purpose returning soon to London you will have the goodness to commission some person to receive what I have brought you from the Dowager Empress of Russia, consisting of a letter and a small parcel, (I believe) containing a ring set in diamonds. I shall probably remain in town until the 15th inst.

I have the honour to be, with great regard,

Sir,

Your most obedient servant,

St. Helens.[50]

It is characteristic of Jenner that he did not immediately rush back to London on receipt of such an honor. He was too deep in his backlog of correspondence, which always accumulated during his absence from Cheltenham. He answered as follows:

My Lord,

I have been honoured with your lordship's letter acquainting me with the distinguishing mark of attention conferred upon me by the Empress, Dowager of Russia. Sanctions like these, my lord, from such exalted personages must necessarily be peculiarly pleasing to my feelings. They not only benefit me individually, but by blending me with the general arguments for universal adoption of vaccine inoculation, the annihilation of that dreadful disease, the smallpox, will be the more quickly accomplished.

May I request the favour of your lordship to make known to the Empress the high value I set upon Her Majesty's present, to express my extreme gratitude and thankfulness for her goodness.

As I shan't be in London for some time to come your Lordship would oblige me by assigning the parcel to the care of Mr. Paytherus, surgeon, No. 13, Norfolk St., in the Strand, who will faithfully transmit it to me.

I have the honour to be, my Lord,
Your Lordship's
Ever obliged, faithful
And obedient humble servant,
E. Jenner.

Cheltenham, 5th October, 1802.[51]

In the meantime, Jenner arranged for a copy of the latest edition of *Vaccine Inoculation* to be presented to Her Imperial Majesty, but again he did not see the ambassador himself about it. This time he delegated his old friend Dr. Ring to be the intermediary. Lord St. Helens replied graciously from his rooms in Old Burlington Street on December 14:

—I have received the honour of your letter and enclosure of the 9th inst.; and yesterday had the pleasure of a visit from Mr. Ring who informed me that the volume of your publication on vaccine inoculation which you intended as a present to the Dowager Empress of Russia, will be ready in the course of a few days.[52]

The short-lived peace with France made continental travel once more available to British tourists, and many of Jenner's friends, including Farington and James Moore, gathered in Paris, where they met Charles James Fox in the middle of September. It was the first time that British and French supporters of the movement had been able to jointly celebrate the triumphs of the cause, and a dinner was held in honor of the absent pioneer. "Jenner's portrait, a print by Smith, was hung up in the room crowned by a chaplet of flowers, and this Motto was attached to it: Viro de Matribus de Puris de populis benemerito." Marshall too was in Paris earlier in the year and had to a certain extent been identified with the victory in Egypt because of his tireless labors in vaccinating members of the armed forces in that theater.[53] Both he and Dr. Walker had been thanked by the two commanders, Lord Hutchinson and Lord Keith. Unfortunately, the high appreciation of the army officers was not echoed by the powers in London. John Ring commented disgustedly: "Our brave soldiers employed in the expedition to Egypt were vaccinated by order from the Duke of York and the Lords of the Admiralty. The smallpox as a consequence was twice extinguished from the fleet and our gallant countrymen were preserved for a contest in which they proved successful." Marshall and Walker, he adds, "received fifty pounds between them."[54] So much for the munificence of a grateful nation.

Ironically, in this reunion of the British and French vaccination forces, Jenner himself was perforce absent. The poor child who could not afford to go to the party, he would have to wait until the gossips returned home to tell him all about it. And there would be a great deal to tell. Fox, that great admirer of Bonaparte, had several audiences with the emperor and probably mentioned his personal acquaintance with Jenner—a fact that his Majesty would have found most interesting. But aside from his financial worries, Jenner was quite happy in his exclusion from the continental festivities. He had Cheltenham with all its amenities more or less to himself. A dead season had a lot to recommend it. Without the usual mobs he had much better access to the libraries and reading rooms. The postal service was markedly improved, and Jenner's daily post could as well be from emperor or ambassador as from grateful peasant. Under the new postmaster, Mr. Smith, everything was much more efficient even though he did everything himself—there being no postman. In the autumn the Entwistles came to Cheltenham and took over the post office. Harriot Mellon, Mrs. Entwistle's daughter, had finally appeared at Drury Lane in June and generously arranged for her parents to open a music shop adjoining the post office premises in the High Street. Another theatrical neighbor of Jenner's, in St. George's Place itself, was the Sadler's Wells Puppet Theatre run by the Seward family and which operated for twenty-five years, until Mr. Seward's death. Writing on the puppets, the printer Ruff commented: "However trivial this sort of dramatic exhibition may appear, it is well known that the countenance of many a high lord and lady has been illuminated with merriment."[55] And, undoubtedly, many a neighboring doctor and his lady.

Despite the small company at the Wells, life in the town went on as usual. One of the first distinguished supporters of vaccination, Lord Ellenborough, was made Lord Chief Justice of England in April and created a baron. On the surface this appeared to be yet another mighty voice to support Jenner in the Upper House.

Powell Snell expressed the enthusiasm of the Cheltenham population when he pointed out how the great lawyer "gaining the sovereign's and his realm's applause, becomes the conservator of our laws." Ellenborough, alas, did not turn out to be quite the ally Jenner and his friends had hoped, despite the protection his huge family received from vaccination. But in this year of the peace and year of the parliamentary grant, no thought was given to defection in high places. Yet another gratifying tribute from overseas arrived at St. George's Place soon after the doctor's return from London. A letter from John Quincy Adams in Boston announced the election of Edward Jenner to the American Academy of Arts and Sciences. The certificate, dated July 13, 1802, was enclosed.

Perhaps it was overconfidence—perhaps the inertia that John Fosbroke occasionally refers to—but one has the feeling that in this important year of recognition Jenner did not take the opportunity to press his advantage the way he might have. Should he, indeed, have been relaxing in Cheltenham at all at this time? A number of his more influential friends were eager to organize the new vaccination association to take the place of the spurious group promoted by Pearson, but Jenner seemed content to sit back and leave everything to them. Great progress was, indeed, made in the capital while he was taking his ease in Cheltenham. Following the example of the Empress of Russia, the entire royal family at home seemed eager to be involved in the campaign, and by the beginning of winter the organizers felt that the final plans could not be completed without the presence of the pioneer himself. On December 3 they called a meeting, presided over by young Benjamin Travers—a pupil of Astley Cooper's at Guy's Hospital. It was voted to urge Jenner to come up to London to take charge of the arrangements. Mr. J. Addington—the surgeon, not the statesman—wrote to Jenner the same night:

Dear Sir,

I persuade myself that you will hear with pleasure of everything designed to promote the extension of the beneficial effects of your inestimable discovery. . . . the gentlemen therefore feel very desirous of knowing when it is probable that they may have the pleasure of seeing you in town, as they are anxious to proceed in the business

without delay. In their name, therefore, I beg the favour of you to give
me this information by an early post. . . . With the sincerest wishes
for your happiness in proportion to your services to mankind,

I remain,

Dear Sir,

Your obliged friend and servant,

J. Addington,[56]

The following morning another member of the company, the
banker John Fox, wrote to him also. "The plan which is in agitation is of the most extensive and liberal kind. It is even expected
that the Royal countenance will be gained, but much depends
upon you; all persons are looking towards you as the only proper
person to lay the foundation stone." But still the reluctant doctor did not respond. To be sure he left Cheltenham—but not for
London. He decided to spend Christmas at Berkeley and actually
kept Addington waiting for a week before answering his letter.
He explained that he wanted a few weeks in the peace and seclusion of his native village after "some years spent, I may almost
say, in constant anxieties." He felt sure that his friends could
well handle the business themselves, although he would go up to
town if they insisted. "Yet I ardently hope," he concluded, "that
my presence will not be absolutely necessary." He explained that
he had written to Dr. Lettsom requesting that he represent him
at the meetings. "I do not think the business will be very complex. The society would perhaps so far indulge me as to permit
my inspecting the outlines of the scheme which may probably be
brought forward at the next meeting; and in the best manner in
my power I shall contribute to its final arrangement."[57] So the
diffident doctor remained in the country while his friends proceeded without him to establish the Royal Jennerian Society.

The inaugural meeting was held at the London Tavern on January 19, 1803, and an impressive affair it was. In Jenner's absence
the chair was taken by the Lord Mayor of London, and a resolution was passed requesting the Duke of Clarence "to entreat His
Majesty that he would graciously be pleased to become the patron of this institution . . . and that he would permit it to be
designated the Royal Jennerian Society for the Extermination of
the Smallpox."[58] At a later business meeting, the complete roster

was announced by John Julius Angerstein, the Chairman: Patron—H. M. The King, Patroness—H. M. The Queen, Vice-Patrons—Their Royal Highnesses the Prince of Wales and the Duke of Bedford. Angerstein actually suggested an annual subscription rate of one hundred, or even two hundred pounds—an enormous sum for those days—but if quite impractical, the suggestion does indicate the note of optimism on which the organization started.

The impecunious doctor finally arrived in London on February 2 and presided over a meeting on the following day, exactly two months after Addington had asked him to join them. By this time, of course, all the work of launching the society had been done, and the real work of promoting vaccination on the widest possible scale was well under way. As a culmination of the social activities, Jenner, with the Lord Mayor, Lord Berkeley, Lord Grantley, Angerstein, Travers, Addington, and Lettsom, attended a special levee at the Court of St. James to thank the King for his patronage. Despite the dogged resistance to vaccination that remained in the capital, the first months of the new society were very impressive. Thirteen vaccination centers were established in various parts of the metropolis, and headquarters with a medical secretary in charge were established in Salisbury Square. The annual rate of smallpox deaths was reduced by almost a half. Jenner was at the crest of his fame and understandably may have felt that most of his worries were over. But perhaps the high point of Jenner's royal year was reached when a future king of England wrote to him in all humility: "[I] cannot but feel proud that my name should stand among those of the patrons of your society."[59] The resumption of the war, however, put an end to the prospect of a brave, peaceful Europe, where new ideas could spread and where even Jenner himself might preside unimpeded over an international crusade against smallpox. By the winter of 1802, three of Jenner's "emissaries" had penetrated every continent, and in many cases they operated through the highest channels. People he met in the bookshops or at the Wells in Cheltenham in the most informal manner would turn up earnestly preaching vaccination at the courts of foreign royalties. Lord Macartney,[60] Britain's first Ambassador to Peking and an elder statesman of vast influence in the diplomatic world, as well as families like the Portlands, Grevilles, and Leinsters, nurtured Jenner's ideas into a kind of invisible export of great prestige value in foreign affairs. People who distrusted "perfidious Albion" grew to revere the gentle West Country doctor, even as they cursed or spat at the names Pitt or Perceval.

Perhaps the most highly developed vaccination network was that of the Elgins; its meshes not only spread over the scattered empire of Turkey—which meant a vast expanse of Europe, Asia, and Africa—with a kind of regional Jenner in the person of De Carro presiding, but at its English end its anchors were even stronger. The Dowager Lady Elgin had the sole responsibility of the heir-presumptive to the throne of Great Britain, and the royal doctors who hovered around the princess, the Baillie–Denman–Croft "family," were all close friends of Jenner's. The secretary of Lord Elgin was John Morier,[61] brother of James Morier, author of *Hajji Baba*, who frequented the Cheltenham Wells, so there might well have been a more direct link between Jenner and Constantinople than the conventional route with all its hazards.

The summer of 1803 was very hot and dry in England, making the Wells more popular than ever to a society once more restricted to its own shores. The great families poured in again just as though the Peace of Amiens had never taken place, and many who were abroad when the rumors of war began to circulate immediately hurried home. Actually there was no real danger to the civilian traveller as such, but an enemy land was scarcely the place to be when hostilities broke out. Most important of all, the Elgins were on their way home, and diplomatic priorities once disposed of, Jenner must assuredly be one of the first people the ambassador would seek out. There might well be a grand reunion with the Aylesbury cousins in Cheltenham, where learned pioneer and noble disciple might meet for the first time while the Dowager Lady Elgin tenaciously held the fort in London. Farington, who had been gossiping with Miss Hayman, Privy Purse to the Princess of Wales, remarked rather cynically on May 10: "The fault of Lady Elgin is *too much solicitude for her own connexions* which warps her occasionally."[62]

But all this became merely academic a fortnight later, on May 28, when on his way home from Turkey Lord Elgin was arrested in Paris and detained, with his wife, as a prisoner of war. For Jenner, the act had serious implications. The people, if any, who could influence the government regarding its reluctance to remit Jenner's grant money were those closest to the royal family; and in the domestic sense no one was closer than the Elgins, Farington's barb notwithstanding. Less than a year before, young Lady Elgin had written enthusiastically from Athens to her mother: "It is astonishing how the *vaxine* has taken here. Dr. Scott is inoculating every day, with the best possible success; he has even inoculated a Turkish child. What an amazing thing it is to have introduced into a country where the smallpox is so fatal!"[63]

The family had left Athens for a leisurely journey home on February 2, but, on arriving at Rome, Lord Elgin made the unwise decision to send the children on by sea and travel overland with his wife. Dr. Scott took charge of the children and brought them safely to England, and, as it turned out, indefinite separation from their parents. The distraught wife wrote to her mother from Paris on May 28: "Dear Mother, You must find out from some of the foreign Ministers, or Coutts, perhaps, could tell you, how to send letters to me,—do all you can that I may hear from you."[64] John Morier, the secretary, had fortunately gone ahead to England before hostilities reopened and was able to give the Elgin relatives there some account of the family, at least up to the time they had left the Ottoman dominions.

For Jenner it was just one more disappointment in the tug-of-war that dogged his campaign. He returned to Cheltenham in the middle of a property speculator's boom that even involved his own quarters. The town had taken advantage of the brief peace and subsequent relaxing of financial pressures to indulge in wide expansion schemes. Joseph Pitt, the banker, now making his £20,000 a year and rapidly becoming one of the town's most active developers, had acquired—or reacquired—the new terrace in St. George's Place,[65] including Jenner's house, together with a great part of the adjacent area. The quack doctor, Colonel Riddell, himself coveted the property and started negotiations to purchase it from Pitt as early as June, though the final manorial release was not granted by Lord Sherborne until October 26.[66] The terrace had been in the market a great deal since its erection and speculators undoubtedly did very well every time it changed hands. In the issue of the *Gloucester Journal* of August 27, 1803, the following announcement appeared (which rather seems as though Riddell was looking for a new purchaser before his own title was clear).

To Be Sold By Private Contract.
The whole of that handsome row of houses called St. George's Place consisting of four capital messuages which are occupied by families of the First Distinction—The most compact and desirable property to be disposed of in Cheltenham. Interested parties are invited to apply to Mr. Hughes the Attorney.

An earlier prospectus for an auction of the four houses gives a detailed description of the arrangement of the accommodation. Since each of the dwellings was identical, it provides an exact picture of the layout of Jenner's home. There were "five good bed-chambers, a drawing room, two parlours, two kitchens, a cellar and a scullery with convenient closets." The site was unenclosed by other buildings save for the stables, coach house, and other offices of each residence. The four houses, according to the prospectus, "all command[ed] most beautiful prospects of the country."

Jenner probably met his new landlord, who was certainly one of the most colorful characters in Regency Cheltenham, during transactions at the Commissioner's office. At this time Riddell was actually living at Enfield, near London, but was deeply interested in the increasing popularity of the western Spa, and saw its potential as a medical as well as a social center. The equally eccentric Sir Francis Burdett was a close friend of his and they were, incidentally, equally distrustful of vaccination. Riddell's knowledge of medicine was, it seems, confined to a belief in potions and semi-magical nostrums. Nevertheless, he was soon to have a wide following among the ladies of fashion. In fact he became "the vogue" and eventually achieved an international reputation.

Thomas Jameson, the only qualified doctor in the town who to some extent supported Riddell's rather than Jenner's views on vaccination, brought out his famous *Treatise on Cheltenham*

Waters and Bilious Diseases in the course of the summer. It was published by Ruff and had an immediate success, eventually running through three editions. This illustrious scholar, far from bearing any ill will to Jenner because of their differing medical theories, actually dedicated his opus to his rival's patron, Lord Sherborne. Young Fosbroke conceded that Jameson's book on the waters "on the whole remains what is considered to be the best work on the subject,"[67] though on the doctor's scholarship in general he had definite reservations. On paper, at least, Jameson's qualifications were greatly superior to Jenner's, but his industry was not matched by his social graces. Through his long professional life he practically worked himself to death, but unlike Baillie, Christie, Boisragon, Newell, and Jenner, he never became Physician Extraordinary to the King—nor did he attend any other distinguished person for that matter.

Sherborne himself kept in touch with Jenner during the latter's absence in London. He intermingled news of the Cotswold countryside with the vaccination controversy. He wrote on April 19:

A woman in this parish has a cuckoo which she has kept in a cage all the winter. If you wish I should make any enquiries as to food, etc. I will do it with pleasure. I hear you are appointing apothecaries in every parish to inoculate for the smallpox. You would oblige me much if you would appoint Mr. Cole, Mount Street. Your friends made a poor business of your application to Parliament, as I think you the greatest patriot that ever existed and you ought to have got at least £30,000. All here unite in most kind regards to you and Mrs. Jenner.

A fortnight later he wrote in a much more militant vein.

I only now wish that the first medical man who can be wicked enough to inoculate for smallpox, and the patient should die, that the coroner's inquest bring in their verdict, willful murder, and that he might be hanged *in terrorem* of his brethren; not as a warning to himself as I once heard an Irish judge tell a man he had condemned to be hanged the next day—"take that my friend as a warning."[68]

Sherborne's letter also reported: "As for the cuckoo it departed this life last Friday." Interestingly enough there is no mention in the correspondence of a family event that could conceivably have helped Jenner during these penurious days. Sherborne's eldest daughter, Elizabeth, married the heir of the Earl of Suffolk on January 14, bringing that distinguished family into a distant relationship with Catherine Jenner[69] at a time when the Suffolks were moving from strength to strength in promoting the growth of the town. In conjunction with Henry Thompson, a wealthy London underwriter, the peer purchased the greater part of the land on the southern edge of the parish from the ancient De la Bere family and laid out the magnificent Suffolk Square and Montpellier Estates in the course of the next ten years or so. The cornfields about Wyatt's Cottage, alas, where Jenner had spent so many happy hours in the company of Michael Kelly and Coutts back in 1796, were to be among the first casualties of the new development. The old Cheltenham was changing.

The Earl of Hardwick gave up Arle Court some time before being appointed Viceroy of Ireland in 1801, but he did not forget his Cheltenham friends. A patron of the Berry sisters' and supporter of Jenner's from the beginning, he was one of the loyal contingent, with O'Hara, Bentinck, and Elgin, who used their administrative authority to forward the vaccination cause overseas. Arriving in Ireland Hardwick found the population in general hostile to the movement. The doctors distrusted it and the peasantry was afraid of it. Hardwick did not arrive in Dublin until late in the year and though vaccination had been introduced some months previously, there was no pressure on the part of the authorities to encourage it. The impact of the Act of Union and the consequent unrest kept the new administrator more than busy for his first year, but on February 18, 1803, he wrote to Jenner and asked for guidance on vaccination, "for extending the benefits to Ireland." Jenner wrote a lengthy reply on March 21, in which Dr. Ring joined him, to prescribe "the best mode of obtaining and preserving the genuine vaccine matter."[70] This letter was later printed in the *Medical and Physical Journal*. The immediate result was a vigorous campaign that within a year made Ireland the most completely vaccinated area in the British Isles, despite the turmoil of Emmett's uprising in the summer. Hardwick was not a man to be trifled with, and he personally dragooned the Irish doctors into line. When the Irish Cowpox Institution was opened in Dublin early in 1804, he became its first patron.

Though they evacuated Arle Court, his family maintained a seat not too far from Jenner's ear at Forthampton Court, ten miles further out, near Tewkesbury.

On the death of old Dr. John Moore in 1802, his son James Carrick Moore inherited the practice and overnight became physician to most of Jenner's vaccination patrons based in Cheltenham, including the Locks and Angersteins. Before this Moore apparently had no interest in vaccination. His brother, Charles, however, was already entrenched in Cheltenham society and would have been the obvious link between him and his new patients and, of course, Jenner himself. Charles followed the Siddonses around on their various occasions and was almost accepted as a member of the family.

After her daughter's tragic death at Bath in March, Mrs. Siddons underwent a complete physical and mental breakdown[71] from the impact of her many sorrows, and, some six weeks later, repaired to Cheltenham with her surviving daughter, Cecilia, to recuperate. Here the faithful Charles remained in constant attendance on the mother, despite the fact that Sally was dead. He remained in the town, on and off, during the entire period of her convalescence, mingling with the leading local figures who gathered around her couch. A number of these were his brother James's patients, including the Chairman of the Royal Jennerian Society, Angerstein.

As a matter of fact, the people who danced attendance on Mrs. Siddons at Birch Farm were mainly members of the Jenner circle, all of whom were eager to help her on the road to recovery. The poet Campbell was there as was Samuel Lysons, who was in charge of her financial affairs. We definitely know that Jenner was a friend of Campbell's, who was then making notes for his biography of Mrs. Siddons, so it is possible that he first met the poet through Charles Moore on this occasion. Certainly had not the latter been so assiduous in his attendance on the actress, he would never have found himself in the midst of all these vaccination enthusiasts during this particular summer. As for the actress herself, she soon regained her strength in the peace and quiet of the countryside. She wrote on May 15:

Our little cottage is some distance from the town, perfectly retired, surrounded by hills, fields and groves. The air of this place is particularly salubrious. I live out of doors as much as possible, sometimes reading under the haystack in the farmyard, sometimes rambling in the fields, and sometimes musing in the orchard, all of which I do without spectators; no observers to say I am mad, foolish or melancholy; thus I keep the 'noiseless tenor of my way' and you will be glad to hear that this mode of life is well-suited to my taste. Rising at six and going to bed at ten brought me to my comfortable sleep once more.[72]

In the middle of June, 1803, completely recovered, Mrs. Siddons left the town for a tour of the Wye Valley accompanied by her brother, John Philip Kemble, her daughter, and Charles Moore.

At Jenner's birthday banquet in London on May 17, the performance of a "Song—Sung by Mr. Bloomfield at the Anniversary of Dr. Jenner's Birthday, 1803," first drew the doctor's attention to this brilliant but shiftless peasant poet. It is not clear whether Bloomfield himself actually sang at the anniversary dinner, as the title implies, but the work itself is deeply sincere. Jenner, a sensitive critic of poetry, recognized that it was immeasurably better than any of the poetic effusions that had so far appeared; in fact, it was the first actual vaccination poetry. Bloomfield's family had suffered seriously from the ravages of smallpox, and he embarked upon a much more serious vaccination poem the following year. The two men became friends via correspondence, and though it was not until 1807 that the poet actually came to Cheltenham to visit Jenner, in 1803 he sang:

> From the field, from the farm comes the glorious treasure
> May its life-saving impulse—all fresh as the morn—
> Still spread round the earth, without bounds, without measure
> Till time has forgot when his Jenner was born.[73]

Another literary event of this year was the appearance of Ruff's *History of Cheltenham*—actually written by Jenner's friend, Dibdin, who was already touched upon briefly. Though the first, it is not a particularly good history, but it is fascinating as a detailed contemporary description of the town as Jenner knew it. In fact the places described were conceivably introduced to the writer's notice by the doctor himself, who knew the town much better than his friend. They used to visit Pruen at the Rectory in Prestbury and undoubtedly drank tea at the Grotto. Like so many of the Jenner coterie, Dibdin fancied himself as an amateur doctor, and his history is full of medical opinions and assertions, possibly because the predominance of the mineral springs would influence anyone writing on Cheltenham. He also comments, as did Powell Snell, upon the rather scandalous dress of the young ladies at the Spa, who went "without pockets and petticoats" and wore "transparent clothing." Dibdin was not, however, concerned about immodesty, but rather about the ladies catching cold and dying of consumption.[74]

Ruff, who had already brought out Jameson's book, was the new key figure in Cheltenham printing circles. He was soon to publish Jenner's own work as well as the first local newspaper. Nonetheless, he eventually went bankrupt.

Another talented friend of Jenner's decided to visit Cheltenham as the summer advanced; it was not from any interest in vaccination, however, but from dire need of Jenner's professional assistance in a totally different area: he had a liver complaint. The painter John Hoppner[75] had been preoccupied for some time with his poor health. He and Farington saw a great deal of each other in July, when it was so hot about London that cattle were dying in the fields for lack of water. They spent some time at the Locks' in Norbury and looked at some of William Lock's pictures, which Farington describes as "miserable performances both in performance and execution." Hoppner left for Cheltenham to consult Jenner on August 19, but Farington, whose elder brother had just died, had certain business to attend to before he could follow.

Despite the splendid weather, Mrs. Jenner was very poorly. Baron reported that Jenner admitted in a letter to Valentin "that the ill-health of Mrs. Jenner entirely absorbing his time he could not write to all his good friends on the continent the way he would wish."[76] Nevertheless, Jenner eventually settled down to a good deal of literary work that was published in the autumn. At least hot weather in a provincial town was a very different thing from hot weather in London. It was cool and quiet in the pleasant back room that overlooked the churchyard. Here one could work in peace. If one had to go out, the streets away from High Street were tree-embowered in all directions, and the little River Chelt ran under St. George's Place some two hundred yards from the Jenners' front door, and was crossed by Jemmy Wood's bridge. The Chelt was, in those days, a sparkling trout stream hurrying down to Alstone Mill; a pleasant oasis where Jenner could work in peace and wait for his London friends to visit him—which they did throughout the summer.

When Hoppner arrived he put up at the celebrated Smiths' lodging house. (Henry Farington, the diarist's brother, and his wife, Marrianne, were also staying there.) He consulted Jenner about the liver condition, which seems to have made him apathetic and lethargic, and in the next week or so manifestly improved.[77]

Also at the Wells were Sir John and Lady D'Oyly, distant relatives of Sir Joseph Banks and, incidentally, old friends of Hoppner's. Probably Banks had sent Lady D'Oyly to Jenner since she was suffering from dropsy, another of the doctor's special fields. She was obviously quite unaware of the seriousness of her condition and led a very active social life. Poor D'Oyly was thoroughly henpecked; though when they had returned from India he had been worth £105,000, his wife had gradually gone through it with her extravagant pattern of living. Be that as it may, the poor woman paid for her follies within a week or two. She died on September 9.

In addition to attending to his health, Hoppner had intended to do some landscape sketching in the neighborhood, but he seems to have been distracted by the surrounding activity. Besides Jenner, Fox, and the Henry Faringtons, there were many of his old acquaintances at the Wells. Because of his association with the D'Oylys, together they were able to visit Warren Hastings at Daylesford House, which was only a pleasant drive through the summer Cotswolds. Of closer interest to Hoppner, perhaps, was the presence of the drawing master and watercolor painter, Claude Nattes, whose picture of Cheltenham's High Street executed that year is the only representation of the town during the period of Jenner's residence—or for a generation more, for that matter. It is a watercolor drawing, taken from the entrance to the church-yard, depicting the old shops, the Market House, and a few private houses just about as far as St. George's Place: a typical eighteenth-century market town with the broad flagstone pavements trodden by Jenner and his great contemporaries.[78]

Fox was back at Vernon House for the summer, after his desertion in 1802, and his walks down the shady side of High Street to Jenner's house were once more resumed. There was plenty to talk about. Unlike most people he did not fear a French invasion and was apparently reassured by his conversations with Bonaparte. Fox had grown very fat, and like Hoppner, suffered from a chronic liver condition.

The renewal of the war brought a great deal of distress to English families, whose relatives, even though unconnected with the armed forces, were detained as prisoners. The Elgins were not the only victims among Jenner's friends. Lord Hertford's son was arrested with his family soon after the outbreak of hostilities and as late as June 5, Mary Berry was still stranded in Geneva.[79] As it happened, Mary was one of the lucky ones who reached home safely, but young Lord Yarmouth, Hertford's heir, appeared fated to imprisonment for the duration, despite his father's pleas "through the highest channels." While France, like Europe and the rest of the world, owed a great deal to Jenner, it was almost winter before it occurred to him that he might be of use to his friend's son. In the meantime the young man had been parted from his wife and sent to the fortress of Verdun. A summer and autumn of increasing national acclaim would eventually stir Jenner into action where diplomacy had failed.

Farington finally arrived in Cheltenham on September 10, after a fast but tiresome trip. His detailed description of this journey, one which was so often made by Jenner, is perhaps worth repeating. He took the Cheltenham and Gloucester mail from the Angel Inn, behind St. Clements in the Strand, which was due to leave at six-thirty in the evening but actually pulled out of the yard fifteen minutes late. They were somewhat behind schedule for the first few hours and did not reach Oxford until four o'clock in the morning, with the steep massif of the Cotswolds still to be climbed. "Here we found a good fire and maid-servant with coffee prepared." After a thirty-minute rest they set out again, presumably with fresh horses, for the worst part of their journey. Surprisingly

enough, they climbed the escarpments in fine fettle. A quick
breakfast at Burford and off they went in the dawn for Cheltenham over the hard, sun-baked roads. The great coach swayed and
lurched behind its six horses down through the waking villages
and finally the long stretch of Charlton Hill into Cheltenham
High Street, to swing into the yard of the George Inn at ten-thirty
in the morning, half an hour ahead of time.[80]

Upon meeting his friend, Farington thought that Hoppner
looked much better than when he was in London, though he still
complained occasionally even after Jenner had put him on a
mercury treatment in conjunction with the appropriate mineral
waters. There was also a number of other interesting and bona
fide invalids staying at Smiths' besides the fashionables who were
in town purely to take the waters. Matthew Baillie did not arrive
until August 8 this year[81]—rather late for him—and by then the
town must have been full of his London patients. Happily, there
seems to have been no one in residence to compete with Jenner
in the treatment of liver complaints.

But fortunately all was not vaccination or liver complaints
during those early autumn evenings. There was an interesting
coterie of music lovers in the town by the beginning of September.
Not only was Jenner himself a musician and singer of some ability,
but his ailing friend Hoppner had been a chorister in the Chapel
Royal until his voice broke. Also present to take the waters was
the celebrated musicologist Dr. Charles Burney,[82] with his wife.
But more important than any of these was the Italian operatic
composer, Francesco Bianchi,[83] who introduced the great English
soprano, Elizabeth Billington,[84] to the Italian stage. He was also the
discoverer and mentor of Sir Henry Bishop. Both Mrs. Billington
and Bishop, indeed, eventually took up residence in the town.
Farington comments on a musical gathering at Smiths' the evening
before he left. "I dined at Smiths with about forty persons—after
dinner Bianchi, who was one of the company sang an Italian air.
—Colonel Heath, —Captain Ogg, and another gentleman also
sang." The following morning Hoppner and Farington went about
the town sketching, or, more correctly perhaps, the latter did.
"Hoppner joined me but did not apply long," wrote the diarist.[85]
In the afternoon they left on a tour of the Wye Valley, though

Hoppner was still a sick man and somewhat depressed. Indeed, his participation in the expedition seems to have been rather halfhearted from the start and after some two weeks of what must have been, for him, tiresome travelling, they made their way to Hempsted Court, on September 25, to visit David Lysons.

While they were resting at Hempsted, Charles Trye—Lysons's brother-in-law—came over from Gloucester Infirmary, and it is possible that the conversation turned toward Jenner and vaccination. There seems to be no other explanation for the ailing artist's decision to change his mind about returning to London with Farington and to go instead to Devonshire to see Lord Borington. This gentleman's family was the pioneer force in establishing smallpox inoculation when Lady Mary Wortley Montague had brought the system back from the Levant. His seat at Saltram, four miles from Plymouth, was, along with his fortune, one of the most magnificent in the country. His prestige had been exerted in the fight against smallpox for two generations. To most people the terms Borington and smallpox inoculation were synonymous, but as yet his lordship had made no public decision on vaccination. So it was that Farington returned to London alone, while Hoppner embarked on the formidable two-hundred-mile coach journey to the borders of Cornwall.

The hospitality the painter enjoyed during his few days in the luxury of Saltram certainly did him no good physically, and he finally arrived in London exhausted from nearly a week on the roads. On the other hand, Lord Borington did change sides on vaccination and became both friend and supporter of Jenner. He had his children vaccinated, though only one reached his majority. The Boringtons became seasonal patrons of the Cheltenham Wells, a social development in which the rather flighty young wife heartily concurred, since the rising Spa, only a hundred miles from London, offered much greater scope for meeting new and interesting people. In particular, they became friendly with the Pagets, who were related to Jenner's friend Bentinck; Lady Borington's sister was married to Lord Jersey's heir, another well-known Cheltenham figure. Whether or not this development was precipitated by Hoppner, the advent of Lord Borington to the cause had a significant effect on the parliamentary history of vaccination. As for the artist himself, the pilgrimage was almost the finish of him. Farington met him on October 2 in London and was not impressed. "Hoppner seems to be uneasy about his thin habit of body," he wrote. "He does not seem to have his spirits raised by having been in Cheltenham—He was at Lord Borington's at Saltram 9 days."[86]

Bianchi and the Burneys remained with Jenner in Cheltenham, where a fresh spate of nobility arrived on September 19, apparently because it was rumored that the Prince of Wales was on his way, and a house was, indeed, being prepared for him. Among the new arrivals were Lord and Lady Ellenborough, Lord Hutchinson,[87] the Earl of Leicester, and the Earl of Suffolk. Hutchinson, who had inherited the command of the army in Egypt on the death of Lord Abercromby, had, with his brother Christopher, seen a great deal of Lord and Lady Elgin, but the friendship had cooled somewhat as a result of what were called the absurdly lenient terms Hutchinson had granted to the French on the surrender of Cairo. Be that as it may, to Jenner he would have been a very welcome visitor. It will be recalled that it was Lord Abercromby's edict that had required the entire Middle East army to be vaccinated in 1800, and, as a result, not a single case of smallpox occurred in the heat and contagion of that unhealthy theater of operations. Elgin's and Abercromby's extremely important roles in Jenner's life's work and the vast area over which their operations ranged would have far outweighed the *social* disapproval emanating from association with the only surviving figure in this triumverate. Hutchinson was described by Sir Henry Bunbury in 1801: "44 years of age, but looked much older, with harsh features, jaundiced by disease, extreme short-sightedness, a stooping body and a slouching gait, and an utter neglect of dress—He shunned general society, was indolent, with an ungracious manner and a violent temper."[88] Hutchinson, though, had been the one to personally thank Dr. Marshall for his work in vaccinating the army in 1801. Whatever question there may have been about the noble lord's social deportment or political wisdom, there certainly could have been none about his personal bravery. One story that went around the salons had great local interest, not the least to Jenner since it related to an old friend. During the Duke of York's campaign in Flanders in 1799, Hutchinson had under his command the young Lord Craven, son of the Margravine of Anspach. In the course of the skirmish, the young officer was thrown from his horse at the head of his party of troops and kicked in the head. Hutchinson fought his way to the temporarily disorganized troops, took command of them himself, and undoubtedly saved the life of the young peer (who was severely injured) and extricated his men.[89] There was, as it were, a common bond between the soldier and the doctor: Jenner had saved the life of the mother and Hutchinson the life of the son.

Jenner did not know Lord Elgin personally when his lordship left England in 1799. The British public was not yet particularly enthusiastic about vaccination, and it was on the Continent that the peer began to hear all about it. His enthusiasm grew after he met Dr. De Carro, who supplied him with vaccine and helped him in every way possible.[90] Much as Jenner must have deplored the imprisonment of such an important ally, he seems to have been too diffident to offer his services to further the ambassador's release. Lord Yarmouth, however, being the son of a personal friend, was a rather different matter, and it was he who became the test case when Jenner finally succumbed to the urging of his followers to intercede for prisoners on the basis of the gratitude that France owed him. He wrote to Lord Hertford in October and offered to solicit the assistance of Count Andreossi in the matter of young Yarmouth's detention. He failed to get a reply from the erstwhile ambassador, however, and addressed Hertford again.

November, 1803.

To the Marquess of Hertford.

My Lord,

Since I did myself the honour of addressing your Lordship on the subject of Lord Yarmouth's liberation, I received a solicitation to intercede in behalf of the Peploes, a family detained in Paris on their way to Spa.

Having made an acquaintance with General Andreossi during his embassy here, I wrote to him, but received no answer. However, I have since heard that his family has obtained permission to go to Germany; so that it is probable, although General Andreossi has not written, that he may have interested himself for them: and not in vain.

On reflexion, my Lord, I think my chance of success would be greater by addressing a body than any individual. My letter I consign to the care of your Lordship. Whether it may be necessary to send it I cannot determine; that it may meet with success is my most ardent wish.

E. Jenner.

The enclosure was as follows:

To the National Institute of France.

Gentlemen,

Pardon my obtruding myself on you at this junction. The Sciences are never at war. Peace must always preside in those bosoms whose object is the augmentation of human happiness.

Permit me then, as a public body with whom I am connected, to solicit your interest in the liberation of Lord Yarmouth, a young nobleman at this time detained with his family in France. Lord Yarmouth is the son, the only son, of my valued friend and patron the Marquess of Hertford. He stands high in my estimation for being among the foremost of those who encouraged my scheme of vaccination when in its infancy, and contending with the prejudice of the world.

There is another family of the name of Peploe in whose behalf some months ago I solicited the interference of General Andreossi, a gentleman with whom I had the honour to become acquainted during his residence in London; but alas! I have received no answer to my letter nor heard anything of my friends.

Should I be so fortunate as through your kind interference to see my friends restored to those who are suffering on their account the most painful solicitude, I shall ever be most grateful to acknowledge the obligation you will have conferred upon me.

I have the honour to be, Gentlemen,
With high consideration,
&c. &c. &c.
E. Jenner[91]

Jenner never had the satisfaction of knowing whether his letter was the cause, but Lady Elgin informed her mother in a letter dated December 10 that "Lord Yarmouth is offered to be exchanged for another French general."[92] It took a year, however, to obtain his final release.

While Jenner was strolling the walks and sipping the waters with the highest in the land, he was not resting as he would have liked. Acclaim continued to pour in from all over the world, and gracious, fitting responses were required from his pen constantly. The year 1803 was for Jenner indeed one of great recognition. During his stay in London, he had made a member of the Society of Medicine at Avignon, and after he returned to Cheltenham the pace increased. First came the Diploma, making him Fellow of the Royal Medical and Economical Society of Madrid, and then, most important of all, his first honorary doctorate from a university. The first week in November, he received the Doctor of Laws from Harvard, dated August 31. Among the signatories was Harvard President Joseph Willard,[93] who was not merely a doctor but a member of the Medical Society of London, and, like Jenner, a Fellow of the Royal Society of Gottingen. Honors were now flowing so fast that had the impoverished doctor received a check with every diploma, his financial problems might well have been resolved. The war itself seemed to make little difference to his admirers, for in rapid succession he received his Diploma of Foreign Associate of the School of Medicine of Paris and the Diploma of the Society of Medicine, Departement du Garde. At home, to round out the scene, he received the Freedom of the City of London, "presented in a gold box worth a hundred guineas,"[94] and the Diploma of the Royal Humane Society of London, signed, among others, by his friend Dr. Lettsom.

Perhaps one of the most interesting tributes of the year came from the least expected quarter—from old Christopher Anstey, who appeared with his family at the Wells as usual in the summer. At the age of seventy-nine, he had, to all intents and purposes, retired—having written nothing of a serious nature since the *Farmer's Daughter* eight years before. It is to his younger son, John, that we are indebted for the details of Anstey's latter years in Cheltenham, where the spate of honors that were flowing in to Jenner from all parts of the world inspired the old poet to add a contribution of his own. He would bring his pen out of retirement one last time to pay tribute to his friend, and he composed what his contemporary, George Cunningham,[95] describes as "an elegant Latin ode" entitled, "Ad Edwardum Jenner, M.D. Carmen Alcaicum." The work was completed while Anstey was at the Wells, but he did not publish it until he returned to Bath in the autumn.

John Anstey was understandably proud of his father's effect so late in life, and describes the work "addressed to Dr. Jenner in consequence of his very important discovery of vaccine inoculation" in the following rather extravagant terms: "A striking example of the *extraordinary* powers of a mind retentive of the impressions made in early youth, and exercising its faculties with more than ordinary vigour and activity at an advanced age."[96] It ran to some nine pages—twenty-three alcaic stanzas of sound, if not inspired, Latin verse of which the following stanza will suffice:

> Jennere, laudes an sileam tuas
> Dum mente sanus, nec cythera careus,
> Turpive succumbeus senectae
> Rura vagour per amoena Cheltae?[97]

All of which Jenner with his "little Latin and *no* Greek" would have no doubt appreciated. The dedicated—and practical—John Ring translated the whole thing into English the following year and donated the profits to the Royal Jennerian Society. Anstey was the first established poet to recognize the pioneer, but Jenner was not allowed to bask in the autumn sunshine for long. In October he was called in by Lord Berkeley whose child was dangerously ill. Berkeley Castle was a good five-hour ride over indifferent roads, but the doctor could do nothing else but answer the unhappy parents' summons. He wrote to Thomas Dibdin on October 10: "An infant of Lord Berkeley's has lately been so ill, as to take me repeatedly from Cheltenham to Berkeley Castle; and this has thrown my general concerns here into confusion."[98] Apparently the pressure of his work would not permit Jenner to stay at the castle until the child recovered—or at his own cottage for that matter. Nevertheless, he somehow coped and by November had an interesting amount of material written relative to the vaccination operation in the Middle East, together with speculations upon using the system against the plague as well as smallpox. Undoubtedly, conversations with Lord Hutchinson were of great assistance in this work. A short piece appeared in *Bell's Weekly Messenger* on November 30 entitled "Edward Jenner to the Public Concerning Cowpox and Smallpox in Constantinople"; but the question of vaccination for the plague petered out when the doctor really examined it and found it impractical. Jenner's friends were far more enthusiastic about the idea than he was.

Lord Fauconberg's demise this summer ended the familiar passage of the great carriages past Jenner's door, and Fauconberg Lodge stood empty and forlorn. Far more tragic was the death of Powell Snell. A combination of the Cheltenham dandy and rugged Cotswold squire, he had graced the scene for half a century. Amateur soldier and amateur poet, his rhyming comments on most of the social events through the years gave a flesh-and-blood character to the lifeless chronicle. Snell had recorded the activities of all the great contemporaries through the years and had been one of the few Cheltenham figures who had grown up with Jenner's fame, and though often the butt of the doctor's humor, always loyal to him. He was buried in the little churchyard at Guiting in the heart of the hills. Then as the year drew to its close, yet another fine mansion fell empty when old Dr. Hooper died at the Great House, in St. George's Place. Strangely enough during this rather melancholy end of the season when people and landmarks of preciously familiar character were passing, the invalid Catherine Jenner became stronger, and had he not had too many financial worries, Jenner himself might have been very happy at the peak of his fame. Indeed, before the year was out, two more great honors fell to his lot; one related to the war; the other was perhaps even more significant. The Commander-in-Chief of the Army, the Duke of York, ordered all the troops to be vaccinated who had not already had smallpox, thus completing the process pioneered by the late Lord Abercromby. The second honor was more related to Jenner's prestige as a man than to his medical achievements.

In the year 1767 a group of peers and wealthy landowners established the Gloucestershire Society in London, under the patronage of the King's brother, the Duke of Gloucester, with the Duke of Beaufort as President.[99] It was described thus in the Abstract of Rules:

The object of this benevolent Institution is to call forth the liberal contributions of such gentlemen as are natives of the county of Gloucester or in any other respect so connected with it . . . for the laudable purpose of apprenticing the children of the deserving poor belonging to the County, who might otherwise be destitute of the means of acquiring a comfortable subsistence through life.

In the nature of things of course, it was a rich man's club, with its annual dinners in town and the gatherings of County families in the interest of charity and conviviality, so much a part of the eighteenth-century scene.

Two stewards were chosen each year, and in 1802 Lysons's friend, Charles Bragg, was named. While this gentleman's successful public career might have been in part due to his being married to Prime Minister Addington's sister, he was, in his own right, a sensitive and intellectual man of some stature. Being a Bathurst on the distaff side, he must have known Jenner who was a mere rank-and-file member of the society. Jenner also knew the Prime Minister, since he wrote to James Moore some years later: "Your friend Lord Sidmouth [Addington was raised to the peerage in 1805] was once a friend of mine and perhaps remains so still. His good humour was an over match for his firmness with the Premier."[100] There was also the familiar community of interest in medicine and literature among this common circle. Mrs. Bragg's father was the celebrated physician to George III, Anthony Addington,[101] who tended Chatham in his fatal heart attack in the House.

There is no evidence that Jenner attended the annual dinner of the Gloucestershire Society in 1803, even though it had been held on the second Wednesday in May when he was still in London. I wonder if the answer lies in a stipulation that appears in the rules, namely that "no . . . member of this Society whose subscription shall be more than two years in arrears can vote at any election of Officers or Boys." At all events, those in the seats of the mighty were apparently uninfluenced by what must now have been Jenner's manifest penury, and he was accordingly chosen to take Charles Bragg's place as Steward of the Gloucestershire Society for 1803.[102] The post thus passed from the Prime Minister's brother-in-law to a penniless provincial doctor.

Another year had passed and another winter had arrived. The Prince of Wales had failed to come to Cheltenham after all, and Jenner's grant money had also failed to come. He was still in no position to buy his own home in Cheltenham, even though renting was such an expensive business. When the captains and the kings had departed, he was left with only his problems.

V

A Leader of Society
1804-1806

The honors and acclaim of the summer resulting in no concrete reward, Jenner's spirits dropped with the passing of the unprecedented sunshine. The grey days of winter reflected only too well his domestic and financial uncertainties. With the new year he was faced with the fact that vaccination practice was not paying. He was earning some three hundred and fifty pounds per annum, and the amount tended to decline rather than otherwise. His London quarters in Hertford Street, Mayfair, to which he was committed for a further eight years, were a constant strain on his resources, but he had still gone there assiduously every spring, always hoping that the tide of prosperity would turn. Instead, the opposite was happening, paradoxically enough, because of his increasing fame. He complained in a letter:

My fees fell off both in number and value, for, extraordinary to tell, some of those families in which I had before been employed, now sent to their own domestic surgeons or apothecaries to inoculate their children, alleging that they could not think of troubling Dr. Jenner about a thing executed so easily as vaccine inoculation. Others who gave no such fees as I thought myself entitled to at the first inoculation reduced them at the second, and sank them still lower at the third.[1]

But what was far more serious, Mrs. Jenner took a grave turn for the worse and began spitting blood. London—with its smoke and congestion—was obviously out of the question, so they would quietly spend the spring in Berkeley. In the summer he could return to Cheltenham, earn some money, and perhaps speak to some of the visiting politicians about his grant.

Lord Hardwick and his lady continued to be very active in
Ireland. Dr. Samuel Bell Labatt,[2] an eminent surgeon of Dublin,
was made Director of the Dublin Cowpock Institution, and the
movement progressed virtually without opposition. Jenner eagerly
cited the case of Ireland when people questioned what the efficacy
of vaccination would be if opposition were withdrawn. The penniless peasant of Erin was safer from the scourge of smallpox
than the affluent English yeoman. The Hardwicks were very
popular in a land still smarting from the bitterness of two insur-
rections. This probably had something to do with the ease of the
spread of vaccination once his lordship had put his heart into it.
Early in March the country showed its gratitude—Edward Jenner
was given the Freedom of the City of Dublin.[3]

In London his friends kept him informed of events and still
urged him to return. Lettsom suggested a fund-raising campaign in
India, and actually spoke to a number of influential people about
it. The project did, indeed, proceed, but like the grant, the money
took several years to materialize and Jenner's situation was getting
desperate. Lettsom was perhaps Jenner's most aggressive and fearless defender; he possessed, like Trye, the zeal of the convert, for
according to Pettigrew,[4] he at first distrusted vaccination.

In contrast to Jenner, his friends appeared to be very prosperous.
The excitement of the war, gossip, and the usual routine of the
London season made for a full life. Farington tells of a meal he
had with Angerstein:

We dined at six o'clock; the dinner consisted of two courses, viz. a
fine turbot at the top and a sirloin of beef at the bottom and vermicelli
soup in the middle, with small dishes making a figure of nine dishes—
the remove roast duck at the top and a very fine roast poulet at the
bottom, marcaroni tartlets, etc., etc. Afterwards a Parmesian and other
cheese and caviar with toast. Champagne and Medeira was served
round during dinner—I noticed that Mr. Angerstein drank very little
wine *after dinner*—while the conversation went on he sometimes slept,
after he woke he eat [sic] an orange with sugar. He appears to consider
his health but he looks very full and well.[5]

Also active in the capital was Rev. Rowland Hill,[6] incumbent
of Surrey Chapel, who was himself something of a rebel within
the church fold. Having adopted vaccination enthusiastically as

soon as it was introduced, he became, like Lady Peyton, one of the leading nonmedical practitioners in the country. In addition to his ministry in London, he had a chapel at Wotton-under-Edge in Gloucestershire (where Jenner had been apprenticed as a boy), and at both places he offered free vaccination after every service. Hill visited the doctor regularly at St. George's Place, not so much for their common interest in vaccination, but to talk. "Jenner was a man of animated conversation with remarkably fine disposition," Hill's biographer relates,—"Whenever he [Hill] went to preach he announced after his sermon: 'I am ready to vaccinate tomorrow morning as many children as you choose.' "[7]

But Rowland Hill, alas, was not a representative example of Jenner's prestige in London. The triumphs of international recognition in 1803 had not had the effect one would have anticipated. Even though it was unavoidable, his absence from the metropolis at this time was most unfortunate. According to Baron, those who were jealous of his fame waxed more bold; his friends became lukewarm; his enemies more united and clamorous. To make matters worse, reports of the failure of vaccination began to come in in increasing numbers, a trend which frightened his friends since Jenner was not there to answer them. He was not to be moved, however. He was in Berkeley to get away from all this. He was able to spend six months in his country retreat for the first time since the publication of the *Inquiry*. To a friend who urged him to return to London he wrote:

You and my city friends suppose me idle—that I no longer employ my time and my thoughts on the vaccine subject. So very opposite is the real state of the case that were you here (where I should be very glad to see you) you would see that my whole time is nearly engrossed by it. On an average I am at least six hours daily with my pen in my hand, bending over writing paper, until I am grown as crooked as a cow's horn and tawny as whey-butter, and *you* want to make me as mad as a bull. But it won't do, Mr. D; so goodnight to you. I'll to my pillow, not of thorns believe me, *nor of hops,* but of poppies or at least of something that produces calm repose.[8]

The last comment was no doubt inspired by his recently deceased friend Powell Snell. The poet having heard of the King's receiving more benefit in his late illness from the hop pillow had written:

Come then, blest opiate—from thy new born power
I claim redress nor dread the midnight hour.
All Hail!—thou broughtest sudden joy from woe.
Our Monarch lives!!! from whom our blessings flow.[9]

Not very good poetry perhaps but typical—and final—Powell
Snell. But Jenner's passing notice of light verse did nothing to
allay the increasing, nagging burden of financial worry. On June 3,
Jenner wrote to a friend, "The Treasury still withholds the payment of what was voted me two years ago; and now there are new
officers, the time may be very long before a guinea reaches me
from that quarter." Undoubtedly he would have to do something
soon in the way of *lucrative* practice. He manifestly could earn
no substantial fees hibernating in Berkeley, nor was there anyone
here to whom he could talk about his grant money.

With the rearrangement of the Ministry in London, Lord
Hardwick's administration in Ireland came under fire. He survived,
at least for the time being, and an increasing number of Irish
nobility were rallying to the cause of vaccination. On July 15, this
movement was helped by the appearance of Jenner's letter on the
progress of vaccination in Ireland in *The Medical and Physical
Journal*. The news from other outposts was not so encouraging,
however. Lord Elgin remained in close confinement in France and
even the loyal Dr. Scott was arrested when he unwisely returned to
Paris to help Lady Elgin in her distress.[10] The dowager still had
the charge of the daughter of the Prince of Wales, but her steward-
ship was now coming under attack in certain quarters. Mr. Coutts
was put in charge of the imprisoned family's affairs until the war
situation changed. Any pro-Jenner activity from the Elgin clan
was, for the time being, completely finished, and Lord Hutchinson's unpopularity, if anything, increased. Farington observes on
July 8: "Lord Hutchinson is respected as a man but not looked
up to as an officer. Among other things he is improperly neglectful
of his *personal appearance*. Hair uncombed,—unbrushed clothes,
&c."[11] This at a time when naval and military leaders were the
lions of society. The spring and early summer were marked by
feverish military activity, particularly in the West of England
where the dusty lanes echoed to the tread of plowboys and shop-
keepers turned soldier. The Cheltenham Volunteers occupied

Gloucester for some reason in May and returned to a royal reception by their townsmen. The sound of drums and barked orders kept many a citizen awake nights. The fear—yet in a way, the fascinating anticipation—of invasion, was in everyone's mind.

In all truth, there was ample besides Bonaparte to keep the doctor awake at night. A new and particularly vindictive adversary appeared in the person of a Mr. Goldston of Portsea.[12] Motivated by an apparent slight he had suffered at Jenner's hands (a private letter was allegedly ignored), Goldston issued a devastating pamphlet that undermined the whole principle of vaccination by, first, declaring it was a purely temporary measure, and second, that it was completely undependable. The writer was a highly esteemed man in his community and his "examples" were expressed forcefully and convincingly. The layman had no way of knowing that his claims were without verification or even sound knowledge of the subject. At first Jenner was contemptuous of the attack, but eventually was so concerned as to offer to meet Goldston and explain the whole matter to him. Needless to say, the offer was declined and the scurrilous sheet continued its tragic work.

When May arrived and Jenner's birthday drew near, his friends urged him at least to come up to town for the annual dinner. He refused, on the grounds of his wife's indisposition, but he probably would have declined in any case. He went through periods when he was completely disillusioned with the capital, and as high summer approached, he began to think of the familiar faces—the confident faces that were much nearer at hand. He would escape London this year. By now the stream of great chariots with their outriders, pomp, and panoply were rumbling westward to Cheltenham bearing the peers of England. It was time for Jenner to end his exile, and on July 22, he added a postscript in a letter to Dunning: "Just setting off with my family for Cheltenham."[13] It might be said that London—or his part of it—was coming to him.

When Jenner's little clan trooped into Cheltenham that July day, the town was like a European capital. The liveried servants of the visiting nobility seemed to have outnumbered the resident population. The great Irish houses were particularly in evidence;

Lord Hardwick had done his work efficiently. The Huntingfields, the Liffords, Ashtowns, Kilkenneys, and the Cootes were already ensconced, and others were expected. Nor were these noble lords and ladies the only representatives of the Emerald Isle. The streets also resounded to the rumble of the emblazoned carriages of the lesser gentry—the heirs and younger sons of the great families—the O'Neils, Fitzgeralds, and, in isolated splendor, the Lord Bishop of Down. Michael Kelly had arrived the week before with Mr. Corry, one of Thomas Moore's closest friends who later moved to the town permanently. Fortunately, among the English arrivals were several of Jenner's earlier and familiar patrons: Lord Spencer, Lord and Lady Rous, Lady Peyton with her two daughters, and, thankfully, the ever-faithful Charles James Fox, with his wife and daughter.

Anstey and his wife arrived on the same day as Jenner and undoubtedly one of the first things they saw, while strolling along High Street, was the notice in the window of Harwood's bookshop:

JUST PUBLISHED, 2/-
A Translation of Anstey's Latin Ode
ADDRESSED TO DR. JENNER
BY JOHN RING.[14]

It was almost like an official welcoming address, and with his own world once more clustered about him, the doctor took new heart. In addition, it was said that the Duke of Bedford, President of the Royal Jennerian Society, was expected the following week, and it is possible that Jenner came to St. George's Place just when he did in order to be in residence when His Grace arrived. Their respective homes were very close.

Successful as the 1803 season had been, the present one outstripped it in every respect. Never had so many of the rich and mighty poured in at once. Never had so much grand building been in progress. *The Gloucester Journal* could not contain itself. Every few weeks it extolled the prosperity and activity of the place. "The great increase of elegant accommodation and the emulation of the inhabitants to render them fit for the reception of their friends have drawn at this early period an unusual number of visitors to this salubrious spot," it observed on May 21. On

July 9, it continued, "Cheltenham has seldom been known to be so much crowded with elegant company as during the present season. The assemblies are numerously attended by beauty and fashion."

As soon as Mrs. Jenner and the children were settled in, Jenner began to sort out his affairs. After his absence of six months, his library was one of the first things he turned to, and he selected a small work to send to Dunning to help reassure him as to the strength of the vaccination case. It was the essay written the previous year by Dr. Yeates of Bedford explaining very succinctly the causes of some vaccination blunders. "Conceiving that you may never have seen this little tract," said the doctor, "I have sent it to you; for like the tracts of *some* folks in days that are past, it was never well advertised and consequently but little known."[15] Jenner was already stimulated by the atmosphere around him, and eagerly fighting the opposition while his friends continued to pour into the town.

A topic of national concern this summer was the "Middlesex Elections" in which the left-wing radical Sir Francis Burdett was fighting the Tory "Pittite" A. B. Mainwaring. Henry Hunt—an old friend of Fox's and, if anything, more radical than Burdett— was in Cheltenham at the time, and both men followed the battle eagerly. Hunt says in his *Memoirs:*

I remember sitting in the library with Mr. Fox at Cheltenham when the news arrived by post that Sir Francis Burdett was elected for Middlesex by a majority of eleven. Fox was greatly elated with this momentary success of the Baronet, but he expressed his doubts about the final issue of an Inquiry before a committee of the House of Commons. This famous contest for Middlesex had caused considerable anxiety throughout the country, and a party of us, including Fox, used to assemble daily on the arrival of the post at the Library to hear the state of the poll.

Perhaps Cheltenham did not after all consist solely of sophisticated but cynical elegance. Hunt, at least, was struck by the domestic bliss of some of the families in the town. Being one of nature's rebels, it is rather interesting that he found the place so much to his liking. Loosely speaking, he was describing the Jenner circle when he wrote:

I was living at Clifton at this period, and during the summer I visited Cheltenham with my family. At the latter place I frequently met Mr. Fox, who was drinking the celebrated waters for his health, which had become greatly impaired in consequence of his attendance so incessantly to his parliamentary duties. He was accompanied by Mrs. Armistead, the lady whom he afterwards married, and to which lady the people of England have had the honour to pay twelve hundred pounds a year, ever since the death of Mr. Fox. Mrs. Armistead appeared to be a very delightful woman with whom this great statesman and senator evidently lived in a state of the most perfect domestic harmony. They were almost always together, seldom, if ever, were they to be seen separate—at the Pump Rooms in the morning; at the library and reading room at noon, when the papers came in; at the theatre or private parties, in the evening; Mr. Fox and Mrs. Armistead were always to be seen together. The Duke of Bedford was then recently married to his present Duchess. Mr. Fox and his lady were frequently of the Duke's party; in fact they were as one family. Cheltenham was then full of very gay company; amongst whom a great deal of dissipation and intrigue was going on. It was frequently made a subject of remark, that Mr. Fox and Mr. Hunt appeared to enjoy more real happiness, more domestic felicity than any of the married persons of Cheltenham, with the exception of the Duke and Duchess of Bedford, who lived a retired domestic life at that time and, from what I have heard, have continued to do so ever since.[16]

Hunt evidently met Fox for the first time this summer, or he would have known that even though his wife was commonly called Mrs. Armistead—on account of some curious whim of the statesman—they had indeed been married for seven years. Fox always put on a brave front, but actually he was extremely ill, and it soon became clear that his liver complaint was growing more serious. He did not, however, appear depressed and was his usual cheerful self in every outward respect. The Bishop of Down, a close friend of his, also suffered from a liver complaint.

On July 22, the day Jenner and his family arrived, a visit was made by Fox and his friends to the Grotto in Prestbury. Humphris included Dr. and Mrs. Jenner in the party, but I can find no verification of this. The incident is described in a rare unprinted manuscript in the Cheltenham Public Library, and gives an interesting contemporary description of that celebrated tea garden. Sarah Fox writes:

I have attempted nothing like pleasure since I came here, once excepted, which was to drink tea in Prestbury, a village about two miles distant, whither I went on a double horse. Our party drank tea in a little garden they call *The Grotto* from there being in it a circular rustic building, decorated with curious stones and shells. Soon after our repast was finished we were informed we must withdraw to make room for another party to whom the apartment was promised. At seven they came when we perceived Charles James Fox, his wife, and others walking towards us, and whom we met on our retiring to make way. I was pleased with the opportunity of again taking a view of one of whom I had heard so much. I say again because I had before met them at the pastry-cook's, and conversed with his wife, who appears sociable, and once, by his speaking, found his voice correspond with his features.

The ones who are unnamed and made up the party were, according to Humphris, Dr. and Mrs. Jenner. The diarist, however, continues:

In consequence of our resigning the apartment we walked about the garden and presently heard, issuing from a cave, the most distressing lamentations from a female voice, as it appeared to me. This so frightened me that I ran towards the house, when Patty Young, who was making her way, as is her custom, to the cry of distress, came after me smiling that it was a ventriloquist who was there for the diversion of the party at Cheltenham and who, I suppose, had come to his garden to divert the honourable assembled.[17]

It sounds like a rather unsophisticated kind of diversion but probably appealed to Mrs. Fox who had very simple tastes, and it would certainly have appealed to Jenner with his well-known sense of humor. Two days later Fox wrote to his nephew, Lord Holland: "The Bishop of Down and his family are here. He looks thin and yellow, but I think him in good spirits, and am, therefore, sanguine that he will do."

Fox had been excluded from Pitt's new cabinet after the fall of the Addington administration; and from the isolation of Berkeley the change of government had made the payment of Jenner's grant seem farther away than ever. Nonetheless, here in Cheltenham, with all these influential politicians around him, his hope rose. As Fox's friend and companion Jenner could meet practically anyone he wanted to, and they were all here—particu-

larly the military and naval leaders so recently under Fox's aegis:
Lord Bridport—better known as Admiral Hood, General Stuart,
General Sherbrooke, the hero of Seringapatam who later became
Governor-General of Canada, Admiral Brisbane, Admiral Pigott,
General Champagne, and Admiral Manir; all of them parading
the walks and probably casting dubious looks at the mere poli-
ticians about them.

Not surprisingly after three weeks in this whirl of activity,
money, and optimism, Jenner's confidence returned. He could
scarcely handle all his patients and was able to write to his apprehensive friend Dunning with all the assurance of a prosperous
man:

Cheltenham, Oct. 25th, 1804.

My Dear Sir,

Before I say anything of your second letter, allow me to notice your
first, when I tell you that I am at this time at least two hundred letters
in arrears to my correspondents, which, as you may suppose, multiply
in every part of the earth to a great extent, you will at once forgive
my not writing sooner to a friend with whom I could take a liberty.
There is not a country in the globe where I do not owe a letter, and
yet all my leisure time is occupied with pen, ink and paper. But you
must be informed that my *leisure hours are very few*; for the company
resorting to this fashionable watering place increases every year in a
most rapid manner, and, consequently, my medical engagements; in-
somuch, that I have it in contemplation to quit it. Should I be compelled to do this, what a hardship I must endure! Shall I not be the
first man in our profession who quitted his post through excess of
business? Vaccination calls imperiously for my attention and to that I
am determined all my other worldly concerns shall yield. But while I
am fighting the enemy of mankind, it will be vexatious to see my
aides-de-camp turn shy.

After continuing for some five hundred words of encouragement
in the face of his friend's fears, Jenner goes on:

Be of good cheer, my friend. Those who are so presumptuous as to
expect perfection in man will be grievously disappointed. His works
are and ever will be defective. Let people if they choose it, spurn the
great gift that heaven has bestowed and turn again to variolation.

What will they get by it? . . . Adieu, my dear friend, and be sure of the unalterable regard of

Yours/
Edward Jenner.[18]

Shrewd speculator that he was, Colonel Riddell, Jenner's landlord, was also busy making money. Mr. Watson purchased a part of Cambray meadow for his new Theatre Royal, which was opened the following year, and also built himself a cottage near by. This entire area had been in the hands of Lord Essex until the Enclosures Act of 1801, when he sold the Impropriation to Joseph Pitt who then developed part of it himself and resold the remainder. Cambray became the "get-rich-quick" area of Cheltenham, and several local people bought sites here, including Mrs. Entwistle, Harriot Mellon's mother, and the lofty Mr. King, Master of Ceremonies at the Spa. Riddell also saw the potential of Cambray as a residential area when he came to live permanently in Cheltenham this year and rented Mr. Watson's cottage in Cambray, which was still not completely finished. Watson had somewhat over-extended himself in his property investments and hoped he could persuade the colonel to buy the cottage. There was one apparent drawback, however: the water supply—the well—was very poor and had a flat unpleasant taste. Unfortunately the day was very hot when the potential purchaser arrived, so Watson instructed his servant to have plenty of fresh water on hand so that no one need go near the dubious pump. A lady in the company, however, grew thirsty and pleaded for some *really* fresh water straight from the well. It was, of course, brought to her and she grimaced the moment she tasted it. Very much alert, Riddell took it from her and sipped himself. He immediately realized that a new mineral spring had been discovered but said no word to Watson when he returned to discuss terms. The poor mummer was no match for the speculator, and only after everything was signed and sealed for the modest price of an unfurnished cottage did he realize that he had sold the spot of the future Cambray Spa. Twenty-four hours after the discovery became known, the remaining properties in Cambray fields *doubled* in value. At least the colonel had the decency to permit Mrs. Watson

free access to the well. She and her husband had long ago found
that the strange water agreed with them; yet it had occurred to
neither that here was a new medicinal spring.

The Duke and Duchess of Bedford arrived as expected on
July 30.[19] This was the first time Jenner had seen the President
of the Royal Jennerian Society this year, since he had not attended
the annual birthday banquet in May. Both his Grace and his wife
were known as kind, responsible people, and Lysons, who arrived
in Cheltenham about the same time, echoed Henry Hunt's sentiments completely, describing the duke as an agreeable, unaffected man.

There appears to have been a general meeting of the vaccination clans, for the first September list of arrivals includes Lord
Hutchinson and Mr. Angerstein and Lord and Lady Macclesfield.
This latter gentleman was, like Jenner, a Fellow of the Royal Society, and a well-known amateur scientist. With the President of
the Jennerian Society joined by the Chairman (Angerstein), serious discussions with the company present apparently resulted
in some scheme to force the government's hand. Jenner's long-
awaited grant was paid within a month. He, too, went into the
property market.

Aside from vaccination affairs, the Whig prejudice was very
manifest in the medical gossip that circulated around the Wells.
The Bishop of Gloucester told Lysons that he was not a bit convinced of the Pittites' assertion that the King was in good health.
His Lordship prophesied that there would be a regency before
November. He obviously did not trust Pitt. On the other hand,
the Bishop felt that Fox was open and a man to be depended
upon. As a matter of fact, despite his jovial front, poor Fox was
now a doomed man. He had developed a severe pain in the side
since coming to Cheltenham, which, according to his nephew Lord
Holland "proceeded no doubt from that affection in the liver
which ultimately brought him to his grave."[20] Dr. Cother also
went to *his* grave this year and his practice was taken over by Mr.
Wood, the surgeon. Wood, apparently a great friend of the Jenners', always took care of Mrs. Jenner's health and, indeed, affairs
in general, when her husband was called away. He lived in Chester Walk, a lane leading to the churchyard off St. George's Place

conveniently adjacent to Jenner's back garden. Dr. Cother left a son William, who eventually became a doctor and practiced from his father's house at Alstone Green.

In the meantime Lettsom, from London, continued to keep the doctor informed of the struggle in the enemy camp. He had deputized for Jenner at certain functions that had taken place, and he gave a most graphic description of a dinner to which he was invited. As Baron truly observed: "He likewise fought his (Jenner's) battles and often signally vanquished his opponents." The following passage is from a long letter written by Lettsom at the beginning of August, when Jenner had been away from London nearly eight months.

I received an invitation to dinner with a party, but could not attend till past eight. When I arrived I found Mr. Alexander, M.P. Chairman of the Ways and Means; the Bishop of Cloyne, Rev. Dr. Parr,[21] Dr. Pearson, Dr. Shaw of the British Museum, Mr. Planter of the Royal Society, Rev. Mr. Maurice, author of Indian Antiquities. Somehow Pearson introduced the House of Commons—their Committees—when he made a Philippic of half an hour's abuse of that committee which recommended Dr. Jenner's discovery, and concluded with severe animadversions on Dr. Jenner. Dr. Parr seemed persuaded of Dr. Jenner's unworthiness; and Mr. Alexander said, had it depended upon his casting vote, as he was Chairman, he would have given it against Dr. Jenner. I then requested to be heard for an absent friend. I then went over the whole ground with a perspicuity I never possessed before. I exposed the whole conduct and mistakes of Pearson and Woodville in so strong a manner that after listening to me half an hour, every person seemed electrified but Pearson. One divine started up, took me by the hand, clapped me on the back, and embraced me, and declared that I had uncontravertably proved Jenner, not merely the promulgator, but inventor and discoverer. Parr exclaimed, "I would have voted Jenner ten times ten thousand pounds." Alexander declared that he now saw the matter in a new and convincing point of view. Pearson then made a reply of above half an hour, and when he concluded, Dr. Parr was appointed to decide upon the facts; and these were his words: "Dr. Lettsom has *convinced* me that Dr. Jenner is the discoverer and Dr. Pearson's defense has *confirmed* me in that conviction." I asked Dr. Pearson if he had anything more to say. He said he had done, and now I trust that he will never again venture, at least in the presence of the company, or any one of them, to broach his unfounded invectives. And I think he has now received his quietus. He little expected that I could have explained his mistakes and Woodville's so clearly. I mentioned facts which thunderstruck him, of which even you are ignorant, respecting this base coalition against you. He seemed confounded. His friend Maurice and his devotee ran about the room:— "Lettsom has conquered, Lettsom has conquered." Parr said he would come and see me, and Mr. Alexander proposes me the same honour. I know that Maurice will talk of this recounter everywhere.[22]

One can readily see from the above, the ground that had been lost by Jenner's staying away from the capital for so long. Thanks to people like Lettsom and the formidable Cheltenham divisions, things seemed to be righting themselves. The Dr. Shaw[23] mentioned above was actually an M.D. of Oxford who had turned to botany and was one of the founders of the Linnaean Society. He came to Cheltenham on August 6, right after the dinner party, and undoubtedly regaled the company with further details of Lettsom's victory. Not that the enemy was completely vanquished. Goldston's tract was sent to France and widely distributed during the autumn.

The combination of an unusually lucrative practice and the arrival of the grant money made Jenner's free vaccination campaign much easier. Since there was no official opposition of any kind in the town, poor people still flocked to his house for treatment. Doctors Fowler and Trye were equally active, and after young Dr. Parry took his Doctor of Medicine in Edinburgh this year he too joined the group. Nevertheless, while every scrap of evidence casting doubt upon the efficacy of vaccination continued to be published far and wide the much more numerous positive evidences were still soft-pedalled. In spite of the resistance, Jenner was not for a moment discouraged. One obstacle to the most efficient operation of vaccine was herpes, and he wrote a paper on this in the August *Medical Journal*. It received less attention than that given to Goldston's diatribe, even though Dunning, Embling, and Trye all wrote letters supporting Jenner.[24] On the other hand, one incident much nearer home gave Jenner a great deal of satisfaction. It was not related to one of his own patients but was given to him by a local doctor "of great respectability" from one of the villages near Cheltenham:

A poor family belonging to Sudeley parish, consisting of a man, his wife and five children, were vaccinated four or five years ago, except the eldest daughter, who had been before inoculated for the smallpox by an eminent practitioner, and pronounced secure. This summer she caught the smallpox when working among the rags at the paper mills, and had a very numerous and confluent eruption. The rest of the family had no fears, and have all escaped, though freely exposed to the infection.[25]

Jenner commented wryly: "Now had this case been reversed, what a precious morsel it would have been for the anti-vaccinationists." He wrote to Dunning November 15 as though the contest was over.

Is it possible that Goldston can appear again in print on the vaccine subject? Your communication is the first that has been made to me respecting it. He had better be silent unless he addresses the public in the humble, yet honourable strains of recantation; for with all the supposed imperfections on the head of *vaccina*, there are ten times as many on *variola*.[26]

The Marquess of Bute was a late arrival this season, and Farington relates an interesting story relative to the marquess and his grandmother, Lady Mary Wortley Montague. Some weeks earlier, when Farington was on the way back to London from his Cheltenham visit, he met a Mr. and Mrs. Hawker at the Lysons' house in Hempsted, who were friends of James Dallaway,[27] editor of *Lady Mary Wortley's Letters* and an alumnus of Jenner's old school of Cirencester. Lady Montague was a somewhat improvident individual and at one time had found it necessary to retire to the Continent because of financial complications. Dallaway's story goes:

Sir Richard Phillips,[28] the bookseller, had somehow been able to purchase a hundred of her letters which had been purloined from the family, for which he paid one hundred guineas, and he intended to publish them. This coming to the knowledge of the Marquess of Bute, her grandson, he, to prevent indiscriminate publication, offered him the mass of correspondence provided that a person he approved should edit them, with liberty to suppress such as might be improper to publish, and in case Phillips should not agree to this proposal his lordship would advertise a publication which would lower the value of anything Phillips might publish. Phillips accepted this proposal.

This story is interesting for two reasons. It is further evidence that Farington apparently revised or corrected items in his diary from time to time, since Phillips was not knighted until 1808. But of more importance was the fact that the bookseller was Jenner's friend. He was a radical in his youth, but after migrating to London from Leicester he eventually became a pillar of society. Having spent some years as a vendor of patent medicines—as a kind of poor relation to the medical profession—he early grew deeply interested in vaccination and at length met Jenner in London. Phillips established the *Monthly Magazine* in 1796, the year of Phipps's inoculation, and became a loyal supporter of the cause for the next twenty years. Both his magazine and his many other publishing activities were concerned with the spread of vaccination propaganda, and he was a main publisher of Dr. Robert Willan's work. When Jenner met Phillips, his early struggles were over and he was a relatively rich man—though not as rich as Bute's father-in-law, Mr. Coutts. It was another case for very careful treading on the doctor's part. If every noble voice in the Lords was precious, so was every friend in the press; and the press, of course, included those who wrote in verse as well as prose.

Robert Bloomfield's major vaccination poem, "Good Tidings or News from the Farm," appeared with very little fanfare this year. It is much more mature than the birthday lines and contains some splendid thought and imagery. Dr. Parr—Lettsom's Jennerian convert—was deeply impressed by the peasant bard as were Robert Southey and Capel Loft, the classical scholar.[29] Many years later, as shall be seen, Southey himself, when poet laureate, wrote in praise of vaccination. Bloomfield's poem was, pathetically enough, based upon the experience of smallpox in his own family. Small wonder he esteemed Jenner.

The account given of my infancy and of my father's burial is not only poetically, but strictly true, and with me it has its weight accordingly. I have witnessed the destruction of my brother's family; and I have, in my own, insured the lives of four children by Vaccine Inoculation, who, I trust, are destined to look back upon the smallpox as the scourge of days gone by.[30]

The description of the little nephew, blinded by smallpox, is as good as George Crabbe at his best. At one point, where the nephew's playmates have unthinkingly left him to run over to the woods, we are shown the childish resilience and quick recovery:

> Yet shorn the pain—
> Soon he resumes his cheerfulness again,
> Pondering how best his moments to employ,
> He sings his little songs of nameless joy,
> Creeps on the warm green turf for many an hour
> And plucks by chance the white and yellow flower
> Smoothing their stems while resting on his knees
> He binds a nosegay which he never sees.[31]

Jenner was profoundly moved and wrote to Bloomfield:

I trust it [the poem] will be as well received and given as high a commendation as *The Farmer's Boy*. It need not obtain more. You must allow me to fix upon some mark of my esteem. Do me the favour, then, to accept a silver inkstand, into which the enclosed may be converted if you will call upon Rundell and Bridge of Ludgate Hill, and use my name. I should like the following plain engraving on it. "Edward Jenner, M.D. to Robert Bloomfield."[32]

By the summer of 1804 Bloomfield's *The Farmer's Boy* had sold twenty-six thousand copies, and in the following year it came out in a German translation at Leipzig. French and Italian versions soon followed, but little of the money stayed in the author's pocket. His family was desperately poor, and he spent his royalties as fast as they came in in alleviating this poverty. "Good News" is a poet's poem. It did not bring in the money its longer forerunner did, but this was more than made up for in the praise of the critics. "The Poem certainly discovers very clearly, the powers of natural, unaffected genius," said the *London Monthly Review*. *Blackwood's*, before whom so many writers trembled, said enthusiastically, "The description of the Blind Boy . . . is worthy of being inserted among the Flowers of English Poetry: graceful, elegant and most deeply affecting, even to tears"—a sentiment the good doctor would have heartily echoed, living as he did with the constant presence of ill health in his own family.

It was when all the crowds had gone home and the town was quiet again that Jenner had time to take care of his own domestic affairs. In the grey cold of a late November day he met Colonel

Riddell at the manorial office in the High Street and arranged
his purchase of the house in St. George's Place. The transaction
is recorded thus in the Sherborne Papers: "Subject, nevertheless
to certain covenants clauses and conditions mentioned and in certain articles of agreement and covenant executed between the
said John Riddell and Edward Jenner bearing the date of the
twenty-seventh day of November last."[33] There were more formalities to be negotiated before the house, now Jenner's own property,
would be transferred on the manorial roll; this would take several
months and it was well into the next spring before the whole
transaction was completed. Nevertheless, the curse of penury
was over, and the restrictions of poverty were, for the time being
anyway, relaxed. Not the least of the year's triumphs had been the
resurgence of confidence in some of Jenner's wavering friends. He
was able to write to Richard Dunning, who had been so worried
at the attacks from certain journals: "You were rallied a little on
your timidity respecting the ugly cases in town and country . . .
and of a little shrinking . . . but all was done in perfectly good
humour and now you will allow me triumphantly to exclaim
'Richard's himself again!' "[34] Perhaps Jenner was a little too optimistic at the temporary discomfiture of his critics. But of course,
happiness is never unadulterated, and this was true for the physician. While the Cheltenham season was still enjoying its late re-
invigoration, rather sad news came from London. Not long after
returning to town, Fox's friend the Bishop of Down collapsed of
his liver condition. He lingered on for a few days at Fox's house
in Arlington Street and died at the end of September. Yet another
face had passed from the Cheltenham scene; and they all seemed
to be succumbing to a common condition.

By December 23 Jenner was in Berkeley, where the family apparently spent Christmas. Reflecting upon the events of the past
year, he wrote another long, forceful letter to Dunning.

Foreigners hear with the utmost astonishment that in some parts of
England there are persons who still inoculate for the smallpox. It
must indeed excite their wonder, when they see *that* disease in some
of their largest cities, and wide-extended districts around them, totally
exterminated. . . . From potentate to peasant, in every country but
this, she (vaccina) is received with open arms. What an admirable

arrangement was that I sent you in my last letter made by the Marquess Wellesley,[35] Governor-General of India, for the extermination of smallpox in that quarter of the globe, contrasted with our efforts here! What pygmies we look like. Did you see the Quarterly Report of the Royal Jennerian Society? . . . how shameful to use a society, constituted for such a purpose, and of which the Royal Family of England bears a part, begging a few guineas of the community for the support of its expenses.

Jenner also mentioned a letter he had recently received from Dr. Christie in Ceylon giving "a charming account of the progress of vaccination there."[36] Christie's almost obsessional concern with the evils of smallpox inoculation undoubtably gave heart to Jenner, and from this year onward his fight against the system dominated his thoughts more and more. There was a tug-of-war in his heart as to whether his energies should be mainly concerned with spreading vaccination ever wider or, vaccination being established, with trying to destroy inoculation.

As a kind of Christmas present, just after they arrived in Berkeley news came of the striking of a medal to celebrate the introduction of vaccination in France. Baron describes it as "one of the most beautiful of Napoleon's series of medals." Initially, one side was left blank (some said to enable a portrait of Jenner to be placed there "as a mark of personal honour to Jenner" by the Emperor), but the striking of such a medal at all while a bitter war was raging between the two countries was remarkable enough. To Jenner it formed a sound reason to attempt another rescue. Dr. Whickham, a travelling Fellow of Oxford University, was detained in Geneva and a young Mr. Williams, apparently of no importance at all but who was in poor health, was also detained. Jenner wrote in the first instance to the Central Committee of Vaccination in Paris. They were helpless to do anything on their own, but they wrote back and suggested that the doctor appeal directly to the Emperor himself. In due course the following letter went forth:

Sire,

Having by the blessing of Providence made a discovery of which all nations acknowledge the beneficial effects, I presume upon that plea alone, with great deference, to request a favour from Your Imperial

Majesty, who early appreciated the importance of vaccination and encouraged its propagation, and who is universally admitted to be a patron of the arts.

My humble request is that Your Imperial Majesty will graciously permit two of my friends, both men of science and literature, to return to England: one, Mr. William Thomas Williams, residing at Nancy, the other, Dr. Whickham, at present at Geneva. Should Your Imperial Majesty be pleased to listen to the prayer of my petition, you will impress my mind with sentiments of gratitude never to be effaced.

I have the honour to be with the most profound deference and respect,

Your Imperial Majesty's
Most obliged and humble servant,
E. J.

Berkeley, Gloucestershire,
February, 1805[37]

Travel and the posts were very slow in those days and the Emperor was in Italy at the time, but Jenner had the foresight to send a copy of the letter to Mr. Williams himself at Nancy. Many months later Napoleon passed through that city, and Williams managed to place the precious message in his hands. A duplicate, or, more likely the original, was also presented to the Emperor by Baron Corvisart, the imperial physician, in June 1806. A month later Mr. Williams was informed by Corvisart that the Emperor had heeded Dr. Jenner's petition, and both he and Dr. Whickham were free to go home. "It was either on this or some similar occasion," writes Baron, "when Napoleon was about to reject the proffered petition, that Josephine uttered the name of Jenner. The Emperor paused for an instant and exclaimed, 'Jenner, ah, we can refuse nothing to that man.' "[38] In supporting vaccination, Napoleon was quite unconsciously balancing the slaughter of his armies. He probably thus saved more lives than he took.

Jenner himself believed the year 1804 "formed an era in the history of variola vaccina," since it was then that the fiction that vaccination merely provided a temporary immunity was planted in the public mind. It mattered little that the statement originated in the mouthings of a completely ignorant man, namely, Goldston. Once spread, a contention of this nature was impossible to disprove save by the passage of time. Nevertheless, a goad will often stir up action where lethargy had interfered with defense, and the incidents that marked this "historic year" were probably, on balance, markedly favorable to Jenner. Not only did the grant money finally arrive, but in buying the house in St. George's Place he became a member of the local establishment. Each successive year saw him progressively entrenched as a leader of the community, and within a year or two Jenner and Cheltenham became almost synonymous terms in medical circles. In addition, it was a year of vindication. Lettsom's splendid performance at Dr. Parr's dinner in London brought a wave of scholarly supporters outside the realm of medicine. One defender, who may be described as a lesser Lettsom, appeared at the very end of the year in the person of James Plumtre[39] of Cambridge. The second of the ancient universities had differed markedly from Oxford in its attitude to vaccination, mainly because of the bitter hostility of the Regius Professor of Physics, Sir Isaac Pennington[40]—one of the men, incidentally, who was particularly active in spreading the allegation that Jenner had inoculated his son with smallpox serum in preference to cowpox.[41] Plumtre, a playwright of some modest reputation in his day, was the nephew of Dr. Russell Plumtre who preceded Pennington in the Regius professorship, and he was the great-grandson of Henry Plumtre, a former President of the Royal College of Physicians. With such highly respectable medical antecedents, he was deeply disturbed at what he considered the betrayal by Pennington. Plumtre inaugurated his defense of Jenner in a sermon before the university at St. Mary's Church, Cambridge, early in February, 1805. Using the great moral advantage of an education in theology, he had a power denied to Pennington and his faction. He cited the Scriptures in delineating the age-long curse of smallpox and the manifest God-directed advent of Jenner and vaccination. It was once more the polished, incisive voice of the literary genius coming to the rescue of the man of science. On March 3, he followed up his university sermon with one of a much more simple character to the parishioners of Hinxton in Cambridge. Though he had no parish he held a comfortable and undemanding university fellowship at Clare Hall, where he was free to devote the greater part of his time to the promotion of vaccination in East Anglia. Addressing the unlettered population on the subject of vaccination, he wrote poems and songs, which he published at his own expense. He was helped by his sister Anne Plumtre, who later achieved fame as the translator of the German dramatist Kotzebue. Plumtre's own literary ability, if modest, was certainly versatile. He ranged all the way from tragedy to comic opera, though his best-known work was a straight comedy, *The Coventry Act,* produced at Norwich in 1793.[42] At the age of thirty-eight, he took his Bachelor of Divinity rather belatedly in 1808, the same year that his cousin became Dean of Gloucester.

The dedication of the university sermon, which Plumtre sent to Jenner on February 25, was marked by a Jove-like thunder perhaps more suited to the stage than the pulpit, and it certainly made short shrift of the enemy. He announced that he "intended to connect the practice of medicine with religion and to set forth the just wrath and power and more particularly the infinite goodness of Our Almighty Father." With such comforting reassurance from Cambridge and elsewhere, the winter of 1804–5 passed quietly on its way; for Jenner the new year opened completely new vistas of possibility after almost a decade of restrictive penury. Even though taxes, fees, and other charges accounted for nearly a thousand pounds of Jenner's grant money, there should have been more than enough to do all the things that had to be done, not only for his family but for those whom he felt depended upon him. But the possession of money again did make him a little rash when there were so many bills to pay. On March 4, 1805— the day after Plumtre's second sermon—Jenner and Colonel Riddell went up to the town offices in the High Street to transfer the ownership of his house on the Manorial Roll. Being now comfortably solvent, Jenner also purchased from Riddell a large piece of land on the opposite side of St. George's Place to use for a garden and a place to turn his carriage. "Edward Jenner," the record tells us, "present in Court prayed to be admitted Tenant to the premises. To whom the Lord by the Steward aforesaid the premises . . . aforesaid with the appurtenances did grant to be had and holden to him, his heirs and assigns for ever."[43] Forever is a long time, but the house did actually stay in the hands of the family for fifty-six years, until Jenner's granddaughter, Catherine, sold it in 1860.[44] It was a handsome and substantial town house with "offices and outbuildings, courtyard and appurtenances," in all respects suited to a man in his station.[45] The ground on the other side of the street extended to something over half an acre— a pleasant enough retreat in the middle of the town, and one which Jenner might arrange as he pleased. One important addition he made to the house, was, in all probability, a surgery. In the earlier sales notice there was no mention of a long room on the ground floor, thirty feet by nine, but a notice later in the century refers to it, and it would be such a room a doctor might need to cope with a large number of patients. The shape would scarcely suggest it as a room for social activities, but it would be ideal to shelter a long line of people waiting to be vaccinated.[46]

In the meantime, Riddell was carefully nurturing the Couttses, Wyndham, and Sir Francis Burdett, all of whom, though sophisticated people, had great faith in his quack medicines. But what was more significant was his hardheaded development of Cambray Spa. In all probability, Riddell gave his "patients" doses of his innocuous remedies while they were taking the excellent iron waters from his new well, so that whatever benefit they derived was inevitably attributed to talents of the "doctor." A striking example was the case of the "miraculous" cure of Burdett after a long period of sickness in the course of this year. Jenner, despite his business dealings with the colonel, had only a good-natured contempt for his ideas. "Quacks," he observed, "go up like rockets but come down like the sticks."[47] Undoubtedly Riddell was aware of this, but he was too thick-skinned to be worried. In any case, his property speculations were doing very well indeed, should his "medical practice" wane. There seemed little chance of this, however, and Riddell was certainly making far more money than most of the Cheltenham doctors. A letter from Sir Francis Burdett's wife in Ramsbury, Wiltshire, gives some idea of his prestige in the highest circles. "I am very faithful," she writes, "to your wishes in regard to my two glasses, though you know I made no promises. Sir Francis and Mrs. Blythe unite in their best remembrances. Little Madame sends her love. She is in perfect health." Apparently Riddell's nostrum was some kind of alleged purgative "for clearing the body."[48] Hence her ladyship's caution about *two* glasses. Needless to say, the mineral waters of Cambray Spa happened to have the same qualities.

Sir Francis's miraculous cure, which caused a great deal of comment, took place in May and June, and the above letter was written in July after he had returned to his country home. His father-in-law Thomas Coutts, however, came to Cheltenham early in the season as was his wont, and stayed all the way through. He was seventy years old, had a wife who was in an advanced state of senile decay, and was popularly known as "the richest man in the kingdom." He probably was. He had been coming to Cheltenham for the last twenty-five years at least but was a retiring man and seldom appeared prominently in society. Yet though he held in his hands the financial destiny of nearly all the grand folk who strolled the walks—from the Royal family downwards—he was lonely and unhappy. After forty-three years of marriage his wife, who was older than he, could no longer comfort him, and his children were grown up. He was a shabby little fellow at this time—a usual enough phenomenon with very rich men—and rather frail.

The Entwistles' music shop was barely a hundred yards from Jenner's front door, just opposite the point where St. George's Place ran into High Street, and not surprisingly that interesting family eventually became his patients. Undoubtedly Jenner's association with such celebrities of the stage as Kelly, Prince Hoare, and, of course, Mrs. Jordan would have made the Entwistles gravitate toward him in any case, but geography made him their neighbor. Mrs. Entwistle was very proud of the fact that her daughter Harriot Mellon[49] was enjoying a full season—albeit the summer season—in London, after eight years on the adult stage. In the provinces this background should surely impress the local managers. She guessed right, and in August Miss Mellon came back to Cheltenham, radiant and happy after her season at Drury Lane, and Watson was delighted to arrange a benefit for her at his new Theatre Royal in Cambray. She and an equally beautiful girl companion strolled the walks in the summer sunshine and demurely requested the nobility and gentry to attend her performance. One of the gentlemen she approached was old Mr. Coutts, though she had no idea of his identity. To her surprise, he remarked that he had already purchased seats as a result of a letter from her mother, the post mistress. He also commended the girl for her efforts on behalf of her parents and implied that he had been observing her from afar. When she returned home her mother greeted her with the news that the great banker, Mr. Coutts, had sent five newly minted golden guineas for a box at her benefit. What had happened was poignantly apparent. The richest man in England had fallen in love with this twenty-seven-year-old woman. It is said that she kept the five gold coins, as a souvenir of their meeting, for the rest of her life. To his credit, Mr. Coutts never attempted to go beyond the bounds of propriety. At his great age and in his domestic loneliness, he was happy to quietly worship this charming young goddess and shower gifts upon her. For her part, she was immensely flattered by his attentions, and grew very fond of him. There was gossip, of course, but no evidence has ever been found of any kind of affair.

Miss Mellon's relationship with the banker was quite unique. While he was alive, she eschewed the company of other men and saw her generous patron whenever her stage commitments would permit. He set her up in a splendid house in London and devoted the rest of his days to her happiness, while still with every husbandly care watching over his poor doddering wife. By the time he died he had given Harriot well over £200,000, and in his will he left his entire fortune to her, making her one of the richest women in the world. But in 1805 all this was yet to happen.

Coutts was noted for his generosity to beautiful women, though, to be sure, he had never fallen so hard as on this occasion. The Duchess of Devonshire was practically his pensioner—on and off—for twenty-five years. She had been an inveterate gambler and lost thousands more than she ever won. People forgave her, however, because she was beautiful and talented. She could turn out a play with the best and wrote excellent verse as an adjunct to her physical and social graces. She married the duke when she was a girl of seventeen and was in Cheltenham constantly in the years before the King's 1788 sojourn; she so dominated society that she became the center of a whole folklore of romantic legend. She lived at the Great House in St. George's Place before Dr. Hooper went there, and enjoyed walking to Swindon Village across the fields to sit under the mighty spread of Maud's Elm, the tree that was supposed to have sprung from the stake driven through the body of Maud Bowen, a suicide buried there. A little boy named Miles Watkins told her the tragic legend of Maud one summer day as she sat there in the shade, and she took him under her wing, educated him, and watched over him for the rest of her life—all because he told her a tender little story.

By the time Jenner had settled in St. George's Place, the duchess was a very sick woman, but not so much so that it would prevent her interest in his cause. Her daughter was married to young Lord Morpeth, who sat in the Commons for the borough of Morpeth and later succeeded his father as Earl of Carlisle. She also had another banker friend who lived in Cheltenham. Old Sir Robert Herries had been one of her earliest financial benefactors and had retired to the town some years before, though he still had profound influence in government circles. Since we know that she and Angerstein discussed Jenner's problems, it is reasonable to assume that she may have also sought the advice of Sir Robert, who lived within a few yards of St. George's Place and probably knew the doctor anyway. There was plenty of support for the cause in the House of Lords but the lower house, dominated by the great world of banking and commerce, was yet to be won. The Duke of Devonshire was inclined to be tightfisted—perhaps as a result of his lady's impulsive behavior, but she was as generous as she was extravagant. When still a young woman, she provided Charles Moore's brother with £500 toward buying his majority in the army. It was a gift which she never regretted and which he never forgot. "Gl. Moore is in the same way one of my works,"[50] she wrote; and well she might, since he became Gen. Sir John Moore, the hero of Curunna.

In the meantime, the subject of all this concern was still in a pleasant state of euphoria over the final change in his fortunes. When his property transactions with Riddell were completed, Jenner went up to London in a much happier frame of mind than he had been in for many years. His main purposes were to discuss the progress of the vaccination cause and to plan future policy. He visited Lord Egremont on May 11 under very different circumstances from his last meeting. His Lordship was concerned about the long travail of penury the doctor had been through and was determined that it should never happen again. As a matter of fact, Jenner had spent a vast amount of money in the purchase of his house and the land for his garden, in addition to many other outstanding commitments, and already he was feeling the pinch less than a year after his grant had been paid. The matter of a public subscription was mooted by his friends, but Egremont felt that a further parliamentary grant would be more just and more dignified. A number of prominent people agreed to this, including yet another great lady who had also become a kind of legend in society—Lady Crewe.[51] Jenner had probably met her through Farington, who wrote in his diary in 1803: "Miss Hayman spoke of Mrs. Crewe's musick parties and of Miss Crewe's singing, and offered to introduce me there on one of her evenings." In the next two years the "Mrs." was changed to "Lady" and Jenner was on visiting terms. Though no longer young, her ladyship still challenged the most distinguished beauties. "She uglifies everything near," said Fanny Burney. "I know not even now any female who could bear comparison with her beauty."[52] Yet she had been a reigning toast in 1784 when, at a banquet to celebrate Fox's being returned M.P. for Westminster, the Prince of Wales gave the toast, "True blue and Mrs. Crewe." Of all women living Fox preferred her, who, he averred, "loved high play and dissipation, but was no sensualist." Her circle was virtually boundless, and Jenner was well aware of her acumen in making the right contacts. He wrote:

During my residence in town, in the summer of 1805, Lady Crewe happened in conversation to tell me how much Lord Henry Petty wished for a conference with me on the vaccine subject; and that she would like to bring us together. We met at her villa in Hempsted: and went so fully into the matter, that his lordship, convinced of the injury I had sustained, expressed his determination to bring something forward in the ensuing session.[53]

Her ladyship's choice was very shrewd indeed. Young Petty was then only twenty-six years old and merely the M.P. for Cambridge; a year later he was Chancellor of the Exchequer.

At the same time Angerstein got in touch with the duchess, who was very grateful for the interest of the great banker. She wrote back:

I had not forgot your kind interest about Jenner. I spoke to the Duke, the Prince and Morpeth, and they will all do what you think best; but Morpeth has undertaken to make enquiries whether it is not possible to bring it again before Parliament. He thinks that if it could be done, it would be more satisfactory than any subscription. I desired him to find out how Mr. Pitt was really inclined in the subject, and I only waited the result of these enquiries to write to you.[54]

Unhappily Mr. Pitt was in his grave before anything could be done, but Morpeth loyally supported his mother-in-law's plan to a successful conclusion.

Jenner left London on August 3 and had twelve days relaxation in Berkeley before proceeding to Cheltenham where a very busy season awaited him. His correspondence had mounted during his absence, and there were untold numbers eager for vaccination. He called himself vaccine clerk to the world, and whatever the genesis of the long room added to his ground floor, it must have been very valuable at this time. "He constantly inoculated all who chose to come," wrote Baron, "and sometimes he had nearly three hundred persons at his door." This would have pretty well blocked the modest confines of St. George's Place, and it is possible that Dr. Fowler at number six and Dr. Newell at number five helped. Miss Humphris does, indeed, mention Dr. Fowler, but she was confused as to the date.[55] We do know, incidentally, that Jenner's manservant, Richard, was an expert vaccinator, and no doubt did his share. All too often, once the inoculation was performed Jenner never saw the patient again, but when he could follow a case through to its successful conclusion, he always felt very happy. One occurrence he related with great satisfaction:

A poor widow and her four children chanced to be under the same roof with a labouring man who had caught the smallpox. They had been exposed five days to the infection, when an humble neighbour happened to step in. The poor woman, it appears, had made up her mind to her fate, not seeing the possibility of her escape from the calamity that threatened her. However, her wise friend prevailed upon her to come to Cheltenham to know what was to be done in such a case; she instantly complied. I happened to be from home; but my servant Richard, who has lived with me many years, exercised his judgement very properly. He soon found out an arm with a fine eight day postule, and inoculated the whole group. They had since all been with me, full of rejoicing at the consequence. All escaped the contagion except one of the children, on whom appeared a few scattered pocks, or rather pimples, for they did not exceed hemp seed in size; nor was the eruption attended with any perceptible indisposition. I have frequently before this disarmed the smallpox of its power on those who had been exposed three days to its contagion; but this fact, with all its circumstances, I own, delighted me.[56]

Though practically all his vaccinations were gratis, outside the nobility and gentry, he was always happiest when he was besieged with people who believed in his system.

While his money lasted, Jenner was able to spend a little on things outside his profession. He had a bust of himself executed by Samuel Manning,[57] a minor sculptor at that time, but it was exhibited in the 1805 show at the Royal Academy and was highly praised by Baron. Jenner himself liked it sufficiently to have replicas made from time to time to give to his friends. But what was of far more interest was a portrait in pencil executed in Cheltenham by John Drayton—an indifferent poet but an excellent artist. To be sure, he *asked* Jenner to sit for him, but the doctor paid one of the leading engravers in the country, Anker Smith, to make impressions from it for private circulation.[58] The fact of the matter was that none of the portraits of Jenner up to then, and indeed, thereafter, really satisfied him, and this reflects upon some very great artists. The first portrait was painted in 1800 by John Raphael Smith,[59] to be followed in 1802 by the first Northcote.[60] Jenner disliked both. "Smith's is a strange likeness," he wrote to Lettsom, "but neither (he nor Northcote) have succeeded in giving my character. Smith's with a few careless touches from the engraver degenerates into an assassin."[61] Nevertheless, after he had sat for the mighty Lawrence in 1809, Jenner decided Northcote's was superior, for what it was worth. Baron commented on the Northcote: "It wants the peculiar expression of Jenner's countenance and does not fully display his manner, but on the whole it is a better portrait than some which have appeared since." Poor humble Drayton had apparently been the only one to capture the correct image. "Done from life," said Baron, "it is allowed to be one of the most exact resemblances of Dr. Jenner."[62] Which I suppose is why the good doctor spent money on having it engraved for his friends. Drayton was poor and scraped a living partly by writing mediocre verse for the local papers, but I know of no other portraits of his. He would certainly have had no studio of his own, so one would assume that the picture was executed in Jenner's house, possibly in one of the light, airy rooms in the mansard roof that towered above all the nearby houses. The artist's intention had been to form a die for a gold medal, but the likeness had been so excellent that, in Jenner's eyes anyway, it remained a simple portrait from which he could take as many engraved impressions as he wished. Drayton became a welcome visitor to the Jenners' and naturally enough had a great esteem for his patron. After the *Cheltenham Chronicle* was established in 1809, his verses appeared there regularly.

In the meantime, the movement so vigorously inaugurated by Lettsom the previous year to rouse support in India had encouraging reactions. By this time Jenner would certainly have met the Russell family of Charlton Kings. There were two manors in the ancient parish, and this family was descended from that of the Prynnes, one of whose seventeenth-century representatives had been a celebrated agitator and scurrilous pamphleteer—William Prynne, who endured untold persecution for his fearless outpourings. The current heir to the estates was young William Russell[63] who after graduating M.D. from Edinburgh had gone to India, where the Governor-General himself, Lord Wellesley, had put him in charge of the dissemination of Dr. Jenner's discovery. He was back in Cheltenham in 1804 or 1805 and, in Jenner's own words, they met there: "Mr. Russell's acquaintance I had the pleasure of making in Cheltenham and renewing in London." Perhaps they also met before he went to India since the young man, only thirty-two in 1805, had been a familiar figure in Cheltenham society eight or nine years earlier. At all events, Russell returned to the East full of crusading zeal following his meeting with the master. Long after Jenner's death, Russell received a baronetcy for his contribution to medicine.

The Foxes and Dr. Saunders arrived in the town together on August 1. It was the latter's first appearance since being made President of the newly formed Royal Medical and Chirurgical Society. He had recently worked with Astley Cooper at Guy's

Hospital, where the younger man was surgeon for the last two years of Saunders's reign as physician (1800-1802). The brilliance of Jenner's circle was augmented later in the month by the arrival of his friend Dr. John Latham, a celebrated authority on gout.[64] This man was not only Physician-in-Ordinary to the King, but he had a son, Peter, who became one of the leading medical scholars of his day and, years later, physician to Queen Victoria.

William Saunders was also physician to William Pitt, who was sinking to his grave as rapidly as was his old rival Charles James Fox, and undoubtedly Coutts, through the ramifications of his government contracts, was kept informed of the day-to-day situation. The old banker was an unusual combination of keen practicality—as his wealth made obvious—and sentimental simplicity. He was the intimate of the greatest medical minds of his day, yet he had the greatest faith in the "witch doctor" Riddell. Talking of the famous "remedy" he comments,

I have witnessed it being used with the most uncommon success, clearing everything away without lowering or tearing, as most purgatives do, and giving instead increased appetite and spirits. I am quite persuaded as far as clearing the body he had hit upon a mode of preparing and administrating his medicines in the most effective and agreeable manner.[65]

Coutts does not ever appear to have retained Riddell's services for his wife, however, nor yet for his beloved Harriot. Of more interest to Jenner, I suppose, than any of this, was the arrival, separately but on the same day, of Lord and Lady Rous—welcome reinforcement for the uncompromising pro-vaccination front. For the first time he could entertain them in a house of his own, and even stroll with them through the future garden opposite.

The death of Admiral Nelson in October and the imminent decease of the Prime Minister, Pitt, cast a shadow over the end of the year. Nearer home, the winter brought new problems. Smallpox appeared in the villages around Gloucester and eventually in the city itself. A notice dated November 28 appeared in the *Gloucester Journal* of December 9:

The physicians and surgeons of the Infirmary are ready to inoculate (gratis) with the cowpox all who apply as a perservative against the infection of the above disease.

Trye and Jenner quietly and undramatically coped with the new
eruption, while their more fashionable friends were engaged in
the capital trying to save a Prime Minister's life.

As Christmas drew near, the local press, as well as the national,
was dominated by the concern over Pitt. Characteristically, his
final decline dated from the disastrous battle of Austerlitz on
December 1. It seems to have broken his spirit completely. He
had gone to Bath under the anxious eye of Farquhar, but the
waters were no relief, and if anything, upset the invalid. Farquhar
called in Dr. Haygarth, the smallpox pioneer (who had obtained
the first vaccine for Dr. Waterhouse from Creaser in 1799), but all
the hapless local man could do, somewhat out of his depth, was
recommend "rest and quiet." Unwisely, Pitt travelled back to
London the same day. On January 22, Dr. Baillie said, "It is all
over with Mr. Pitt, that his inside had gone." Later the same day
Dr. Saunders added, "The constitution of Mr. Pitt is breaking
up." He was right; the poor man died at a quarter past four the
next morning.

The tragic passing of a great man did have its compensating
repercussions: the new Ministry chosen after the Prime Minister's
death was remarkable in that Jenner's friends were elevated to
such exalted places. Fox became Foreign Secretary; Spencer, Home
Affairs; Addington (now Lord Sidmouth), Privy Seal; and Lord
Henry Petty (soon to become Lord Lansdowne), Chancellor of the
Exchequer. True, Lord Hardwick was dropped from his position
of Lord Lieutenant of Ireland, but he was succeeded by none other
than the President of the Royal Jennerian Society—the Duke of
Bedford! It seemed that everyone, *outside* the medical world at
least, had finally lined up with Jenner. It is not surprising that he
assumed his main opposition problems were ending, and on
February 21, when the town was empty of all its crowds and the
streets were cold, he wrote a long letter to Dunning. There was
so much to talk about after his most busy year, and his friend
had been silent for six months. "My dear Sir," he wrote, "It is a
long time since you have written to me. Why did you drop your
correspondence?" He went on to talk of mundane things; in-
fluenza; family and, inevitably, the activities of the enemy in
London, where there had been six thousand cases of smallpox from
the London curse.

So little have the people round me (though only a hundred miles from it) felt it, that since August last, I have vaccinated within a few of 1,500; and I certainly must deem it a piece of good fortune that out of the many thousands I have vaccinated no failure or accident of any sort has arisen to my knowledge. . . . My communications from various parts of the world are very encouraging. 800,000 cases from India. Adieu![66]

With everything at last running smoothly, Jenner was able to do a great deal of writing during the winter. He completed a letter to Robert Willan[67] on February 23, which was printed as an appendix in that author's *On Vaccine Inoculation* and came out later in the year. But there must always be a break in any period of happiness, and very sad news came just over a month later. His good friend the Duchess of Devonshire died on March 30 in her forty-ninth year.

Though a relatively young woman, she had been a familiar figure in Cheltenham for longer than anyone except, perhaps, Mr. Coutts, and her delightful retreat beside the Chelt, Georgiana Cottage, marked her memory until comparatively recent times. Her sponsoring of Jenner's cause with the Prince of Wales was the last generous act in a life of spontaneous kindness and adventure. Despite her vivacious manner and appearance she had suffered for years from the awful curse that perhaps drew her to the Cheltenham Wells long after her youthful escapades. Like Hoppner, the Bishop of Down, and Charles James Fox, she had been sinking under a liver complaint. A fortnight after her funeral Farington heard the whole story from mutual friends. (Toward the end she had still been tormented by the extent of her debts.)

Lord and Lady Thomond I dined with; no company. Lady Thomond spoke to me of the Duchess of Devonshire. She said that her liver was decayed and had also a positive disorder in it. Her pain was great and in a state nearly approaching to insensibility of what passed. The Duke not knowing how much her mind might be affected by her circumstances, which had long been distressed, desired her to dismiss from her mind any uneasiness on that score, assuring her that as soon as it could be, her debts should be discharged.[68]

To round out the Devonshire saga: many years later her son the Marquess of Hartington, by then Duke of Devonshire, came back to Cheltenham. A sensitive boy and very close to his mother, perhaps an early hero worship of Mary Berry had put thoughts of romance permanently out of his head. At all events, he never married, and devoted his life to ameliorating the condition of his tenants and spontaneous acts of generosity. In the hours he spent at his mother's knee, she had undoubtedly told him of the early days in Cheltenham before it became such a Mecca. So he came back and wandered around her early haunts where, alas, so much was changed and so much was gone. He went to Maud's Elm, had a drawing made of it, and even endeavored to find the little boy who had so enchanted his mother. He was delighted when Miles Watkins was discovered—a very old man and probably a very surprised one. Like the good prince in the fairy tale, the duke provided him with enough money to live the rest of his life in comfort. Georgiana Cottage was demolished some years ago, and Maud's Elm is no more, but there is a quiet little street at the lower end of the town that perpetuates the memory of the Duchess of Devonshire. It is only about half a mile from the home of the great man in whose interest she made her last great benefactions. Tragically enough, she did not live to see her plans bear fruit.

When winter died and spring began to light the countryside, Jenner went down to Berkeley for a couple of weeks before his annual visit to London. At long last Dunning had answered his letter. On March 14 Jenner wrote back, "Your letter of the seventeenth arrived which had at length found me in my cottage in old Berkeley. I was happy to find that you had been corresponding with Mr. Moore. He is an excellent man and has produced an excellent book. I presume you know that J. Moore is brother to the general."[69]

Jenner arrived in London at the beginning of May where the seed sown by the good duchess was about to bear fruit despite the usual bitter resistance from the enemy. On June 27 Farington mentions the growing concern among responsible people about the continuing attacks on vaccination. Dr. Grant said that owing to a prejudice excited by pamphlets against vaccine inoculation . . . "the consequences are so fatal that the Bills of Mortality show that there are now more deaths by the Smallpox than there were before the Vaccine Inoculation was known."[70] A bitter pill, indeed, for Jenner to swallow after ten years of dedicated work. It was obvious that though his personal affairs grew more secure, the campaign against his system and approach was as vindictive as ever. Nevertheless, honors continued to come. Measures for the easier spread of vaccination were debated in Parliament, and the Royal College of Surgeons was instructed to investigate the matter, which resulted in their rather stiff endorsement and promise of cooperation. On the other hand, the Royal College of Physicians in Edinburgh, presided over by the celebrated William Wright, was much more cordial and to show its own feelings made Jenner an Honorary Fellow on May 20.

A few weeks later Lord Henry Petty was able to arrange for the motion for a further monetary grant to come up for debate in July. There would obviously be far less opposition this time, but actually the business was so drawn out that no decision was made until the following year. On the eighteenth of the month Jenner received a long letter from the Duke of Bedford referring to their conversations the previous summer, and expressing gratification at Petty's activities in the House. But he also expressed great alarm at the hesitancy of Parliament in enforcing measures to stop the *spread* of the disease. There was too much tolerance of the non-conformists.

This surely cannot be consistent with good government, or even of a free one; and without it, I fear, we shall never effect that great object the Jennerian Society has in view, the extermination of the smallpox. I have written my sentiments to Lord Granville freely on the subject; and took occasion to mention my anxious hope, that you would at length receive that just reward from the public which in my opinion has been too long withheld from you. I trust the enquiry will extend to Ireland. With the assistance of Dr. Yeates[71] (whose zeal in the Cause you well know) I am endeavouring to obtain some information on the progress vaccination has made in this part of the United Kingdom which I hope will be useful.

He signed his letter "Your very sincere well-wisher and faithful servant,"[72]—a little balm to compensate for the degrading filth that was being exhibited in certain bookshops of the metropolis. On display were prints of people gradually assuming the appearance of cows as a result of the hideous, unnatural vaccine. Emotional legends on these publications drew attention to "Master

Jowles the cow-pocked, ox-cheeked young gentleman, and Miss
Mary Ann Lewis, the cow-poxed, cow-manged young lady." The
author of this enlightening work was none other than Dr. William
Rowley,[73] who was not a semi-quack like Moseley. He was a man
who should have known better, with his Oxford background and
L.R.C.P. Strangely enough, Rowley died in the course of the
year while his masterpieces were in full circulation. In England,
the prints reenforced the hostility toward vaccination, but fortunately these machinations seem to have had little effect overseas.

In India, it was the vicissitudes of politics rather than medical
opposition that temporarily disturbed the smooth progress of
vaccination. The governor, Lord Wellesley, in ordering the system
for the vast eastern empire, saw considerably more people treated
in that part of the world during his term of office than were treated
in England during the same period. The Wellesleys, as a family,
were an impressive force in the subcontinent at the turn of the
century. The governor-general's secretary was his younger brother,
Henry, who was in 1801–2 governor of the ceded area of Oudh,
and his other brother, Sir Arthur Wellesley, was in command of
the army. Some years afterward, the governor-general's natural
daughter, Anne, married the brother of Jenner's friend Bentinck,
then Governor of Madras. But, unfortunately, in 1805, when the
cause appeared to be well established, the government decided to
replace Lord Wellesley, having recalled his brother Henry two
years earlier. At this Sir Arthur resigned all his appointments in
disgust, followed his brother to England, and got himself elected
Member of Parliament for Rye the following year. But there
were other problems both physical and emotional at the time
which eventually guided his steps to Cheltenham. His fiancée had
contracted smallpox during his absence abroad, and though she
had survived, she was disfigured for life. In addition, Sir Arthur
himself was thoroughly rundown and needed the "cure" at the
resort favored by his family. However, during this particular
spring none of them had yet arrived, nor was Dr. Jenner present,
so the gallant soldier turned to his sister-in-law, Lady Mornington,
and asked her if she could help him. As it happened, she could.
Her friend Madame de Gontaut, one of the ladies of the French
court in exile, was at that moment resident in the household of

Lady Templeton, a leader of Cheltenham society. Madame tells the story delightfully in her *Memoirs:* Lady Mornington had painted a pathetic picture of the lonely young man—he was then thirty-seven—which no kindhearted French matron could resist.

"He knows nobody," pleaded her Ladyship, "and it will be a charity if you will pay him some attention; so I trust him to your kindness and your friendship to me." She had no reason to worry as the ensuing account by Madame de Gontaut reveals.

He was to arrive that very day; and in visiting me he would have the pleasure also of making the acquaintance of Lady Templeton and Miss Upton. . . . Nothing on earth would have induced me to fail in honouring the recommendation of my friend. I announced my intention of setting off at once to find this person, who was brother-in-law to all the Wellesleys, of whom I was very fond. My companions, however, were very far from sharing my enthusiasm. Lady Templeton's indolence took alarm and Miss Upton's jealousy awoke. They were both greatly disturbed at having this man *whom-no-one knew, imposed upon them.* . . . Without listening to their grumbling, however, I set off for the Pump Room to look for the arrival. With great difficulty I at length persuaded Miss Upton to accompany me. I proceeded straight to the Pump Room, where I went to look at the list of new arrivals. . . . I found the name of Wellesley and read it aloud, so that Miss Upton could hear it, but she did not say a word. A stranger standing beside me was also reading the list, he put his finger on a name, smiled, and, looking at me, said "Madame de Gontaut." Nothing could be more piquant; we had never met and yet we knew each other at once.

So the great lady immediately took the diffident, future "Iron Duke" under her wing. She continues:

During one of our walks he confided to me a trouble which was disturbing him greatly, but I will give it in his own words.

"In a few days I shall leave Cheltenham on account of a very grave matter which will decide my whole future life. When I was very young I became attached to a Miss Pakenham, a very nice person, pretty and sweet, and we became engaged. We were both very young. I had an ardent desire to enter the army, and I was obliged to leave her though we both cherished the hope of one day being re-united. Years passed and in the meantime Miss P. had smallpox. She wrote to me that, remembering our promise, she must warn me that she had lost her beauty. It appeared that the smallpox, while destroying her beauty, had not destroyed her memory."

His manner of saying this was so peculiar and so like him that I could not help laughing; "But she has my promise and my honour demands that I should keep it; it was rather fine of her too, to write me with so much simplicity and truth, so I shall start for Ireland at once. I have very little time to lose. Perhaps I shall come back this way, alone or with her."

He went and they returned together, she in the carriage alone and he on the box.[74]

There is something very upsetting about this anecdote—perhaps in the cold way Madame de Gontaut relates it. Catherine Pakenham was the third daughter of Lord Longford and, it was said, a lovely young woman until smallpox struck her. Wellesley married her in Ireland on April 10, so that when he brought her back to Cheltenham the season was in full swing. It must have been a humiliating ordeal—the young pock-marked bride riding alone in the gloom of the carriage, hidden from the gay and animated crowds, while her new husband apparently preferred to sit beside the coachman. The following year Wellesley returned to active service and left England once more, so his wife scarcely saw him until the general peace in 1815, the year in which her brother, General Sir Edward Pakenham, was killed at the battle of New Orleans.

As a postscript to the above I might quote one sentence from Lesley Blanche's excellent selection from Harriet Wilson's *Memoirs*. "The Duchess of Wellington, loaded with the honours of her husband's glory, was often to be seen driving alone, buried in a book; she was so short-sighted she could not recognise a face, and so shy she could never greet anyone."[75] It could have been much worse, indeed. Smallpox all too frequently left the patient totally blind as well as disfigured.

Fortunately Cheltenham continued to be uncontaminated by the anti-vaccination fever, except for a rather amusing advertisement that appeared in Mr. Sheldon's "elegant shop in the centre of the High Street," in September. He apparently had a commodity that might be considered to be competitive with Jenner's system—Tyce's anti-scorbutic drops, which will be found an excellent cure for the scurvy, pimples, foul festering eruptions, evil, scrofula, leprosy, old venereal ulcers, (where mercury had failed), the scaldhead in children, and those eruptions that frequently appear after the smallpox, COWPOX. Price 2/9. One bottle frequently effects a cure.[76]

A bargain indeed. It is not clear why, of all these horrors, cowpox should be capitalized.

In addition to new products there were new faces, many of which were undoubtedly rich curiosity mongers anxious to see the remarkable cowpox doctor; a steady proportion came, saw, and were convinced. Very late in the season—October 13—the very anti-Jenner M.P. for Hereford, Mr. Shaw Le Fevre, appeared at the Wells, but he seems to have behaved himself. To balance him, there were the new vaccination people, including several members of the Eyre-Coote family, relatives of the last Earl of Mountrath who died in 1802 without heirs. The following year Angerstein bought the vast Mountrath estates in Norfolk and Suffolk. Mountrath was so terrified of catching smallpox that he had relays of horses at five places between his seat in Devon and his lands in East Anglia, so that he would not have to sleep at an inn and thereby risk infection. He led the life of a recluse and rarely saw anyone except on business. Charles Moore was also on the list of arrivals and though Mrs. Siddons, for a wonder, did not appear, Lady Jersey with her family and Lord Hutchinson were all back, taking the waters and gossiping. Nevertheless, there were still a few people left in the capital as the weather grew warmer, and Jenner's friends continued to promote his interest far into the summer, even after he himself left for Cheltenham.

On July 19 William Wilberforce[77] gave a dinner at his house to which Farington, Thomas Bernard[78] and a Mr. Baker were invited.

He (Baker) is in a state of much acquaintance with Wilberforce and appeared to come now for the purpose of engaging him to meet some other gentlemen on the business of Dr. Jenner and vaccination. He said he had brought the matter forward to Lord Henry Petty who on his first application to him appointed a time for the consideration of it after the public finance business should have been discussed.—He spoke handsomely of Lord Henry in which Wilberforce concurred.—

Mr. Bernard said that what he had proposed to Lord Henry was to grant Dr. Jenner a pension of a thousand a year for his life, and six thousand to recompense him for expenses he had been at in consequence of his having promulgated his discovery of vaccination.[79]

They went on to talk of the losses the doctor had incurred. How, penniless from his activity in London trying to launch his discovery, Jenner had returned to Berkeley only to find that "during his absence one or two other physicians had established themselves." Wilberforce pointed out that "the vaccine inoculation had spread much more considerably in other countries than in England. Even in remote countries and even in China, a country in which innovation is jealously opposed, it had been admitted— In India it is used. . . . "[80]

The reference to China is of particular interest since the geographer, John Barrow[81]—then Secretary to the Admiralty—had written to Jenner shortly before, enclosing a Chinese work on vaccination. He wrote:

I have great pleasure in being able to enclose for your inspection a short treatise in the English language, translated by my friend Sir George Staunton, and published by the Chinese in the city of Canton. . . . As the smallpox in China has usually been attended with the most fatal effects, there is little doubt that the same willingness which has manifested itself at Canton, to receive so mild and effectual a substitute, will be felt in every province of this populous country.

The letter concludes with the reassuring comment so similar to sentiments expressed everywhere outside of the British Isles: "Public confidence there [in China] is not likely to be shaken by that kind of illiberal and undignified opposition which has been so industriously employed elsewhere."[82] Sir George Staunton had been with Barrow in Lord Macartney's embassy to China, and, in 1805, introduced vaccination to that country. In later years he used to visit the Cheltenham Wells regularly so in all probability he and Jenner met.

With these encouraging signs of a new parliamentary grant being on its way, there was nothing further to keep Jenner in London, so he returned to Cheltenham and his domestic circle. Perhaps the most appreciated gesture from his friends after all these years of uncertainty was his appointment to the Town Council, or as it was then called, the Board of Commissioners. He and his circle, in effect, now ruled Cheltenham; for on the board with him were: Dr. Trye, Colonel Riddell, the Earl of Suffolk, Dr. Jameson, Rev. Thomas Pruen, Watson (proprietor of the theater), Dr. Newell, and of course Lord Sherborne. It was fitting that in the year Jenner took his place among the rulers of the community, a Cheltenham publisher should issue one of his works. *Varieties and Modifications* was based in part upon an article that had appeared in the *Medical and Physical Journal* two years earlier. As Le Fanu describes it: "The same year Jenner published it as an independent pamphlet in Cheltenham with a few slight verbal changes."[83] Apparently he preferred not to publish in London on the heels of Dr. Rowley's masterpiece. Inevitably, the publisher was his neighbor, the ambitious Mr. Ruff, who would never again have such an exalted name on one of his title pages.

There had been some sad moments but on balance, 1806 had been kind enough. The town continued as pleasant as ever though much building was going on—in fact far too much from Jenner's point of view. It had been eleven years since he came to the small resort looking for security as well as health. "Cheltenham is much improved since you saw it," he wrote to a friend. "It is too gay for me. I still like my rustic haunt, old Berkeley, best; where we are all going in a fortnight. Edward is growing tall and has long looked over my head. Catherine, now eleven years old, is a promising girl, and Robert, eight years old, is just a chip off the old block."[84] Fortunately the two younger children were robust and happy. Little Catherine is the subject of several of her father's verses, which are sufficiently indicative of the poet's nature to merit quotation. For example, the poem "To a Tomtit Who Was Fed Every Morning at the Bedroom-Window of Catherine Jenner, at Cheltenham," was, within its limits, a most charming thing:

> I peeped at eight, at nine, at ten,
> And then I peeped and peeped again.
> But oh! my heart, my pretty bird,
> Was neither to be seen or heard;
> Untouched, the breakfast I had spread—
> Yes, and the cup I'd early dipped
> In the clear Chelt remained unsipped.

Just when she is convinced that some "Murderous hawk or ravenous kits" had eaten poor Tommy, all ends happily with his appearance.

> The joy I felt I cannot utter,
> When I beheld thy charming flutter;
> Heard thy sweet voice upon the tree,
> And saw thee look, and look for me:
> But I must chide thee dearest bird,
> Indeed I must upon my word.
> Well, well, it shan't be now—but then
> Tommy ne'er serve me so again.[85]

I suppose the clear Chelt was a popular spot for the younger children. Under the anxious eye of Mlle. Montier, the governess, one could play at will and without fear its entire length. It was never more than two feet deep from Barreett's Mill to Alstone Mill, and there was well over a mile between flowery banks and not a jarring note. When the Jenners went to Berkeley, of course, there was the great River Severn entering the channel, but that was no place for little children, even though it was near the sea— a never-ending wonderland. The eldest child, Edward, was in a somewhat special situation, despite his father's brave comment. The boy, now sixteen, was probably outgrowing his strength; he had the seeds of tuberculosis and was manifestly backward in his studies.[86] He would certainly never be suited to school life—nor could he well come under the ministrations of Mlle. Montier. A solution would have to be found; at least there was money for such things now.

One familiar figure was still tragically tied through sickness to the heat and dirt of the capital. Charles James Fox had been reconciled to ill health for several years, but he seems to have realized his coming demise this year and was sure that nothing could be done. He was marooned at the Devonshire's town house, where he had collapsed, refusing to be seen by any doctors for some time and only wished to be left alone. By the end of August the situation was critical. "Aug. 31—Mr. Fox at the Duke of Devonshire's at Chiswick, was tapped a second time (the first was on August 8th) by Mr. Cline, when 29 pints of water were taken from him. Drs. Moseley and Vaughan, and Mr. Taggart, surgeon, also attended, also Charles Hawkins." The patient was unable to get to Cheltenham, of course, but Coutts was pathetically convinced that Riddell held out the only hope! We have no date, but he wrote to Mrs. Fox from Luton Hoo, the Marquess of Bute's seat, and urged her to ignore the doctors and put her spouse in the hands of the quack: "But there could be no hope of his trying it if the regular physicians were to be consulted. It is impossible they should advise his trying, though there is conviction that there is no danger in the trial." Coutts mounted a last-minute campaign to secure Riddell's services to save his friend. The Colonel had apparently been in London but had left for Cheltenham before they could catch him. "Lady Holland called in the Strand yesterday, with Mr. Pigot, and proposed going to Morris Hotel, Oxford Street, opposite Bond Street to enquire after Riddell. I do not know if she found him or if he is still in town, for he was here in the morning yesterday and talked in my shop of his leaving it. The bearer of this is going to enquire——."[87] But Fox was beyond help now, and he died just four days later on September 13, five months after Pitt. He had never been able to leave the Duke of Devonshire's home after his tapping and so died there. When the sculptor Nollekens came three days later to take a cast of the face, Dr. Vaughan warned him that the change as a result of his last hours would make the impression unrecognizable; the sculptor was inclined to doubt him. He had actually taken a cast of Fox some time before and was in a position to make a comparative measurement. When Nollekens saw the corpse in the coffin, however, he was shocked—Fox's face had so shrivelled that the head measured an inch and a half less in width from ear to ear "and other parts in proportion."[88] One would suppose that all the water came away from the bloated body in death; nonetheless, the shrivelling of the head is surely an extraordinary medical phenomenon.

Bereavements and disappointments notwithstanding, life went on and the matter of young Edward's education had to be faced. In the course of the summer Jenner had heard of an unusually promising young man in Bristol who would possibly make a suitable tutor for the boy. When the family went down for their promised visit to Berkeley, the doctor proceeded to Bristol to see the recommended youth, whose remarkable precocity must have impressed Jenner. He immediately engaged the tutor, and it was arranged that the youth take up his duties in the autumn. The boy's name was John Worgan and he was fifteen years old—two years younger than his pupil. Nor was this his first teaching post. He had spent the summer tutoring the son of Mr. Richard Hart Davis, M.P., a wealthy Bristol banker, at Clifton.

John Dawes Worgan was born on November 8, 1791, and was in his way as remarkable a prodigy as that other young Bristol genius, Thomas Chatterton. Contrary to Baron's assumption, the boy did not come from poor parentage. The Worgans had been clock and watchmakers as well as goldsmiths in Bristol for upwards of half a century, and several of the leading eighteenth-century clockmakers had been apprenticed to the firm of Worgan and Son.[89] The fact that the boy helped his father in the learned craft of clockmaking fitted in the general practice of "sons of the firm" in those days, and had no relationship to poverty. Among the friends of the family in Worgan's childhood were the poet William Hayley and the distinguished theologian Thomas Biddulph[90] who moved from the village of Bengeworth, some fifteen miles north of Cheltenham in 1799 to become vicar of St. James, Bristol. Worgan was sent to the school run by the United Brethren at Fullneck, Leeds, but returned home before the death of his father at the beginning of April, 1803. It was then that he announced his decision to enter the ministry of the Church of England, and the fact that Mr. Biddulph relinquished the living of Bengeworth the same year (he had held both parishes up to this time) might suggest that there was more opportunity for association between the two. Baron seems to have assumed that the Worgans' clockmaking business would have perished had not the boy been willing to give up his ambition and take it over (at the age of eleven!), but actually the firm was carried on by other members of the family at Castle Ditch. There were at least five Worgans who were well-known clockmakers in Bristol in the eighteenth century, and there are references to the firm well into the nineteenth.

Since Jenner already knew Hayley it is possible that the poet was among the many who may have introduced him to John Worgan, though it could also have been through Biddulph who had a number of friends in common with Jenner. Be that as it may, in September we find the lad at Berkeley prior to being established at the house in St. George's Place. His transition from the relatively colorless home of a solid Bristol tradesman to the glamour of the doctor's circle in Cheltenham is movingly expressed in a letter to his mother soon after he arrived.

> Cheltenham, 27th Sept.
> When I reflect on the mercies I have received and the advantageous situation in which I am placed I cannot but fall with humble gratitude at the feet of Him whose guardian love has protected me and I trust will still be exerted in my preservation.[91]

A sonnet he had written the previous month accompanied the letter. Unquestionably, the boy was an adult in every but the chronological sense. He had read voraciously, wrote good verse, and had a keen, incisive mind. He was probably a case history to Jenner, as well as a tutor for his children. Part of the doctor's intention was to have a resident companion for Edward rather than a mere teacher, but as it developed Worgan became a valued companion to the whole family. He was deeply interested in theological discussion and speculation, which was not the doctor's strong point, but Mrs. Jenner, so often housebound by her health, was delighted. She was more concerned with the hereafter than most people—a common characteristic of invalids in those days. On the other hand, the boy's facility at poetry suited his employer very well. His was a welcome new face among the Cheltenham singing birds of whom Jenner remained by far the best. The household had expanded considerably since the parliamentary grant arrived, and the fourteen rooms at St. George's Place were none too many for Dr. and Mrs. Jenner, the three children, Mlle. Montier, Richard, the manservant, Worgan, and the three female servants.

Soon after he had settled in Cheltenham, Worgan received a long letter from Hayley suggesting that he write an epic poem on the great odyssey of Balmis, surgeon of the King of Spain (of which more later) and the vaccination cause. It never came to anything,

however. Worgan was too impetuous and active in his new life
to sit down to such a long project. To him Cheltenham was Ely-
sium. He flitted from task to task, always active, but always changing direction. Perhaps his short life was the fuller for the many
fields he entered. One long major effort would have been too
prodigal for the little time he had. Inevitably, John Drayton—
who had been writing since he was ten years old—struck up a
friendship with him despite a great disparity in age (the former
was some seven years older), and they compared notes in their
several poetry projects. But even in these first glorious months
of his new life, Worgan felt the dull secret pains of his deadly
malady—he was tubercular like his young pupil. He had periods of
dramatic melancholy. "Though I am young in years," he once
said to Hayley, "I am old in the school of adversity."[92]

Aside from Hayley's suggestion that the subject offered scope
for a poem, the safe return to Spain of the Balmis expedition in
September was not surprisingly the main topic of interest in
Jenner's circle. In due course a copy of the *Madrid Gazette* dated
October 14 was sent to the doctor across a war-torn continent.
Jenner knew no Spanish, but fortunately his friend Petty (now
Lord Lansdowne) did, and translated the paper for him. It was
accompanied by a letter from his lordship which contains the
oft-quoted comparison of Bonaparte's and Jenner's conquests.

Cheltenham, Nov. 18th, 1806.

Dear Sir,
    I send you a translation of the official account of the vaccine expedi-
tion undertaken by command of His Catholic Majesty, which will, I
hope, be found to possess the merit of fidelity. The importance of your
discovery will be much better comprehended by those who have been
in the habit of occupying or frequenting countries characterised by
heat of climate than by those who have constantly enjoyed the advantages which belong to a temperate region. You have conquered more
in the field of science, than Buonaparte had conquered in the field of
battle; and I sincerely congratulate you on so glorious a testimony of
your success, as that which the Spanish narrative affords.

I am,
Dear Sir,
Yours very sincerely,
Lansdowne.[93]

The saga that the paper celebrated was breathtaking in its scope. Starting in November, 1803, the Balmis expedition had spent nearly three years circumnavigating the globe and establishing vaccination all the way. Baron's chronicle of events is as good as any:

The important narration alluded to in his Lordship's letter, stated that on Sunday, 7th of September, 1806, Dr. Francis Xavier Balmis, Surgeon Extraordinary to the King of Spain, had the honour of kissing His Majesty's hand on the occasion of his return from a voyage round the world, executed for the sole object of carrying to all the possessions of the King of Spain beyond the seas, and to those of other nations, the inestimable gift of vaccine inoculation. The reader will recollect the expedition of which Don Balmis was the director sailed from Cadiz on the thirtieth of November, 1803. It made the Canary Islands first; it then proceeded to Puerto Rico and the Caraccas. On leaving the port of La Guira, it was divided into two branches, one part sailing to South America, under the charge of the sub-director, Don Francis Salvani; the other, with Balmis on board, steering for the Havannah, and thence for Yucatan. There a subdivision took place. The professor, Francis Paster, proceeded from the port Siral to that of Villa Hermosa, in the province of Tobasco. The rest of the expedition traversed the Vice-Royalty of New Spain and the interior provinces, and thence returned to Mexico, the point of reunion. This being accomplished the next object of the director was to carry the preservative from America to Asia. After surmounting various difficulties, he embarked in the port of Acapulco for the Philippine Islands, carrying with him from New Spain twenty-six children to be vaccinated in succession, the cowpox having been thus disseminated through the islands subject to His Catholic Majesty. It was originally designed the expedition should then terminate. The Director, however, and the Captain-General, concerted the means of extending the beneficence of the King to the remotest confines of Asia. Setting sail, therefore, for Macao and Canton, they introduced the preservative to the Portuguese settlements, and to the inhabitants of the Empire of China. Balmis returned from Canton to Macao, and embarking in a Portuguese vessel reached Lisbon on the 15th of August, 1806. In his way he touched at St. Helena; and, strange to say, was the first to induce the English inhabitants of that settlement to adopt the antidote; and this even though it had been discovered in their own country and sent to them by Jenner himself.

The fate of that part of the expedition destined for Peru was disastrous, having suffered shipwreck in one of the mouths of the river La Magdalena. Fortunately the sub-director, the members of the faculty and the children, with the fluid in good preservation, were saved. It was thence carried to the Isthmus of Panama. Another part of the expedition ascended the river La Magdalena. When they reached the interior they separated, to discharge their commission in the towns of Teneriffe, Mompox, Ocana, Secorro, San Gil-y-Medellin, in the valley of Cucuta, and in the cities of Pamplona, Cuenca and Quito, as far as Lima. In the August following they reached Guayaquil.

Not one of the least remarkable events in this expedition was the discovery of the indigenous cowpox in three different places; namely in the valley of Atlixo, in the neighbourhood of Valladolid de Mecheacan, and in the district of Calabozo, in the province of Caracca.

The conductors of the expedition were everywhere welcomed with the utmost enthusiasm. It was to be expected that the representatives of the Spanish monarch and all the constituted authorities would gladly co-operate, but it was scarcely to be anticipated that the unenlightened minds of the Indians would soon appreciate the value of the mission. It is, nevertheless, most gratifying to know that the numerous hordes which occupy the immense tract of country between the United States and the Spanish Colonies, all received the precious fluid with the utmost readiness. They acquired the art of vaccinating and soon performed the operation with great dexterity.

Fame had preceded the arrival of Salvani at Sante Fe. On approaching the capital he was met by the viceroy, the Archbishop and all the civil and ecclesiastical authorities. The event was celebrated with religious pomp and ceremonies, and in a short time more than fifty thousand persons were vaccinated. Similar honours awaited the expedition throughout its whole course. At Quito they were greeted with boundless joy and festivity. Such expressions well became them. The people of this country, the Indians more especially, having been often scourged by the horrid ravages of smallpox, regarded it as the most terrible affliction which Heaven could send them. On its first appearance in a village, panic seized every heart. Each family prepared in an isolated hovel, to which those who were supposed to be infected were banished. *There* without succour, without remedy and with an insufficient supply of food, they were exposed to the alterations of a very variable climate and left to their fate. In this way whole generations perished. Under the Viceroy Teledo the population of the native Indians had amounted to seven millions and a half. At the time of this expedition the number was supposed to be reduced to one fifth.[94]

To say that Jenner was gratified by this momentous saga is a gross understatement. It seems to have moved him more than any other development of his life's work. A month after he had received the *Madrid Gazette*, when all the company had gone from the Wells and he was pretty much alone with his family, he wrote ecstatically to Dunning:

What a delightful narrative is here! What lover of vaccination can feel himself at war with His Catholic Majesty after its perusal! I must tell you that from several countries where Balmis and his philanthropic companions touched, I have most satisfactory accounts of the result. From Manila and the Philippine Islands they send me an account of 230,000 successful cases. From Canton I have a most curious production; a pamphlet on vaccination in the Chinese language. Little did I think, my friend, when our correspondence first began, that heaven had in store for me such abundant happiness. May I be grateful!

Present my best compliments to Mrs. Dunning and the family, and believe me with best wishes.

Yours truly,
E. Jenner.

Cheltenham, Dec. 10th, 1806.[95]

Such abundant happiness indeed. Perhaps now the cruel libels of Rowley could be forgotten.

The town was quiet with all the sounds of creaking chariots and clattering of hooves stilled until the spring came round again. Now there were only the street vendors' cries and the occasional carriages of the resident nobles—including the Suffolks who perhaps visited St. George's Place now and then when all their mighty friends were gone. Lord Sherborne, also, would be in and out attending to town affairs and projects, not the least of which was Dr. Trye's railroad in which Jenner and most of his friends had purchased an interest. Welles and Gwinnett, the solicitors, announced on September 29 that parliamentary application had been made for a railroad between Gloucester and Cheltenham. It took three years for the road to materialize, however, after which horse-drawn wagons operated from Leckhampton Quarries through the southern outskirts of the town and so to Gloucester. Nor was this the only project of public works in which the good doctor was involved. A sewage system in the town was almost nonexistent, despite the fact that the population had doubled since he had settled there. There was, indeed, but one sewer pipe and

that was in St. George's Place. Jenner's first utterance on the
Board of Commissioners was to request that he be allowed to
open a drain from his house into this sewer—at his own expense,
of course.[96] He subsequently took an important role in planning
a system for the whole town. The matter of public health was a
vital one to him in terms of eliminating incubation areas for
smallpox, cholera, and other diseases. Another problem he took
up was that of the road surface in St. George's Place. Since his
property extended at one point to both sides of the thoroughfare,
he had a proprietary concern. The surface was badly drained,
among other things, probably due to the camber, and after rain or
snow pools of water formed over large areas. This latter problem
was resolved in Jenner's day, though the complete sewerage system only came after his death. Unfortunately the position of town
surveyor was in the hands of an enthusiastic amateur named
Colonel Brissac, whose services, though they cost nothing, provided virtually nothing. Jenner changed all this by tactful persuasion and introduced a professional—Thomas Morhall.

Morhall, a man with neither literary nor medical background,
soon became a valued friend of the Jenners' through his loyalty
and dedication to his work. While the doctor, as a town commissioner, was to some extent his employer, Morhall exerted himself
far beyond his civic obligations. He was a combination of family
aide and man friday, and with his advent St. George's Place became perhaps the best-maintained street in the town—particularly the High Street end where the Jenners lived. There are accounts of deep steps from curb to road being neatly bridged and
pavements made passable for the delicate Catherine and her like.
To be sure, as Morhall was the town surveyor one might assume
that these things were part of his normal duties, but, if anything,
they composed the smaller part of his work. For the rest of his
life, Morhall was in the forefront of every cultural and civic activity with which the doctor was associated. He found time to be
secretary or treasurer of the various literary and musical groups
that sprang up in the ensuing years—particularly after Jenner's
gradual withdrawal from London and his increasing involvement
in local affairs. And while there were still great triumphs ahead,
there were already signs that the patient doctor's local adulation
would never necessarily be reflected in the country as a whole.

ILLUSTRATIONS

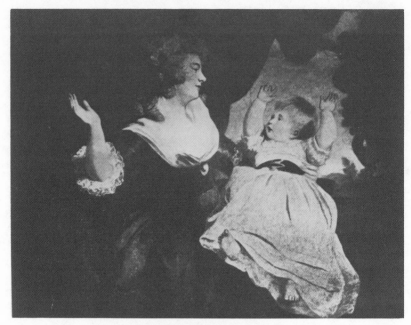

Georgiana, Duchess of Devonshire, and Lady G. Cavendish

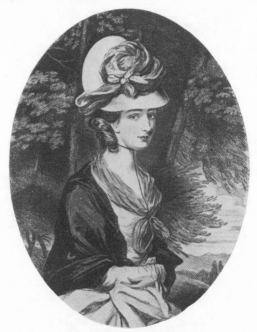

Lady Crewe *from an engraving by*
Thomas Watson at the British Museum,
after the portrait by D. Gardner

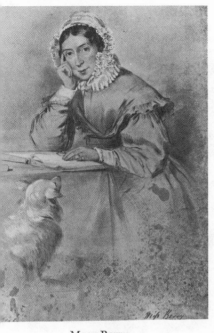

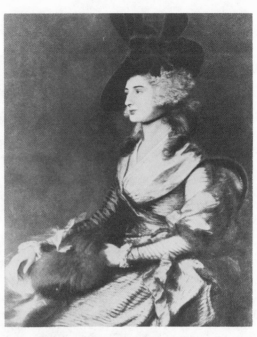

Mary Berry   Mrs. Sarah Siddons *by Gainsborough*

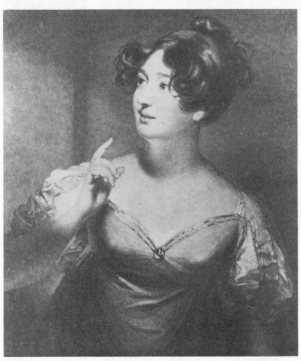

Harriot Mellon *as Volante in* The Honeymoon, *after
Sir William Beechey*

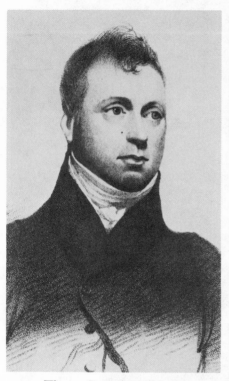

Thomas D. Fosbroke at 46

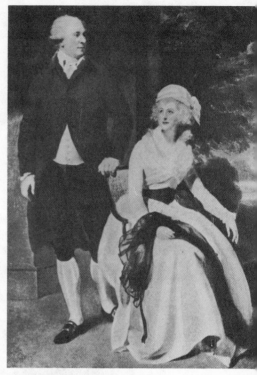

John Julius Angerstein and his second wife

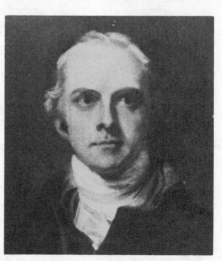

Samuel Lysons, the antiquary,
a portrait by Sir Thomas Lawrence

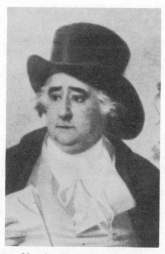

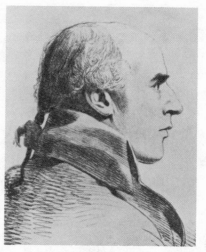

Charles James Fox *from
the portrait by K. A. Hickel*

Joseph Farington *from the
drawing by George Dance*

THE GREAT DOCTORS

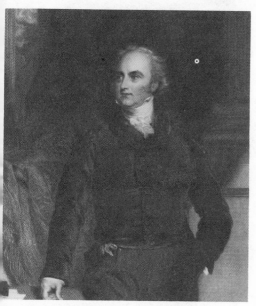

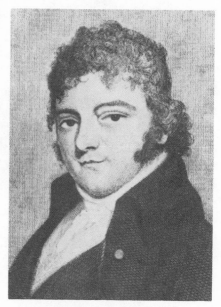

Sir Astley Paston Cooper

Caleb Hillier Parry *from an
engraving by Philip Audinet*

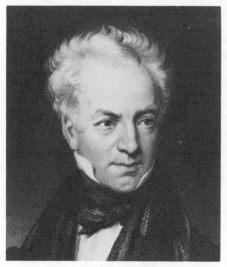

John Baron

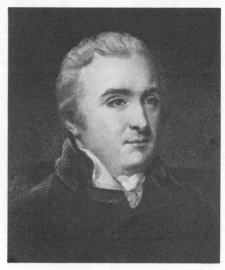

Matthew Baillie

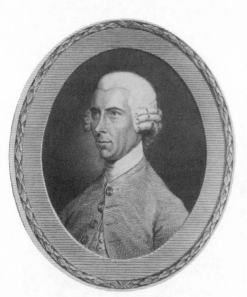

John Coakely Lettsom

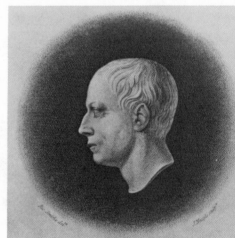

Charles Brandon Trye

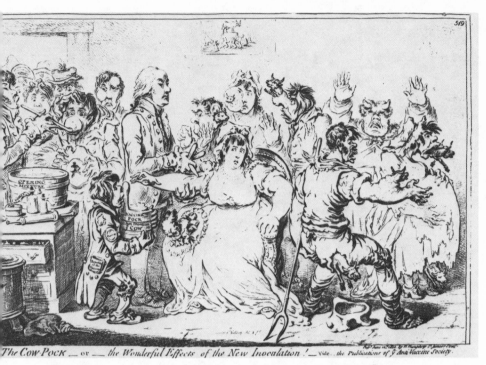

"The Cow-pock—or—the Wonderful Effects of the New Inoculation,"
a cartoon by the anti-vaccinationists

ON THE

VARIETIES AND MODIFICATIONS

OF

THE VACCINE PUSTULE,

OCCASIONED BY AN

HERPETIC STATE OF THE SKIN.

BY EDWARD JENNER, M. D. LL. D. F. R. S. &c.

Cheltenham,
PRINTED BY H. RUFF, HIGH-STREET.

1806.

Title page of *On the Varieties and Modifications of the Vaccine
Pustule occasioned by an herpetic state of the skin* by Edward Jenner
autographed by the author with best regards to
Dr. Waterhouse of Harvard

AN

ACCOUNT

OF THE

Ravages committed in Ceylon

BY

SMALL-POX,

PREVIOUSLY TO THE

INTRODUCTION of VACCINATION;

WITH

A STATEMENT OF THE CIRCUMSTANCES ATTENDING

THE

INTRODUCTION, PROGRESS, and SUCCESS,

OF

VACCINE INOCULATION IN THAT ISLAND.

By THOs. CHRISTIE, M.D.

MEMBER OF THE ROYAL COLLEGE OF PHYSICIANS, LONDON, AND OF THE ROYAL MEDICAL SOCIETY, EDINBURGH; AND LATELY MEDICAL SUPERINTENDENT-GENERAL IN CEYLON.

"But now Providence has conferred on the Inhabitants of Ceylon, a
"milder and more sure relief—by the introduction of the Jennerian
"improvement."
Cordiner's Description of Ceylon.

CHELTENHAM,
PRINTED BY J. AND S. GRIFFITH, PORTLAND-PASSAGE;
AND SOLD BY
MURRAY, 32, FLEET-STREET, LONDON; J. BLACKWOOD, EDIN-
BURGH; AND GILBERT AND HODGES, DUBLIN.
1811.

Title page of *An Account of the Ravages committed in Ceylon by Small-pox, . . .* by Thomas Christie

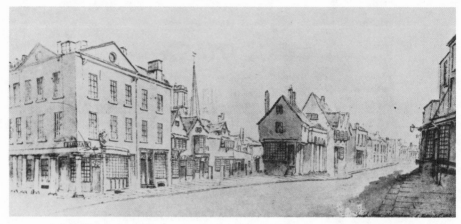

The High Street, Cheltenham, *from a drawing by John Claude Nattes*

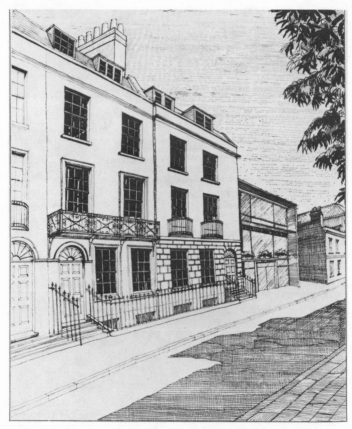

Architect's impression of what Jenner House (third from left)
would have looked like today if it had been restored

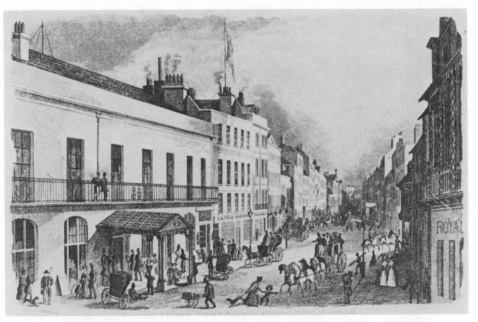

High Street, Cheltenham, published by R. Edwards, Stationer, Bookseller, and Binder, Cheltenham

EDWARD JENNER

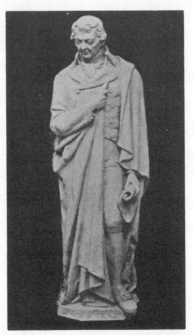

Edward Jenner statue in Cheltenham College Chapel

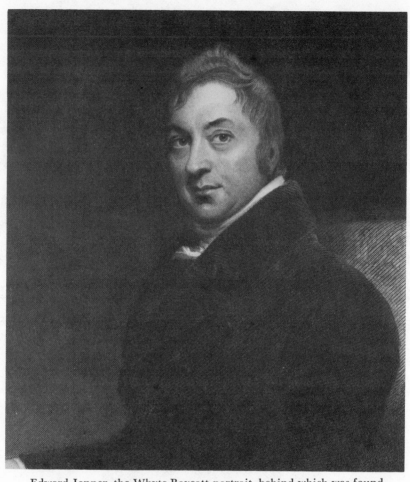

Edward Jenner, the Whyte-Boycott portrait, behind which was found in 1971 a letter from Jenner to a lady asking for her intercession with Sir Hugh Inglis (see page 265)

✍ VI ✍

The Fortress Assailed

1807-1809

Just as the town fathers of Cirencester had lamented in 1758 that there could be no more smallpox in the place because there was no one left to have it, Jenner was able to look around him in Cheltenham at a town in which there were no more left to vaccinate. "I have inoculated such multitudes in this place and its vicinity," he wrote on January 13, 1807, "that a patient . . . rarely approaches me." It was not a pompous boast but a mere statement of fact. In the one community where he had been allowed to have his way, smallpox had been completely eradicated. Given such freedom on a national scale, he reflected wryly, the entire country might have been in like case. He enclosed for his correspondent a copy of the Spanish report and hoped it would be read with pleasure in appreciation of the "full philanthropic spirit of the Catholic King. What a noble enterprise"; he went on "How strange that this should be the only country in the civilised world where vaccination is not held as a blessing." Strangely enough he still had faith that legislation would take place in the not-too-distant future. His supporters were more enthusiastic than ever and their numbers tended to increase. It just seemed that through some inexplicable pattern in the machinery of government, his system was not adopted—even in the face of his being assisted with a financial grant. Still worse, variola inoculation continued to flourish, and with it smallpox itself—except in Cheltenham. But Jenner was sure the situation must change soon. "I trust the day is not far distant when we may see the energies of the British Government employed in establishing it among the British people."[1]

All in all, he was enjoying his quiet winter in the almost deserted town. Here he could forget the denigration and malice outside and bask in the homage of the vaster world beyond the seas. Consequently he was less than enthusiastic when he was asked to go to London. In the capital the somewhat frigid confrontation of Phillips, the publisher, with the noble house of Bute had no adverse effect on Jenner's relationship with either party; a few days after he wrote as quoted above to the unknown correspondent, he received a letter from Phillips begging him to vaccinate his new baby. Jenner's reply continues the thought of the previous letter and reveals the fact that the impact of the Balmis expedition was still very much with him, combined with a strong disinclination to interrupt his peace for a visit to London.

Dear Sir,

I congratulate you and Mrs. Phillips on the addition to your family. It is my intention to be in Town soon; but how soon I cannot at the moment positively say. My movements will be regulated by those of the College of Surgeons and the House of Commons. The former have not yet finished their Inquiry, which will, when completed, be laid before the House. This Inquiry will lay all those troublesome ghosts which have so long haunted the Metropolis with their ox-faces, and distant mooings against vaccination. However,—tis all for the best—you may depend upon it, the New Investigation will prove the touchstone of the vaccination discovery.

I have not yet seen your monthly mag: for this present month. Probably you may not have inserted the curious and interesting piece of intelligence I received from Madrid. The supposition induces me to enclose it. What a glorious enterprise! I have made peace with Spain, and quite adore her philanthropic monarch. Could not this be touched up by some of those who *through* you introduce pathetic stories into this world?

A word more respecting your little one. Although I should be happy to shield it myself from the speckled monster, yet I advise you not long to rest my coming to town. I will just add that I consider the vaccine lancet in the hand of John Ring just as safe as in my own. Please present my best wishes to Mrs. Phillips and tell her I have not forgotten her civilities.

Yr. very faithful dr.,
E. Jenner.[2]

Jenner did not get up to London until the middle of March so, in all probability, Ring did perform the operation.

But when he did arrive there, in 1807, the capital seemed much more bearable. The birthday dinner, in particular, was exceptionally gratifying with so many of his personal friends present, and the Duke of York in the chair. His Royal Highness made the usual flattering speech, followed by Rowland Hill and Dr. Lettsom. In his remarks Jenner was still full of the international scene. "After the very animated speech of the Duke of York," he said, "and the important information conveyed by his friend, Dr. Lettsom, he had very little to say on the subject. He continued to receive the most agreeable information respecting vaccination from all parts of the world, from Greenland to the Cape and from the Mississippi to the Ganges."[3] John Ring, that excellent classical scholar, translated a moving letter from Dr. Reiss of Makow, Poland. It was written in Latin and referred to Jenner as "the Illustrious exterminator of that pestilential disorder the smallpox." Accompanying it was a handsome silver cup that had once belonged to a man named "Jenner."[4] But most moving of all was the request for a portrait of the doctor and a small sample of the cloth that he wore so that his Polish friends might wear a similar attire at his birthday festival on May 17. Jenner was so delighted that rather than send a mere print he ordered the sculptor Manning to prepare a bust for his Polish friend.

In the New World while vaccination flourished so prosperously in the white community of the United States, there had been no parallel development among the Indian tribes of Canada. During the preceding four years there had been sporadic efforts to introduce the system, but it was in this historic year of 1807 that the seed was finally sown. As Baron put it: "After various attempts to disseminate vaccination among the native tribes of North America, Dr. Jenner at length had the happiness of finding that his efforts were successful."

Baron's description is very garbled, however, and we are indebted to the researches of Le Fanu for a succinct narrative of the business.[5] As far back as 1803, John Chew, superintendent of the Indian Department in Montreal, received a plea from Father Le Noir, a mission priest, to send a doctor to inoculate him and his Indians at St. Francis against the smallpox. Whether this referred to smallpox or cowpox inoculation is, of course, not clear, but a year later at Jenner's birthday dinner on May 17 a report was made to the effect that "the Canadian Indians came down the country many hundred miles to procure the matter, and most of their tribes escaped the smallpox." After this things seem to have remained in abeyance until May 15, 1807, when Lieutenant Governor Francis Gore of Upper Canada addressed the Indians at the Head of the Lake and urged them to adopt vaccination since smallpox had recently appeared among them. He told them of the "safe and easy method of Inoculation lately found out on the other side of the Great Waters." His appeal failed because it was the time of the great hunt. A month later, however, when the Indians were home again, Colonel William Claus, Deputy Superintendent General of Indian Affairs, approached them again and strongly urged them to adopt the system. This time the plea was apparently listened to sympathetically for we find Jenner writing to the Indians—presumably at the behest of the colonial authorities. He sent the letter to Lieutenant Governor Gore, together with a copy of the "Address to the Royal Jennerian Society for 1803." It is dated London, August 11, 1807, so he must have sent it about a week before he left for Cheltenham. It did not arrive until November, at which time Colonel Claus addressed the Indians after showing them the doctor's message addressed to "The Chief of the Five Nations from Dr. Jenner."

Brothers! I have now the satisfaction to deliver you a book, sent to you from England, from that great man, Dr. Jenner, whom God enabled to discover so great a blessing to mankind: it explains fully all the advantages derived from so great a discovery. . . . I therefore Brothers, at his request, and in his name, present this book to the Five Nations, as a token of his regard for you and your rising generation, by which many valuable lives may be preserved from that most dreadful pestilence, the smallpox.

The presentation took place at Fort George, Upper Canada, on November 8, in the presence of Colonel Proctor,[6] the commandant of the garrison, with his officers. The ten chiefs present—of the Mohawks, Senecas, Cayougas, and Oneidas—were deeply impressed and replied to Jenner the same day.

We shall not fail to teach our children to speak the name of Jenner: and they thank the Great Spirit for bestowing upon him so much wisdom and so much benevolence.

We send with this a belt and string of Wampum, in token of our acceptance of your precious gift; and we beseech the Great Spirit to take care of you in this world and in the land of spirits.

The letter concluded with signatures in Indian hieroglyphics of the ten chieftans.

I have continued the narrative straight through the year 1807 in order to preserve its unity. It will not be out of order therefore to point out that the letter from the chiefs arrived in Cheltenham in December following the most prosperous, and perhaps the happiest, year Jenner had spent since he came to the town. After the glitter of the highest society in England, "such tokens and assurances of regard from the unsophisticated children of the wilderness were highly acceptable." He wrote a long letter to Lieutenant Governor Gore (though, typically, Baron gives us no date or address), thanking him for his services in the matter. "You, also, Sir, are entitled to the most grateful acknowledgements, not only from me, but from every friend of humanity for the philanthropic manner in which you originally introduced the vaccine among these tribes of Indians."[7] But a tragic aftermath of this ceremony in the wilds of the Canadian frontier, dedicated to the cause of saving lives from the greatest of nature's killers, came five years later. When the war with the United States broke out in 1812, Fort George was the center of some of the bloodiest fighting throughout the three long years. Colonel Proctor, by then promoted General, was himself wounded, and many of the officers present at the 1807 celebration were undoubtedly killed.

This was, however, far in the future, and the present scene was made even happier for Jenner when Caleb Parry's boy, Charles, set up his practice in Cheltenham later in the year. Now twenty-eight years old, the young man had finished his extensive travels, had taken his M.D. in Edinburgh in 1804, and only the previous year had been elected L.R.C.P. Despite the difference in years, Charles Parry and young Fosbroke became good friends. John Worgan, in the meantime, was adding a great deal to the Jenners' domestic scene. Catherine, housebound a great deal of the time, now had a splendid new companion with whom to discuss her theology. In fact, Worgan made himself an active member of the family and shared all its interests. In January he completed a Latin poem on vaccination addressed to Dr. Ring, *"Ad Illustrum Johannem Ring,"* and he was soon recognized by many of his employer's intellectual friends as a serious and mature colleague. Unhappily, he was sophisticated in other respects besides literature, and the constant passing of beautiful young women at the Wells disturbed—or inspired, depending upon the way one regards it— his poetic concentration. He appears to have fallen in love on at least one occasion during his first autumn with the family and grew depressed when he found his passion was not returned or— more likely—not noticed. Nevertheless, he was able to write to Hayley that he had completed "a century of sonnets" and early in the new year wrote a delightful poem (considering his sixteen years) entitled "Recollections of a Summer's Day."[8] In the spring, however, while at Berkeley, Worgan contracted typhus and was forced to return to his family in Bristol until he recovered. After some six months of savoring the fascinations of the Jenner home and the Jenner circle, he was forced back to the kindly but intellectually desolate atmosphere of his parental roof. But it was only a phase—the doctor eagerly awaited his return and, as it were, kept his bed aired at St. George's Place. He was much too valuable to lose.

Local literary activity continued apace, and Ruff did very well out of the Jenner "school." Pruen completed his vaccination contribution: *A Comparative Sketch of the Effects of the Variolus and Vaccine Inoculation*[9] dealt in particular with the Jennerian Society's 1804 report on the campaign among the Canadian Indians—of which we shall hear more later. Everyone in Cheltenham seemed to be writing. Parry produced his descriptive and, in places, excellent poem on Cleeve Hill, which he entitled "Winchcombe Hill"; it was not published until some years later. Perhaps the young man accompanied Jenner on his walks on the hill to collect vaccine, and since most people do not associate that dangerous, cliff-broken mountain with grazing cattle, I quote his words:

> And honied herbage fluttering, passes by,
> Makes not unpleasant music; not the sound

Of shrill sheep bell on the turfy down;
Nor low of herds that wander on the brink
Of the steep precipice . . .[10]

Returning from the muses to the more prosaic facts of vaccination, however, early in the year Ruff brought out a leaflet, the *Supplement to the Madrid Gazette of Octotber 14th 1806*. There is not an author or editor mentioned, but as Le Fanu observes, it was "presumably" issued by Jenner, who returned home briefly in the early summer to take the now recovered Worgan back with him to join the family in the capital. Here, according to Worgan's biographer, "he met many literary characters," and one can well imagine the unsophisticated boy's reaction. He arrived during a period of unusual literary activity and feuding among the authors. Hoppner made a scathing attack on Richard Payne Knight[11] in Prince Hoare's magazine, *The Artist,* at the end of May. Hoare had been involved in a dispute with Thomas Bernard in January relative to a projected periodical called *The Director.* It seemed that Bernard had offered Hoare the editing of it in order to get him interested in helping; but as soon as it seemed that this was achieved, the wily philanthropist announced that he would handle it himself—with Hoare as his assistant. The latter's angry reaction was to start a paper of his own—*The Artist*—and by the time summer came round the action was well under way.

The first issue came out on March 14. It was a weekly and Hoare described it as "a collection of essays relative to painting, poetry, sculpture, architecture, the drama, discoveries of science, and various other subjects." It was a pathetic enough little sheet of eight pages, and though it ran for three years it is understandably forgotten. What is of interest, however, is the distinguished company of contributors it attracted. In addition to Hoppner at least two other of Jenner's friends wrote for it: James Northcote and Anthony Carlisle.[12] While its title suggests that it was primarily an arts magazine, the man who contributed the most essays was the scientist Tiberius Cavallo,[13] who was a pioneer in the therapeutic aspects of electricity. Carlisle contributed an essay to the July 4 issue entitled "On the Connexion Between Anatomy and the Arts of Design."

Two weeks later Hoare published Jenner's essay with the extraordinarily long title "Classes of the Human Powers of Intellect—Hints for the Classification of the Powers of the Human Mind as They Appear in Various Descriptions of Man." It is not a very good piece of work and seems to take the most unusual view that insanity is the final upward expression of the mind. His seven classes range as follows: the Idiot, the Dolt, Mediocrity, Mental Perfection, Eccentricity, Insanity, and the Maniac. The grading of the first four seems logical, but surely one would treat the three latter as aberrations or deviations from the pattern. Jenner must have been fairly proud of it, however, for many years later he had it published in Cheltenham as a separate pamphlet.

It is hard to see how a magazine like *The Artist* could pay, though it may have been subsidized by the wealthy art collector Thomas Hope, who was himself a contributor to its pages. It certainly had its critics. Between the publication of Carlisle's and Jenner's essays, on July 14 Nathaniel Marchant,[14] the painter, attacked it mercilessly to Farington—perhaps because he had not been asked to contribute.

He spoke with great contempt of the publication called *The Artist* and said he had never heard it mentioned by anyone. Prince Hoare, the editor, is watergruel mixed with salt. He has the power of meeting the types; his work is stillborn;—Northcote wrote in it and makes the Artist first a puppy, next an ass,—and then horse,—He read only three or four of the numbers and then threw the rest away.

Carlisle, on the other hand, seems to have been proud to have contributed to it, for two days after Jenner's paper appeared, he reminded Farington of some observations he had made on anatomy in his own article a fortnight earlier.

Where did Jenner take young Worgan, in the course of meeting the literary figures? Banks was in poor health; though thanks to a vegetable diet imposed by Carlisle, his gout had manifestly improved. When he was fit, he usually had an interesting coterie at his house and Hoare himself, who was the center of a huge circle, as was Bernard, with whom Jenner must have been in touch relative to the gout. It is interesting to speculate upon the manner in which the doctor rationalized writing for his old friend Hoare's magazine without offending his new friend and patron, Bernard, who was a somewhat volatile and erratic type.

Fortunately these feuds between authors had no effect upon the grant itself, and it seemed fairly certain that the money would now be forthcoming—it was mainly a matter of how much. Lysons returned to Cheltenham in the middle of July, but Jenner and the family preferred to wait, despite the summer heat, until the suspense was over. On Wednesday, July 29, the question finally came up in the House.

Mr. Spencer Perceval, Chancellor of the Exchequer, moved that £10,000 be granted to His Majesty to remunerate Dr. Edward Jenner, as a further reward for promulgating his discovery of Vaccine Inoculation; to be paid without *any deduction*. Mr. Morris moved an amendment, that £20,000 be inserted instead of £10,000, and Sir John Sebright seconded the motion.

> For Mr. Morris's amendment   60
> Against it   <u>47</u>
>   13

Farington, whose account is given above, added that "Mr. Perceval persisted in his proposal to give only £10,000." But of course the sum voted by the House stood, and Jenner got his £20,000. It is interesting to note that the only well-known figure to oppose the grant was Shaw Le Fevre, M.P. for Hereford, but his case was greatly weakened by the fact that after maintaining that vaccination was of little value, and getting no support, he changed his approach and asserted that Jenner had not discovered it anyway. It will be remembered that Sir John Sebright,[15] seconder of the amendment motion, was related by marriage to Mrs. Jenner. Lord Lansdowne had faithfully pursued his commitment to the Duchess of Devonshire, and the long struggle for Jenner's solvency seemed to be over. When the doctor returned to Cheltenham with his family it was a triumphal homecoming in more respects than one, and he travelled in noble company. The town had been filling up with national celebrities all through the month of July, and just two days before Jenner's grant was decided, the first member of the royal family had arrived—the Duke of Gloucester. He came this time not as a visitor but as a seasonal resident with his own home, and he continued thus until his death in 1834. The Prince of Wales was due at the end of the month, and part of his "court" had preceded him. The most magnificent ball in the town's history, "an unprecedented assemblage of elegance and beauty" to the number of twelve hundred, was presided over by Gloucester himself. Mrs. Siddons was at the Theatre Royal, while Cramer and Bianchi were at the Assembly Rooms. A brief note in the *Gloucester Journal* announced:—"Fauconberg House is preparing for the reception of H.R.H. the Prince of Wales who is expected at Cheltenham about 25th of August." It was to this festive atmosphere that Jenner and his little caravan returned in August 1807.

Certainly his financial security for the foreseeable future appeared to be settled. Twenty thousand pounds *without deduction* was a lot of money and the season ahead of him looked extremely promising, especially since Catherine's health seemed to be going through a relatively easy spell. Poor Worgan was an occasional source of worry, but he was one of the family now and the matter of his medical care was, to Jenner, no more of an imposition than looking after young Edward or, indeed, Catherine herself. All things being equal, there was no reason why he should not enjoy the social pleasures of this brilliant season while maintaining his professional and domestic commitments.

Leaving London was always a relief to the family—passing, as it were, from the land of the enemy to the security of their provincial fortress. This was particularly true since Jenner was now one of its rulers. Probably the nearest thing to hostility in Cheltenham was the increasingly strong cult of Colonel Riddell. He was not a particularly talented man, and his one or two half-hearted sallies on vaccination in the local press were more likely attempts to take away a little of the doctor's limelight rather than serious intellectual challenges to the vaccination principle. Trye from Leckhampton replied very effectively in each case, and Jenner never personally crossed swords with his erstwhile landlord. Perhaps the doctor's disciples were more concerned than he. A fortnight before Parliament voted the second grant, but when everyone knew it was imminent, Sir Francis Burdett in a "professional" letter to Riddell wrote, "I am still unable to move without crutches, and cannot sit in a writing position without some, though not much pain. I think with you, that if you can extinguish fever, you beat the cowpoxers all to nothing."[16]

None of which should have given Jenner much concern or detract from his pleasure at meeting all the distinguished company.

There was, however, one unfortunate shadow that rather tempered the grant. Before leaving London, Jenner had seen Perceval and begged him to initiate some kind of parliamentary action to prevent the continuance of *smallpox* inoculation, but the statesman had not felt that he could do anything. "Alas," wrote the doctor to Lettsom, "all I said availed nothing; and the speckled monster is still to have liberty that the Smallpox Hospital, the delusions of Moseley, and the caprices and prejudices of the misguided poor, can possibly give him. I cannot express to you the chagrin and disappointment I felt at this interview."[17] Perhaps Perceval suggested the possibility of discussing the matter further in Cheltenham. He had his summer residence in the town and would certainly be there shortly with the Prince. Jenner thought that since Perceval's wife and young daughter would be with him at their house in Constitution Terrace, it might be easier to talk in an informal domestic atmosphere. In addition, Perceval's brother, the Earl of Egmont, was in and out of the town throughout the season and was a lavish as well as gregarious entertainer. Jenner moved in such society these days, and at Egmont's one would sooner or later meet everyone who mattered, inside the huge Perceval clan as well as outside.

Among the great figures of the stage and concert platform who helped to crowd the salons this season was Louisa Brunton who played at the Theatre Royal the week preceding Mrs. Siddons's appearance, and whom the great actress conceded to be her only serious rival in tragic roles. The young woman, however, was being avidly courted by one of Jenner's most licentious friends, Lord Craven, and she gave up a most promising stage career at the age of twenty-three. She was greatly loved by the Cheltenham audiences and her departure was a matter for much concern and gossip. For Catherine Jenner and her like it was, of course, a moral tragedy as well as a loss to the stage. Louisa Brunton never returned to the Theatre Royal, but within two weeks of her departure an artist of a somewhat different character started his roundabout journey from London to meet Jenner, whom he "knew" but had never seen.

Robert Bloomfield was the one English poet to whom the phenomenon of vaccination was the stuff of poetry. Coleridge promised much in later years, but we never saw the fruit of his inspiration; and Anstey, of course, was essentially a satirist. Undoubtedly, Bloomfield's interest continued to be stirred by the impact of the disease in his own family: "My method of treating it has endeared it to myself," he wrote; "for it indulges in domestic anecdote."[18] Once, despite his financial straits, Jenner impulsively gave the poet an expensive present—a gesture that attested to Jenner's awareness of real poetry as opposed to the well-meant verses of his first admirers. Bloomfield's genius, as a matter of fact, was appreciated widely, but he was one of those poor souls who somehow do not flourish under patronage, and every gesture left him as poor as before. With the peasant poet becoming a fashionable interest, the vaccination poems caused a mild stir in Gloucestershire medical circles. In addition, when the bard, sick and well-nigh destitute, published a volume called *Wild Flowers* late in 1806, one poem moved Bransby Cooper profoundly. It was a slender little verse entitled "Shooter's Hill" in which the ailing poet laments—sincerely enough—that he may never see the beauties of his own country.

> Of Cambrian mountains still I dream,
> And mouldering vestiges of war,
> By time-worn cliff or classic stream
> Would rove but Prudence holds a bar
> Come then, O Health, I'll strive to bound
> My wishes to this airy stand,
> 'Tis not for me to trace around
> The wonders of my native land.[19]

As it happened, Cooper was organizing one of those fashionable rituals of the eighteenth-century gentleman—a tour of the Wye Valley with a group of his friends. The party was to consist of Cooper, his wife and young son, and Mr. and Mrs. Thomas Lloyd-Baker, plus one or two others whose names have not been preserved. Interestingly enough in later years one of these Lloyd-Bakers married into Sir John Sebright's family and so became distantly related to the Jenners. The poignance of Bloomfield's lines struck Cooper profoundly, and he decided to invite the poet to join them so that he might actually enjoy those grandeurs of Gloucestershire and the Wye Valley, which he had despaired of ever seeing. "It was not in the power of this happy party," wrote Bloomfield, "to falsify such predictions, and to render a pleasure to the writer of no uncommon kind."[20] They would, indeed, drop from the Cotswolds across the vale through the very lanes that Jenner had trodden so long, and, after the Forest-of-Dean and the Wye Valley, go into Cheltenham to visit Jenner himself.

The party left Ferney Hill, Cooper's house in Dursley, at 10 A.M. on August 17 in two carriages with seven horses. In addition to some poetic aspirations, Cooper had some concrete talent as a draftsman and brought along sketching materials, so that he might illustrate the descriptive poem Bloomfield intended to write in the course of their travels. In addition to the poem, "The Banks of Wye," he also kept a journal that is of great value, recording, as it does, the visit to Jenner.

They journeyed through the Forest-of-Dean where the first impact of forest and mountain grandeur made a deep impression; Bloomfield loved the rural peace and happy beauty of the country-side just as much. London was another planet; traffic and postboys seemed gone forever. As is seen in these splendid lines, Bloomfield's poetry is more like Rupert Brooke's than Cowper's, with which it is often compared:

> Harmless we passed and unassailed
> Nor once at roads or turnpikes railed,
> Through depths of shade oft sunbeams broke,
> Midst noble Flaxley's bowers of oak;
> And many a cottage trim and gay,
> Whispered delight through all the way;
> On hills exposed, in dales unseen,
> To patriarchal Michel Dean.[21]

Bloomfield was entranced every mile of the way, and at some points, poet though he was, he had no words to express his feelings. "A ditch along the ridge of the hills marks the boundary between the counties of Gloucester and Hereford. I think if I lived on the spot, I should climb the hills about twice a week for six months, and then be able to give a tolerable account of the scene;—delightful Malvern." As a matter of fact, the view he had in mind is between the counties of Gloucester and *Worcester*, but no matter, he made his point and each new vista brought him nearer and nearer to Cheltenham and Jenner. Not that the impact of the human herd, in the middle of the season at a fashionable watering place, would be all he desired; but he would see the great benefactor who had been such a major figure in his thought and inspiration for the past three years.

The party reached Cheltenham at eleven o'clock on August 27 direct from the contemplation of Tewkesbury's battlefield and the awe of medieval history, but entering the town among the shabby cottages of the Tewkesbury Road was not the happiest of choices. It was as opposite to the grandeur of Norman Tewkesbury as one could possibly conceive. The tranquility of the promenades and murmur of polite conversation were markedly missing, for this was no ordinary summer day in Cheltenham. The poet might have thought himself back in London. With the Prince of Wales in residence, even the great width of the High Street was filled with the type of vehicle that demanded six or eight horses and as many outriders, and where the postillions of great noblemen shouted impatient epithets at those of great actresses and mistresses. One wonders about the problems of precedence in a place like Cheltenham at the height of the season, when so many nobles of similar rank jostled to be nearest to royalty. No doubt Sir Isaac Heard, as Garter King of Arms, was one of the most courted men in town, and he may even have found these annual contests stimulating. One swarm had departed when the Duke of Gloucester left, and now a new swarm had come in to dance attendance upon the heir to the throne.

One gets the impression from Bloomfield's comments that his fleeting impression of Cheltenham was a very disappointing one. Where was the peace of the "Hallowed bowers"[22] that meant so much to the Berrys and the Locks? Where in this maelstrom could "the poet court the shade!" In another mood and at another time, he would no doubt have loved the classical grandeur of the new palaces and ornamental gardens in contrast with the Gothic dignity he had just left behind in Tewkesbury—but now he would look up his friend Jenner and then be on his way. The seething, laughing crowds had jolted his mind from the tranquility of time and antiquity in the countryside. Now he was conscious of coming back to earth.

> Muse, turn thee from the field of blood,
> Rest to the brave, peace to the good,
> Avon with all they charms adieu!
> For Cheltenham mocks thy pilgrim crew;
> And like a girl in beauty's power,
> Flirts in the fairings of an hour.[23]

Of his visit, he wrote: "I proposed calling on Dr. Jenner, who joined our party in the walks, and sent a Cheltenham gift for my wife which shall remain in my family with his former tokens between us." This use of the plural is interesting, and suggests that the doctor had presumably made other gifts beside the inkstand. Of the town itself, Bloomfield observed, "Cheltenham appears to be an increasing town, full of dashing shops, and full of what is often called life, i.e., high life. I am not qualified to judge of high life, and may be laughed at for my strictures; but as I never feel happy in Bond Street, I see no reason that I should here."[24] They spent about three hours there, and then went on to Gloucester, where there were no crowds to contend with, to dine at the King's Head before going home.

There is a little suggestion of the anticlimax here. Jenner could spare gifts, but not, it would seem, time. Three hours was not very much after a journey across the breadth of England. Perhaps Catherine was having a poor day, or possibly the poet's hosts were tired and impatient to get home. Jenner, of course, would be no novelty to them. Nevertheless, Bloomfield was very grateful. "I have imbibed the highest degree of affection for all the individuals of the party," he wrote, "from the most natural cause in the world —because they all seemed glad to give me pleasure, and I shall forget them all,—when my grave is strewn with flowers."[25] When his book was published in 1811, Bransby Cooper's four drawings composed the illustrations. As far as it is known, Bloomfield never came back to Cheltenham, but the doctor and the poet remained in sporadic intercourse until 1823, when they both died within a few months of each other.

There is no question but what Jenner was, indeed, more swept up in the social whirl than he had ever been in his life, and he would have been foolish not to have taken advantage of it. He was, in effect, living at court and a part of everything. The sojourn of the Prince of Wales was the greatest royal occasion since the residence of George III in 1788. If you date it from the arrival of the Duke of Gloucester on August 10 to the departure of the Prince of Wales and the Duke of Sussex on September 5, the royal presence in Cheltenham lasted for twenty-six days. It was an exciting time for the Jenners when royalty was in residence at Fauconberg Lodge, situated as they were in St. George's Place, which was still the only entrance to and from the mansion. Every chariot and every courier on state business going back and forth must needs pass the house. Here the children in particular might stand on the delicate iron balconies and timidly wave perhaps two or three times a day as His Royal Highness swept by. And on one occasion they did not have to wait until the appointed time before this very special treat. The Prince of Wales was due on August 25, but something apparently developed that required him to be there long before the people were ready for him. It was near midnight on the twenty-second and most folks had gone to their beds, when a great cavalcade came rumbling unannounced down the silent High Street and turned into St. George's Place. The good people no doubt wondered what it was until they pulled back their casements and saw the score or more great chariots, outriders, footmen, and sweating horses. There would be shouting and releasing of scraping brakes after the run down High Street and new orders for the last brief climb up Bayshill. The coat of arms emblazoned on the dusty doors of the first chariot explained the commotion—the Prince had arrived in Cheltenham three days early. But Jenner, who always went to bed very late, would certainly have been up when the great vehicles rolled past his front door, and perhaps the noise woke poor Catherine, who never slept very well. But for most of that large household, it would have been a spectacle well worth waking for—the bobbing lamps, the swaying and creaking of leather, the shouting of postillions, and the thunder of so many iron-tyred wheels over the cobbled surface of St. George's Place to disappear into the summer darkness with only the fading sound in the distance to recall their passing.

As though unwilling to compete, the Duke of Gloucester had left for Sidmouth as soon as his royal cousin's imminent arrival had been announced, but most of the brilliant company had remained—except Mrs. Siddons. After a gala performance under the duke's patronage of *The Grecian Daughter* (which had reduced the entire audience to tears), she left the town soon after His Grace. A noteworthy absentee this season was the popular Mrs. Jordan, but she had been in very poor health since her last daughter had been born at the end of March.[26] After a long tiresome summer, the mother had to think of the child's vaccination. "Knight (Dr.) has advised the postponing of little Amelia's inoculation till the weather is decidedly colder," she wrote to the Duke of Clarence. "The dear children were all eager to send their love."[27]

The Milbankes were in and out of the town most of the summer, and when the Prince arrived Sir Robert was his main companion in the walks, together with the first equerry, Colonel Bloomfield, and MacMahon. Anne Milbanke—then a young girl—eventually married Byron, whom she met at Cheltenham, a few years later, and a very tragic business it turned out to be. An even more tragic young woman was also at the Wells; one of Coutts's many protegées—Lady Hester Stanhope.[28] She may well have been there to see Charles Moore, who had arrived earlier, since she was passionately in love with his brother, Sir John. She had been keeping house for her uncle, William Pitt, and when he died in 1806, Coutts took her under his wing and more or less watched over her for the rest of her life. Moore was her one great love, and when he was killed in 1809, she never wished to see England again. She had money at the time, and travelled widely in the Levant, where she chose to live out her life.

When the Prince of Wales recovered from his travel exertions, he joined fully in the social life of the Spa, and in a few days the local press was able to say, "We are extremely happy to report that the Prince of Wales has already derived considerable benefit from the salubrity of the air of Cheltenham and its celebrated springs." The town was crowded and everyone did very well indeed, from pastry cooks to fashionable doctors. When the Lord Chief Justice of Ireland, with the Duke of Beaufort, Mr. Perceval —Chancellor of the Exchequer, and the Archbishop of Canterbury were joined by the other royal brother, the Duke of Sussex, the gathering of regular peers was outshone. The highlight of the month was the special state performance at the Theatre Royal on September 3. It was what one would today call a "double bill," and it departed from the old tradition of presenting tragedy on great social occasions. The celebrated comedy actor Samuel Russell came down from London and appeared in his greatest role, *Jerry the Sneak*. The *Gloucester Journal* rhapsodized as usual. "H.R.H. the Duke of Sussex, the Earl of Leinster, Lady Rose Boughton and others have arrived at Cheltenham Spa. On Thursday last (3rd Sept.) Cheltenham Theatre was honoured by the presence of the Prince of Wales and the Duke of Sussex who were received with enthusiasm by one of the most numerous and brilliant audiences it has ever boasted." What is more important for this record, however, is that included in the list of distinguished guests on this great occasion was the name of Dr. Edward Jenner[29]—a mighty sparrow among the modest peacocks. One can imagine his going home that night to tell Catherine, Edward, and young Worgan all about it, with the faithful Richard, perhaps, listening at the foot of the basement stairs. He probably also told them that the great Mr. Russell had started his stage career as a juvenile under the family friend Charles Dibdin. This was also the first occasion, as far as can be determined, upon which Jenner met the Duke of Sussex, by far the most intellectual of the King's sons. The following Saturday, the royal brothers left Cheltenham for Ragley Hall in the company of the Marquess of Hertford.

When he was not busy with young Edward, John Worgan spent the autumn busily studying the Italian language. He was enthusiastic, as his mastery of the tongue enabled him to read and enjoy the poetry, and he decided that he would translate the sonnets of Petrarch into English. On the other hand, he was still distracted by unrequited love. It is uncertain whether this was a new passion or a lingering memory of the past, but it touched off periods of melancholy that affected him profoundly. He was probably working too hard in any case, but he still had dreams of entering the university the following year. He had a very respectable circle of friends in Cheltenham and was patronized by Thomas Pruen, who spent a great deal of time at the Jenners' home.

It gave the doctor a great deal of pleasure to once more be able to spend money on the things he felt were important. Even though his new grant money had not yet arrived, its magnitude made it possible to plan for the future as well as move in the upper circles of society without embarrassment. In November the first substantial reward from his supporters overseas arrived—some £4,000 from the grateful people of India. With the considerable earnings of the Cheltenham season, plus his government grant, 1807 was to be the most lucrative year of his life. His loyal friends in India— Russell, Bentinck, and others—had effectively broken the logjam. Certainly one of the things that could be done, now that there was real money, was to secure the young tutor's entrance to the university.

The lovely Miss Brunton's summer romance came to its happy conclusion and caused still more comment in the town when she married the Earl of Craven early in December. This wealthy nobleman was the son of Jenner's good friend and patient the Margravine of Anspach. The young actress was endowed with great physical beauty. Fitzgerald refers to her as "that beautiful Louisa Brunton," while the more prosaic Farington calls her "extremely handsome and striking," and records the happy event in his diary. The romance seems to have been swift and spontaneous. On December 8 he writes, "Miss Brunton the actress a few days since sent in her resignation to the manager of Covent Garden Theatre, preparatory to her nuptials with the Earl of Craven, who by the marriage articles has settled £5,000 a year upon her." When the fortunate Louisa returned to Cheltenham it was no longer to the Theatre Royal.

We have already noted Jenner's aplomb in this scarlet world of the Regency rakes. Craven had been the first "protector" of the celebrated courtesan, Harriet Wilson, in 1802. She was then fifteen years of age but eventually became a kind of uncrowned queen of the demimonde. Wellington, in the bitterness of his obligatory marriage, sought her embraces, as did Lord Yarmouth on his return from bondage in France. She was also mistress to the most notorious rake of them all and probably the closest friend of Jenner's—Colonel Berkeley, the earl's eldest son. Harriet Wilson's younger sister Sophia, incidentally, married another noble patron of the town, the Earl of Berwick, in 1812. The Duke of Argyll, who fell passionately in love with Harriet after she broke with Craven, later married the daughter of Cheltenham's arrant Countess of Jersey, the long-time mistress of the Prince of Wales. Such was the lush world that seethed around the unruffled doctor and his very proper wife.

The Prince himself after a sojourn at Ragley spent a few days with the Berkeleys. Whatever the enthusiasm he met with in Cheltenham, it was not echoed in other parts of the country. He grossly upset the countess in not approving the room she had allocated to him, and he was indifferent to the meal arrangements. Possibly the meeting with Lady Hertford at Ragley had not gone off to his liking.[30] "At Bristol, at Gloucester and wherever he went, people were dissatisfied with his behavior," wrote Farington on November 23.[31] No doubt the forthright countess told her doctor all about it herself when she arrived in Cheltenham later in the season. Jenner was a patient and sympathetic listener.

It was Catherine's invalid condition that undoubtedly saved Jenner from an almost permanent state of social embarrassment. Scarcely one of the vast circle of grand dames who patronized him could possibly have been received by his pious wife, particularly since these ladies were not at all discreet in their adventures. The Duchess of Devonshire had two illegitimate children while she was married to her lord, Mrs. Jordan presented her duke with no less than ten (having previously borne four others by two different fathers), and Lady Craven lived openly with the Margrave of Anspach for eight years without bothering to divorce her husband. Lady Berkeley, Lady Crewe, and Lady Spencer were not quite so outrageous, but they were nevertheless far too abandoned for Catherine Jenner. Even the innocent doctor's respectable patrons in the peerage—there were a few—could scarcely have brought their ladies to St. George's Place. Lady Elgin, Lady Bellasye, and Lady Borington all ran away with their lovers in due course. As for the remaining gentlemen of Jenner's camp, they were extremely "progressive"—Berkeley, Egremont, Hertford, and Craven being among the most extravagant rakes of the age. So it came about that Jenner seldom entertained these people at his own house, and since Catherine was unable to go out in the evenings, he mingled alone with this scarlet entourage, uncontaminated and unshocked, while benefitting mightily from their powerful support. There was not a moralistic bone in his body, and he obviously enjoyed the company of his friends without feeling that he was endorsing their sexual morals. In a rather poignant sense, Catherine's ill health actually benefitted the vaccination cause. Had she been free to accompany him on his social occasions, he may have been restricted to less profitable pastures.

But the gay season of 1807 was actually the lull before the storm. The Peninsular War was about to explode on the world, and the sporadic campaigns since 1803 were to level out into the long, bleak, and bloody struggle that ended at Waterloo. The French armies entered Spain late in the year, and the Spanish vainly tried to buy safety by cooperating in a Franco-Spanish occupation of Portugal. The British government swiftly acted to counter these moves, and men who had been enjoying the royal month at Cheltenham were sent straight to the war. General Beresford,[32] second only to the great Wellington, left his strolls with Lord St. Vincent—Nelson's old commander—and went directly to the Portuguese island of Madeira to prevent its falling into the hands of the French. St. Vincent himself and General Tarleton were called back to London while many a dashing young officer who had never smelled powder before left Well Walk for a lonely grave in the Torres Vedras.

Since the tragic death of Jenner's nephew in 1795, the tide of war had not swirled too near to him, but now things began to change as one after another of his closest friends became involved in the war. George Berkeley was sent to the Portuguese coast to command the naval forces there, and Rowland Hill's nephew, *Sir* Rowland Hill,[33] covered himself with glory in the first battle of the Spanish campaign at Rolica, where he commanded a brigade. Both of James Moore's brothers were immediately posted to the front; Captain Moore to the Tagus and Sir John to command the first British expeditionary force. The old order was changing. Serious as the Napoleonic threat had always been, with the actual opening of a land campaign on the continent of Europe, the war was brought home to everyone with a much greater impact. Even before the eruption in the peninsula, Jenner had been getting more involved in attempts to help friends who were un-lucky enough to be caught in the war zone. But now appeals came to him from friend and stranger alike.

Lord Somerville and Sir John Sinclair, both important sup-porters of Jenner's in Cheltenham, were bitter enemies. Each had been Minister of Agriculture with the successive changes of gov-ernment, and on the death of Pitt, Somerville once more ousted his rival. A most delicate situation indeed developed for Jenner, who not only knew the archenemies very well but must have been constantly running into them in Cheltenham. Sinclair's son was cut off by hostile armies in Vienna where he was a student, and it was to Jenner that the father immediately turned. Without hesitation the doctor made contact with the French Emperor, and passports were secured for the young man's safe return home.[34] Somerville, however, did not become disenchanted with Jenner; in fact the peer became increasingly active in the vaccination cause, and after the peace he worked closely with Jenner in Cheltenham local affairs.

Two other gentlemen were liberated on direct appeal to Napo-leon—Mr. Gold and Mr. Garland—though I can find no con-nection between them and Jenner. There was another case, how-ever, of a completely different nature that did not involve the French government at all. Nor did it concern an innocent stranded civilian. Charles Murray, then secretary of the Royal Jennerian Society, came to Jenner with a tragic story from a kinsman in the colonies—W. D. Powell, Chief Justice of the Court of the King's Bench in Upper Canada. Powell's young son got involved in an insurrection against the King of Spain. His real intention had been to escape from Santo Domingo, where he had unwisely been persuaded to engage in a mercantile enterprise. The various moods of the dictator Desalines made the boy frightened for his life, and he agreed to join a ship under the command of the revolutionary leader Miranda, who put in at the island on his way to Venezuela. Young Powell, who was only twenty, felt that once free of Desalines he might contrive to get passage back to Canada. However, the expedition failed and while Miranda es-caped, the youth was among the "rebels" captured by the Spanish forces. After a trial, he evaded the death penalty but was sentenced to ten years' imprisonment with hard labor at the notorious fortress of Omoa on the Mexican coast. It was at this point that the stricken father asked Murray to enlist the help of Dr. Jenner. The good doctor, bearing in mind the Balmis expedition of the previous year, hoped that perhaps the Spanish ruler would have sufficient interest in the discoverer of vaccination to listen to his plea. Baron writes:

To obtain the remission of his [Powell's] sentence, Jenner directly memorialized the King of Spain; and it is to the honour of all parties to be able to say that the appeal was not made in vain. After lamenting that it could not be presented through the medium of an ambassador, he stated that he was encouraged to hope from the magnanimity that had recently been shown by His Majesty in the glorious expedition to disseminate through every quarter of the world, alike to friends and enemies, the discovery which he had the happines of introducing, that his petition on behalf of the unfortunate object would be received with clemency.[35]

Like Napoleon, the Spanish king was unable to deny Jenner his prayer, and the young man was released from his living tomb to be restored to the arms of his family in Canada. From York (now Toronto) on February 19, 1808, Powell was able to write a moving letter of thanks to his benefactor in Cheltenham, announcing his safe arrival home.

Somehow or other across the war-torn world Jenner's correspondence reached him eventually, although some of it took a very long time. To be sure, the service had vastly improved since 1805 when the Post Master General had established a government post office in Cheltenham with a regular postman to make daily deliveries. The fact that it was in the charge of the easygoing Mr. Entwistle eventually caused problems in efficiency, but it was a great improvement on the previous "amateur" service. Jenner's mail, from abroad at least, was generally encouraging. Dr. Sacco wrote a long, detailed letter from the heart of the war zone at Trieste on January 5, and the record it revealed undoubtedly gave considerable pleasure to its recipient.

During eight years I reckon more than 680,000 vaccinated by my own hand, and more than 700,000 by my deputies in the different departments of the kingdom. I assure you out of a population of six millions, to have vaccinated one million three hundred thousand is something to boast of; and I flatter myself that in Italy I have been the means of promoting vaccination in a degree, which no other kingdom of the same population has equalled.[36]

Nor was Jenner the only one in his household corresponding on vaccination business. We find young Worgan writing to his friend Henry Biddulph in Bristol.

> Cheltenham, Feb. 27th, 1808.
>
> . . . On communicating to Dr. Jenner your description of the appearances that followed vaccine inoculation in the arm of your little girl, he requested me to inform you that he is at present fully satisfied that the former inoculation was properly effective;

But later the letter inevitably takes up the theme of his love affairs, though in the deserted condition of Cheltenham in the winter the appearance of new beauties must have been very rare.

> . . . My thoughts as you know have been harassed in the most distressing manner, particularly by one of a tender nature which has probed my heart to the bottom. I stand in a painful dilemma, between doubt and hope, between appearance and uncertainty, between duty and inclination.

But Worgan never mentioned the names of the maidens to whom his heart so repeatedly went out. At the end of his letter he proudly returns to the subject of vaccination.

> The printed poem which I have taken the liberty to enclose is to be read before the Royal Jennerian Society, on their Anniversary festival, May 17th, which is Dr. Jenner's birthday, and is regularly commemorated by a splendid dinner at the Crown and Anchor Tavern, at which the Duke of York ordinarily presides.[37]

Though the boy may not have attended some of the more sophisticated routs, he would certainly have socialized in many a drawing room of visiting intellectuals. Jenner had an excellent library at St. George's Place, and the three local book salons, Seldon's, Harward's, and Mrs. Jones's were readily accessible. Then of course, Mr. Ruff's library was right at the doorstep, so to speak. Worgan found Cheltenham's resources satisfying to his almost boundless appetite for learning. In contrast, the family visits to

Berkeley, where there was practically nothing, were difficult for Worgan.

As a member of the local authority, Jenner now had the power to regulate public health medicine, a subject dear to his heart. He was preoccupied with the incubation potential provided by unsanitary housing relative to cholera and typhus, besides smallpox. In 1808, he proposed a sewerage system for the whole town that would stem from the single pipe in St. George's Place. He was one of the committee set up for the purpose, which included Thomas Pruen, Rev. Hugh Williams, and Colonel Agg of the Hewletts. There was little chance of a financial venture of this magnitude being viable until the war was over, but it reveals an interesting social relationship between the latter gentleman and Jenner. Colonel Agg was a colorful character who had made his fortune in the East and had returned, as did so many who followed him, to live graciously at Cheltenham. In his big house almost at the top of Cleeve Hill he entertained many of the great figures of the age. He became a kind of Cheltenham legend and there are stories relating him to Byron and Shelley. Colonel Agg put his vast wealth into local commercial ventures when his sister married John Gardner, a brewer and half owner of the Cheltenham and Gloucester Bank. One might indeed call Colonel Agg the prototype Cheltenham Anglo-Indian, and Jenner, it will be recalled, had been the first local doctor to seriously study the problems of Europeans returning from the East. The two men undoubtedly had a great deal in common besides sewers. In March, workmen excavating a courtyard adjoining Jenner's garden uncovered an earthenware jar containing a hoard of gold coins dating from Philip and Mary (1553–58) to Charles I (1625–49). The work was described as the digging of a "vault" but it was probably exploratory work on the sewer project.[38]

While the doctor was going about his civic duties and medical affairs through the winter in Cheltenham, the open season for abuse resumed in London. There were two periodicals in particular that kept up the attack: the *Medical Observer* in rather restrained terms, depending upon misinformation rather than crude abuse, and the *British Forum* which was frankly vituperative. An example of the intelligence level of the latter's readers is well illustrated in a leader on March 28. It demanded, "Which has proved a more striking instance of the public credulity, the gas lights of Mr. Winsor or the cow-pox?" There was another sheet entitled the *Cowpox Chronicle or Medical Reporter*. Says Baron who in 1807 becomes a first-hand reporter:

This was printed on stamped paper and circulated through the post office. I have understood that the indulgence of their humour became at last rather too expensive for the proprietors. They put forth their lucubrations in the shape of advertisements in which they parodied all the ordinary topics that fill the columns of a newspaper; but they were not aware that the duty for the advertisements would fall upon them. This weight, however, was not required to sink the publication. Its atrocious falsehoods, its course and disgusting ribaldry, and its impious scurrility must soon have caused its destruction.[39]

One might well assume that with the endorsement Jenner's campaign was receiving all over the world, this grotesque vilification at home would have been better ignored. By any reasonable standard his case had been proven—the growing pains were over. However, with vested interests of the medical establishment still under assault, there was little chance of the vaccination battle being won by default; and the loyal forces did not handle the situation very wisely. Some of the sincerest of Jenner's friends flattered his enemies by taking them too seriously. Debating with these people was a waste of time, and after the first few years of bitter experience, Jenner himself concentrated purely upon the spread of vaccination and the abolition of smallpox inoculation. He believed in actions rather than words and showed not the slightest interest in personally meeting, arguing, or dealing in any way with his opponents. All his writings were aimed at explanation, elucidation, and repudiation of charges of failure. He *never* conceded in the remotest way that his system was open to debate, and he would himself painstakingly and patiently run down every individual case that had allegedly failed. Nevertheless he was at times embarrassed and even discouraged when men like Dunning appeared apprehensive about the strength of his position over some particularly vicious attack. Since Goldston's humiliating refusal to meet him, Jenner was not interested in personal confrontations. For this reason he was very upset when the Royal Jennerian Society agreed to meet a group of doctors at Ringwood in Hampshire to discuss vaccination failures in that area. "An excessive alarm had been caused by false and exaggerated reports in newspapers and various periodical publications. The authors of these statements were the same individuals who had distinguished themselves by a blind and inveterate opposition to the strongest evidence." To even suggest such a meeting in the face of the worldwide proof of vaccination's efficacy was an insult to its discoverer. But unfortunately, Mr. George Rose,[40] a most loyal worker in Jenner's interest, incidentally, besides being Vice-President of the Board of Trade, was also deputy warden of the New Forest and M.P. for Christchurch. He apparently felt that he was only being loyal to his constituents when he persuaded the society to cooperate. Jenner, of course, would have no part in it, but extraordinarily enough, Ring, Blair, and several other of the doctors accompanied Rose to Ringwood. There was actually no tangible evidence at all to form the basis of a conference; it was quite plainly a ruse to get Jenner in a position where he could be personally abused and perhaps subjected to mob behavior. "I have no doubt," said Baron, "that they would have made it the occasion of personal insult to him." As it was, the meeting held at Ringwood Town Hall was something of a fiasco. Without Jenner present there could be no sport, though the *Medical Observer* tried to convey the appearance of public apprehension by solemnly announcing "that the deputies carried pistols to defend themselves against the astonished people of Ringwood." These same deputies humiliated themselves by spending two whole days with the hostile doctors, going through over two hundred cases without finding "one person in Ringwood or its neighbourhood who had caught the smallpox after going through regular and complete vaccination." Since the whole business had been arranged by the anti-vaccination forces, there was no way in which these gentry could explain away the result, and no way to distort the conclusions since the investigation took place in front of an audience of the townspeople. Nevertheless it was unfortunate that the society stooped so low as to be part of what had obviously been planned as a personal attack on Jenner. Nor was the "vindication" of much value, since everyone of intelligence realized that there had never been any real evidence to investigate.

The melancholy picture of the London scene was not all related

to the invective against Jenner. The war also brought its tragedies
in the most indirect ways. The marriage of two of vaccination's
staunchest pioneers foundered on the rocks of wartime separation
and loneliness. On December 22, in the Sheriff's Court, Lord Elgin
was awarded £10,000 in damages against Mr. Ferguson of Raith for
"criminal connexion" with Lady Elgin.[41] This was followed by
divorce the following year, and both parties remarried soon afterward—Lady Elgin to the partner of her intrigue. In the period
of her exile from England and her separation from her husband,
she had lost her little son, William, whom she worshipped. Undoubtedly kindness and consolation were desperately needed.
Mr. Ferguson, as it happened, was detained in Paris with her
while her lord was confined in the south.[42]

With the opening of spring, young Worgan worked urgently,
almost as though pressed for time. He had taught himself Italian,
Hebrew, and French in addition to the classical tongues, but this
hard work, much as he loved it, was too great a strain; also, at
the age of sixteen (his birthday was not until November 8), he
was allowing his physical condition to be sapped by his preoccupation with the gentler sex.[43] The work and the emotional strain
combined were too much. Jenner took him down to Berkeley for
a couple of weeks, before going to London in May, and left him
there when he proceeded to the metropolis. The village apparently
did not agree with Worgan—either its quietness after the stimulating intellectual adventures in Cheltenham or, more likely, the
climate and the low-lying lands along the estuary. He once more
succumbed to typhus, and when he was well enough to be moved,
had to go to Bristol to be again cared for by his mother. Jenner,
when he left for London, must surely have sensed that the poor
lad did not have much longer to live. Catherine, of course, would
not have been able to take care of him even though, according to
Baron, he was "Companion to the delicate and religious Mrs. Jenner." On May 17 the annual dinner was held, and the boy's poem
was read to a fitting acclaim. It would have been so much more
moving, however, had Worgan attended himself—which was naturally what Jenner had hoped for.

Aside from the scurrilous journalism and anxiety about poor
Worgan's health, Jenner was fairly contented about the way things
were progressing in London, where his friends had worse problems

than he. Actually, society was in turmoil. Since he seldom came out of his provincial cocoon during the winter, the spring emergence always revealed a new social panorama. This year he was not terribly affected—except for the domestic problems of his most powerful supporters, which might deter them from continued efforts on his behalf. And there were also the problems of growing old. As he himself drew nearer to his sixties more and more of his colleagues sank by the wayside. The domestic tragedies that afflicted Jenner's most important allies at this time did naturally reduce his support in the Upper House.

All the royal dukes who patronized him were having their difficulties. The Duke of Clarence (who maintained so openly his menage with Mrs. Jordan) was growing increasingly worried about his critical financial condition. He was hoping for a naval command now that the war had taken a more serious pattern, but the government was coldly unsympathetic.[44] And when Jenner met the Duke of York, as usual, at the birthday banquet on May 17, he had no inkling of the heartache that was disturbing that royal breast. The poor man was in much more serious trouble in his domestic affairs than his brother the Duke of Clarence. His mistress, Mrs. Mary Ann Clarke, was slowly but surely ruining him.[45] Not being able to obtain the £1,000 a month he had earlier undertaken to pay her, she evolved a form of corrupt military patronage that was possible only because the duke was Commander-in-Chief of the army. The duke, who was perhaps more foolish than criminal, suffered greatly through trial by public opinion long before the matter was investigated officially in 1809. These troubles did, indeed, eventually interfere with his activity in the vaccination cause, and eventually he faded out of the campaign completely.

The Duke of Sussex, not only a friend but soon to be a patient of Jenner's, was still smarting from the complications of his alliance with Lady Augusta Murray in 1793, which had been nullified under the terms of the Royal Marriage Act. The lady in question, herself descended from the Kings of Scotland, England, and France, was not easily disposed of. Law or no law, she styled herself a princess and insisted upon the royal status of her son. There was no doubt but what she was abominably treated, particularly since Sussex, initially loyal and brave in her support, eventually gave up the struggle. Needless to say, this made him extremely unpopular among the people as well as among his erstwhile friends. He became very run down and unhappy. But the heartache and sorrows suffered by certain members of the royal family were nothing compared with those of one who outranked them all.

The unfortunate Princess of Wales had terrible financial as well as domestic problems. Not only had her husband finally and completely rejected her and taken her daughter from her, but a powerful faction was endeavoring to prove adultery against her— a capital offense if pursued to its ultimate end. On top of this her debts were mounting to the point where some tradesmen would no longer supply her. She scandalized more and more people by pretending to seduce certain prominent men from their wives, and on a more serious note, did actually have an affair with George Canning. Indeed, even the rather frigid Thomas Lawrence was whispered about in connection with her. By and large Jenner's friends were loyal and sympathetic to her owing to the abominable treatment she had received from the Prince of Wales. So, at first, was Lord Eldon, who was no friend of Jenner's. But her fondness for the doctor himself is rather puzzling. It is very hard to imagine him at one of her outrageous drawing rooms where she occasionally stripped to the waist. Yet it was while he was in London this summer that Baron tells us: "The day before I saw him (Jenner) he had had an interview with the Princess of Wales and he showed me a watch Her Royal Highness had presented to him on that occasion."[46] This at a time when she could scarcely pay her grocery bills!

But the complications of London society and the disasters befalling his friends were increasingly disenchanting to the basically unsophisticated doctor, and he disencumbered himself of the rashly acquired lease of a house there. When he came up in May for the birthday banquet he stayed at Fladong's Hotel in Oxford Street. Just around the corner from the hotel, off Portman Square, lived Hoppner's friend Lord Borington—not a royal duke to be sure but a peer who as earnestly as Jenner himself saw variola inoculation as the most important social issue of the day and was dedicated to bringing about its abolition through parliamentary legislation. It was the very day after the Jennerian banquet— indeed, Borington probably attended it—that society was stunned by the news that the peer's wife, Augusta, had run away with Sir Arthur Paget. The Boringtons and the Pagets were now well-known figures in Cheltenham society, and both were valuable allies to Jenner. Lord Borington was a serious, scholarly type who had been at the same Oxford College as Paget, though he was a year his junior. Like Jenner he was a Fellow of the Royal Society and was one of the more aggressive supporters of vaccination. His great wealth was no doubt the reason why his lady married him since she was the younger and poorer daughter of the Earl of Westmorland. (To complicate matters for Jenner, her elder sister, Sarah, was the daughter-in-law of the celebrated and wealthy Lady Jersey of Cheltenham.) His lordship obtained a divorce on the following February 14, leaving the lovers free to marry. In this particular family tragedy, however, Jenner may well have bene-fitted, since seven months after the divorce his lordship married Frances Talbot, a far more serious young woman than the flighty Augusta. In the typical Cheltenham bluestocking tradition, his new wife was, among other things, a connoisseur of painting and vitally concerned in the interests of her intellectual husband, in-cluding vaccination. The strong ties between the Jerseys and the Egremonts on the one hand, and Jenner's urgent need for Borington's parliamentary support against smallpox inoculation on the other, again made his role a very delicate one when the scandal broke; but, as usual he somehow managed to cope.

Then on April 7 a tragedy far greater than the domestic wrangling noted above took place. Lord Hardwick's son and heir, Lord Royston, was drowned when his boat was sunk in a storm off Lubeck, within a month of his twenty-fourth birthday. When the news reached England, Lady Hardwick was so prostrated with grief that her friends failed to recognize her. Sir George Beaumont visited them,

and found a circle of several persons. He did not perceive Lady Hard-wick till, on enquiring of his lordship of her, she lifted her veil, and showed her face which was reduced to apparently half its natural size and her eyes *"looked like beads"* having lost all lustre. When she first heard of Lord Royston's death, she was for three days *silent* and as one in a state of stupefaction. At the end of that time she was relieved by tears.[47]

But this, alas, was not the end of the tragedy. The new heir, and recipient of the courtesy title of Lord Royston, was their second son, Charles James. He died exactly two years later, in April, 1810, within three months of his thirteenth birthday. This was the last of the Hardwick sons, and on the earl's death the title passed to a nephew. The impact of all this on Jenner was disastrous, coming as it did at a time that he needed every ally he could get. The Hardwicks completely withdrew from the vaccination cause, sold all their Cheltenham holdings, and retired from public life. Never had the doctor so desperately needed support in the House of Lords as in the years following 1810, when he was without Lord Hardwick's support.

It was while he was in London this somewhat chaotic summer that Jenner first met Dr. Baron. Again no date is given—not even the month—but the occasion may be described in Baron's own words.

He was living at Fladong's Hotel, Oxford Street in the summer of 1808 making arrangements for the national vaccine establishment. I was introduced to him at that place by Dr. Maton[48]—I little thought that it would so speedily lead to an intimacy and ultimately to a friendship which terminated only in his death and placed me in a relationship to his memory that no-one could have anticipated. . . . He condescended as to an equal; the restraint and embarrassment that might naturally have been felt in the presence of one so eminent vanished in an instant. . . . Though more than twenty years have elapsed since this interview took place, I remember it and all its accompaniments, with the most perfect accuracy. He was dressed in a blue coat, white waistcoat, nankeen breeches and white stockings. All the tables in his apartment were covered with letters and papers on the subject of vaccination, and the establishment of the new National Vaccine Institution.[49]

Baron was twenty-three years old and had taken his M.D. at Edinburgh at the age of nineteen.

Dr. William George Maton was a physician at Westminster Hospital with Thomas Bradley, who probably introduced him to Jenner. He was only thirty-four when he brought young Baron round to Fladong's Hotel but he had already achieved some stature in his field and ultimately went on to become physician extraordinary to Queen Charlotte, the Duchess of Kent, and—much more interesting—many years later, the young Princess Victoria. Baron asked Maton to arrange the meeting—"impelled by a desire to do homage to a man whose public and private character had already secured my warmest admiration." His knowledge of Jenner's private character undoubtedly came from Baillie who took the young man under his wing when he came down from Edinburgh in 1806. "Dr. Baron was also in constant intercourse with Dr. Baillie," writes Baron's biographer, "who took an interest in his welfare and selected Cheltenham as the place where he should commence practice in 1808."[50] So to Cheltenham he went and stayed there for just under a year. There is no trace in the records of his initial stay in the town, and it is, indeed, ignored by most reference books. Of course, Baron did return there in 1832 to spend the rest of his life and to complete his biography of Jenner.

In the spring of 1809 the position of Physician to the Royal Infirmary at Gloucester fell vacant through death, and Baillie immediately entered a request that the post be allocated to Baron. His wish was granted and the young man assumed the post the same year. Here he worked beside Dr. Trye for the next two years and was, of course, only nine miles away from Jenner to whom he became increasingly attached. Both Jenner and Baillie seemed to have had an urge to attract likely doctors to Cheltenham and the years 1809 and 1810 were exceptional in this respect. It is interesting that Baron says nothing of the kindness and help he received from Baillie at the beginning of his career—before he had even met Jenner—but the meeting at Fladong's Hotel so swept him off his feet that he described its impact even thirty years later with an extravagance that is awesome. It is quite obvious that he did not anticipate a lifelong friendship when he came into the idol's presence. "The greatness of his fame, his exalted talents, and the honours heaped upon him by all the most distinguished bodies of the civilised world, while they made me desirous of offering my tribute of respect to him, forbade the expectation of more than such an acknowledgement as a youth, circumstanced as I was, might have expected."

Jenner was still detained in London when what was to be an important vaccination center was inaugurated on his home ground. On Tuesday, July 11, the foundation stone of Cheltenham Chapel in St. George's Place was laid by Rev. Rowland Hill. The site chosen adjoined Jenner's garden and was formerly in the possession of Colonel Riddell. On account of Hill's being a national figure, the ceremony attracted wide interest. Some three thousand people packed the narrow thoroughfare and the little lane leading to the chapel. Jenner's house looked straight down this lane, and it was to be a well-trodden path to his friend's pulpit for many a long year. The two men had the highest respect for each other, and though Jenner differed in his religious views, he thoroughly enjoyed Hill's sermons. On one occasion Hill introduced Jenner to a nobleman, saying, "Allow me to present to your Lordship my friend, Dr. Jenner, who has been the means of saving more lives than any other man." To which Jenner replied, "Ah, would I, like you, could save souls!"[51] Hill's elder brother Richard died in the course of the year, leaving his considerable fortune to the clergyman, and incidentally, making the cost of the chapel a negligible matter.

Nor was the learned clergyman the only new neighbor. The environment of St. George's Place was further enriched by the advent of at least one celebrated painter—no doubt reminding Jenner of the halcyon days with the Hunters. Adjoining the site of the chapel a new terrace of houses named St. George's Square was being built, facing a small field. In the course of the summer, the miniature painter, John Engleheart[52] the younger, moved from London to occupy number seven—the end house nearest to the chapel—and actually overlooking Jenner's garden. Engleheart had a great following in his day and exhibited regularly at the Royal Academy from 1801 to 1828. He must have known both Hill and Jenner, living, as it were, cheek by jowl with them.

For one of those present at the opening of the chapel, however, it was to be a farewell visit. Sir Henry Mildmay died four months later, leaving eleven children, several of whom married into families prominent in local society—the Radnors, Bouveries, Radstocks, and others. He was only forty-four years of age, and with Mildmay's death Jenner lost yet another of his bulwarks in Parliament. Years later the Radnors sold their local mansion to Matthew Baillie when he moved to Cheltenham.

Toward the end of the year 1808 the Royal Jennerian Society unofficially came to an inglorious, almost unnoticed end. Its demise was probably owing to a clash of personalities between

Jenner and Walker. The latter had ideas of his own about vaccination, and once ensconced as medical director, had gone his own way. He deviated in too many ways from the orthodox principles for Jenner or indeed many of the other members to be happy. There was a small faction who felt that it would be unwise to stir things up, particularly since public support was not all that it might be. After Walker ignored repeated admonitions between 1804 and 1806, the committee decided that they would have to consider introducing a new medical director. Strangely enough, Jenner's earliest London supporter, Dr. Cline, joined Bankes and the minority in trying to come to some accommodation, but they were overruled and a ballot was arranged for August 8, 1806. Angerstein, Lettsom, and William Blair, the surgeon, solidly supported the ballot, but Walker solved the problem himself. He sent in his resignation the very day of the voting in order to avoid the humiliation of being discharged.[53] But the Royal Jennerian Society was finished. Subscriptions were not paid and the royal patrons were alienated by the petty bickering that had taken place. The society dragged on, in name at least, for a further two years and then closed down for lack of funds.

Riddell's book, *The Riddellian System or New Medical Improvements,* came out in 1808, but it was published in London, not Cheltenham, which indicates that the quack enjoyed more than just local celebrity. Jenner's latest pamphlet, *Facts . . . Respecting Variculus Contagion,* was published by Gosnell of Little Queen Street a few months later on November 18. The image of rivalry for the Cheltenham medical patronage was probably very much in the prosperous Riddell's mind. Jenner, however, had new problems and was in no mood or condition to dispute with quacks—no matter how high up in the social scale. There was every sign that his few years of happiness were drawing to a close. A chapter of sorrow started with the sad reports from Gloucestershire at the end of the summer. John Worgan was dying.

The young tutor had spent a very melancholy summer away from his patron and friend. He apparently never came back to St. George's Place after his partial recovery under his mother's care, and he remained in the cottage at Berkeley where he would be free of work and responsibility, but also free of everything he had learned to consider essential: good conversation, literature, and most of all, his friends. Under the circumstances it is little wonder that his condition did not improve. Worgan wrote some very dejected letters from the village toward the end of the year after he had been alone for some considerable time. On November 24, he mentions that Dr. Jenner just returned to Berkeley the night before. It was apparently a short visit, however, since three weeks later (December 15) Worgan was still alone. He wrote to Rev. Biddulph (not the son), "In a few months the period of three years I engaged to remain with Dr. Jenner will have expired. . . . I propose to enter (university) the first term after the long vacation."[54] He goes on, rather pathetically, to enquire about possible financial aid. On February 16 he is unmistakably depressed. He wrote to a Mr. D. C. Wait:

It is with much reluctance that I make myself so troublesome to you, but in this outlandish corner of the globe we have no learning, either ancient or modern, foreign or native. . . . I have postponed the furtherance of my progress in Italian and my intended acquisition of Spanish, till I have met with some congenial soul to accompany me in my studies. It is the most heartless of all employments to engage in learning a fresh language without a fellow student *or trot* by your side. I shall therefore abandon my projected pursuit of modern continental literature until I have quitted the solitary cells of Berkeley.[55]

It is conceivable that the doctor, realizing the boy's tubercular condition, was not very happy having Worgan living with the family but did not have the heart to send him back to Bristol. The natural companion for his studies of course would have been young Edward, for whose instruction he had been employed. Certainly Jenner tended Worgan whenever he could, and we know the doctor was in Berkeley on February 9; but no family and no *trot*. It is a shame that no books were brought from Cheltenham to help his morale. As the winter gave place to spring his condition became increasingly poor, and the only kindness to be done for him was to arrange that he at least die at home.

"At the end of March," wrote Worgan's biographer, " a copious spitting of blood confined him to his room, where his mother, called from Bristol, nursed him under the tender care of Dr. Jenner. He appears to have improved sufficiently to be moved to

Bristol in the doctor's carriage about the end of May." His death was now just a matter of time. He actually lasted another two months but suffered considerably—emotionally as well as physically. His aesthetic soul had been shown paradise while he was in Cheltenham, with everything a young romantic could desire: books, conversation, beauty, music, and—most of all—companionship. Then came his sickness and it was all snatched away; and now he was dying—abysmal tragedy in a boy of seventeen.

On the thirtieth of June he requested that his copy of the poems of Rev. Henry Moore[56] be given to Mr. T. S. Biddulph after his death. He had been very concerned about his reputation as a literary man surviving his passing, though he tried to conquer this vanity as being too worldly in one facing death. . . . John Worgan died on the twenty-fifth of July 1809. In the course of the night he frequently enquired the hour and was much employed in private prayer. At one o'clock he desired to be supported in his bed, saying "This is about the time." Within the hour he haemorrhaged badly and said, "Gracious Saviour, support me." Then being speechless, he smiled at his mother and expired.[57]

So ended the brief sojourn of poor Worgan. His poetry is nowhere outstanding except in individual lines, which indicates that he had not yet mastered his craft. Yet he was undoubtedly a genius, and was taken seriously by the important men who knew him—Jenner, Hayley, Pruen, Biddulph (senior), and John Ring. As soon as he had news of the boy's death, Jenner wrote to his informant.

Your letter came too late for me to make any observations upon what you drew up for insertion in the Bristol paper, respecting our dear departed friend—I beg you will present my best wishes to Mrs. Worgan and tell her, unless she particularly wishes it, I should be sorry to put her to the expense of a ring; but yet I should like to have something in remembrance of poor John. A book would be acceptable.[58]

Worgan's "intimate acquaintance," Mr. Pruen, wrote an excellent appreciation in the new *Cheltenham Chronicle*—and his friend Drayton wrote a poet's tribute. The latter had a great respect for the brilliance of the dead boy and made no secret of his feelings; "though Worgan's senior by several years [he] has candidly acknowledged, that whatever refinement and polish his slender vein of poetic ore has attained, he owes it to his young friend's superior judgment and taste."[59]

But while the ordeal of the boy's death was dragging to its close, tragedy just as deep had happened to others of Jenner's friends. Taking up the thread of events at the beginning of the year once more, we find that the war was not progressing at all well. News from the Spanish front indicated that after the initial victories at Rolica and Vimiera, the British forces threatened to be overrun by the massively reinforced French armies. At the end of the year Sir John Moore's troops began to retreat toward the coast with an eye to an evacuation by sea. For a time the maneuver seemed to be going according to plan, and the French were defeated whenever the forces made contact. Farington related on January 11, "The British cavalry had had several engagements with the French cavalry and had been successful in all of them—General Lefevre was taken and brought to Plymouth." Then on the sixteenth came the bloody victory of La Caruña and the subsequent safe evacuation of the British army. But General Moore was killed in action.

Jenner had returned to London in February, not only because he was concerned about the way the Vaccine Institute was going, but also because he was due to have his portrait painted by Lawrence. The sad news from Spain, however, somewhat changed his plans, and he felt that this was no time to bother James Moore. "As for yourself, my dear friend," he wrote to Moore on February 9, "It cannot be expected that you can at present coolly exercise your correct judgement on anything of the kind."

Lawrence had by this time painted most of Jenner's friends, and it is likely that the doctor's commitment to sit for him was the main reason for his going through with the London arrangements once he realized that it would be out of the question to bother the Moores. Perhaps under the circumstances Lawrence also would have welcomed a postponement, since he was still being badgered by the enemies of the Princess of Wales and his reputation was paying dearly for his loyalty to her. More than ever she seemed to lack common sense in all her vain activities, and alienated many of her remaining friends. She even shocked poor Lysons for instance when she seduced—or pretended to seduce—the husband of one of his friends in Gloucester. As long as one's intrigues were confined to the capital they might be ignored, but when the tentacles of the aging and rather gross princess reached out to the Gloucestershire countryside it was too much for the virtuous antiquarian. Jenner and Lawrence, though Gloucestershire men, apparently took a more charitable view. They visited the Princess at Blackheath this winter when the un- happy woman's fortunes were at their lowest ebb. (She was in a state of bankruptcy to the extent of £75,000 despite the fact that she received an income of some £17,000 per annum.)[60] Jenner as it happened was very concerned about London's foul atmosphere during the winter months, with hundreds of thousands of chimney pots contributing their quota of pollution. A remark made by Lawrence in this context reveals at least one trip to Blackheath. Farington recorded that Jenner "could by smelling his handker- chief on going out of London ascertain when he came into an atmosphere untainted by *London* Air." And Lawrence relayed to the diarist Jenner's procedure:

His method was to smell at his handkerchief occasionally and while he continued within the *London atmosphere* he could never be sen- sible of any taint upon it: but, for instance, when he approached Blackheath and took his handkerchief out of his pocket where it had not been exposed to the better air of that situation—his sense of smell- ing having become more pure he could perceive the taint.—His calcu- lation was that the air of London affected that of the vicinity to the distance of three miles.[61]

The "for instance" in the above paragraph could possibly suggest several visits to Blackheath. After all Lawrence was a close enough friend of Her Royal Highness's to be suspected of an affair with her. Ridiculous as this is, there is no question but what he was quite intimate with her and might occasionally have had Jenner accompany him on any visits made during the period of the sit- ting. From the point of view of prestige, the Lawrence portrait is by far the most important one we have of Jenner, but according to contemporary opinion, it is not one of the more exact like- nesses. Like most of the fashionable painters of the day, Lawrence was not above a little flattery. It is a formal, half-length portrait, and though the doctor was approaching his sixtieth birthday, he looks younger than in the earlier portraits. As Le Fanu correctly observes, "the face is somewhat idealized with the features less blunt."[62]

Jenner's visit to London, however, had another purpose, and Baron sums up the situation very well.

The adjustment of the second parliamentary grant, the increasing importance attached to vaccination, and the decay of that institution which had been formed for its support, called for the adoption of other measures better calculated to give stability to the practice. It was therefore resolved that the influence of the government should be exerted in founding an establishment for the propagation of vaccination throughout the British dominions. The late Rt. Hon. George Rose took the lead in this transaction. Dr. Jenner was requested by him to draw up a plan and give an estimate of the expense.

Notwithstanding his somewhat poor judgment in the Ringwood affair, Mr. Rose, vice-president of the Board of Trade, was a new type of vaccination supporter. Neither a member of the medical profession nor a nobleman, he was a keen economist and an authority on finance. At the age of sixty-five he was an elder statesman in the government, having been made a privy councillor in 1802. Jenner had accordingly drawn up his set of proposals, dispatched them to London, and had immediately been requested by Mr. Rose himself to come up to town for consultations. He was there for some five months altogether, returning from time to time to John Worgan's bedside. It was a tiring and anxious period, since Rose, with the best of intentions, had used his high government office to conscript the support of the President of the Royal College of Physicians, Sir Lucas Pepys, who was manifestly not an enthusiastic supporter of Jenner's. A number of the most influential doctors in the metropolis—while shrinking from the stupid and ignorant attacks on vaccination itself, which disgraced so many of their colleagues—were still not happy at the acclaim this poorly qualified provincial doctor was receiving in the highest places. It was for this reason that the discussions were stretched out for such a long period.

Not but what there was plenty for Jenner to do in London

much as he detested the place. On March 21 he delivered one of the season's first lectures at old Dr. Saunders's Medico-Chirurgical Society (of which he was a founding member). The lecture was entitled "Distemper in Dogs" and was based on firsthand observations of the Earl of Berkeley's foxhounds.[63] Strangely enough, Jenner did not dwell on the possibilities of vaccination procedures to combat distemper, a new disease that was only about fifty years old in the British Isles, but in later years he developed this line of research extensively. On April 4, he delivered a second lecture, "Smallpox-in-Utero," based upon two cases of fetuses being infected in the womb.[64] But these occasions were overshadowed by the increasingly obvious efforts that were being made for effectively excluding him from any status at all in the new vaccination institute.

Notwithstanding Mr. Rose's request to Jenner for an estimate of the expenses of the new vaccination authority, the estimate when presented, and most of the rest of the report, was simply ignored. The Royal College of Surgeons was brought in and a plan was drawn up to suit the combined colleges. The institution was to be governed by a board, from which Jenner, not being a member of either college, would be excluded; but he would be *named* director of the whole. He heatedly protested that he could direct nothing if he had no place on the governing board, whereupon they agreed, as though humoring a child, that he should be admitted. He also pointed out that they had initially informed him that "no person should take any part in the vaccinating department who was not either nominated by [Jenner] or submitted to [Jenner's] approbation before he was appointed to a station." To which Sir Lucas[65] smoothly replied, "You, sir, are to be the whole and sole director. We (meaning the board) are to be considered as nothing. What do *we* know of vaccination?"

This soothed the doctor's feelings for the time being, but it was soon apparent that the wily Sir Lucas was indeed placating the director. Of eight names Jenner submitted, the board, without consulting him, rejected six. Even Dr. Ring was turned down, and only the bereaved James Moore was accepted from among the expert vaccination pioneers. Perhaps the colleges selected Moore on the assumption that, being preoccupied with his late

brother's affairs, he would turn it down. In fact, it is surprising
that he did not do exactly this. The attacks on the general since his
death continued to cause upset in the family, as well as bitterness
about the ingratitude of it all. At this tragic time, Moore must
have understood his friend Jenner's feelings through years of such
abuse. To make matters worse, in the spring Charles Moore had a
complete mental breakdown from which he never recovered. No
more would he faithfully wait on Mrs. Siddons and her remaining
daughter or meekly watch the great folk in Cheltenham from afar.
As for Graham Moore, he was at sea and probably knew nothing
of his brother's death until much later.

As midsummer approached, and with the shock of Worgan's
death fresh upon him, Jenner was forced to wait upon the whims
of the Royal College in the sweltering heat, which was almost as
bad as the winter fog. Then came the news from Catherine. The
family was at Berkeley and the deadly curse of the Jenners'—the
typhus—had once more struck as it had poor Worgan the year
before. First of all Edward, who was in delicate health in any case,
fell sick, and then the healthiest child, Robert, caught it from
his brother. It was the worst possible time for such a complication,
since by the early autumn final arrangements for the new institution would definitely have been completed under Jenner's eye,
had he been able to remain in town. As it was he was forced to
leave the field to the enemy. Perhaps, indeed, he left his departure *too* long, for Edward, at least, was in extremis: "He
found him on his return home," says Baron, "quite a wreck with
little hope of recovery."[66]

The chronology of events during this confused summer is
difficult to follow, but it would seem that on leaving London to
go to his son, Jenner stopped briefly in Cheltenham. Since the
vitally important moves afoot in the capital were not able to keep
him from the sick bed one would have thought that affairs at St.
George's Place could have also taken care of themselves for the
time being. However, the Master of Ceremonies list has him arriving on August 31, and it is possible that the list of the previous
week has the explanation—perhaps the only one that would allow
him to steal a few precious hours from young Edward's side.
Among the arrivals for August 24, flanked by people of rank and

title is the simple name Mr. Clinch.[67] We have no record of any correspondence between Jenner and his friend in Newfoundland after August 1805, but in that last letter Jenner had written, "had it not been for a fierce catarrh that harassed you for two months in spring, everything would have gone on well with you. If this malady should dare to molest you next year, retreat, seek the milder shores of Old England, and leave the land of snows and ice to the bears, for whom nature made it."[68] Clinch is a most uncommon name and it would be nice to think that the schoolboy friends had met again after more than thirty years. On the other hand it may have been a son or other relative of the missionary's. Whatever the situation, it was an inauspicious time for *any* visitor to arrive. It is hard to believe that anyone but John Clinch could have drawn Jenner's attention just then unless, of course, it had been a member of the royal family.

The Duke of Sussex was suddenly taken ill at Gloucester during the first week of September. Jenner, who was just about to leave for Berkeley, was immediately called over from Cheltenham and, after a day or two, had the royal patient out of danger, but far from well. On the twelfth they both travelled to Berkeley where His Royal Highness spent two weeks' convalescence at the castle under the kindly eye of the countess, and Jenner was able to care for young Edward while waiting upon the duke daily. During this period the visits to the castle afforded some respite from the melancholy vigil at the cottage. The duke was well informed in the vaccination field, and hours were spent chatting about its aims and aspects. In particular he reassured Jenner on a matter that was then causing the doctor some heartache. A Portuguese named Corneiro had written a scurrilous pamphlet, which it was feared might stir distrust in a part of the world that had had virtually no anti-vaccination movement—the Iberian peninsula. Jenner wrote afterwards:

This gave me the opportunity of bringing up Corneiro and going fully into the subject of his abominable pamphlet. The Duke understood the matter so well that *he* could refute every charge that related to Portugal and explained many things very minutely, particularly that respecting the Royal infant who, he assured me, was vaccinated (I think he said by Domeyer) in spite of all remonstrances.

There were other common interests as well. Sussex had been at Göttingen in Blumenbach's time, and he was also a prominent freemason (Grand Master in 1811). In due course, completely well, he was able to resume his interrupted journey to Cheltenham, where he arrived on September 28, while Jenner returned sadly to the bedside of young Edward. The duke left with profound expressions of gratitude to his benefactor that manifested itself in tangible form a few weeks later. He sent Lady Berkeley a hookah, which he requested her to give to Jenner in appreciation of his kindness. In his reply the doctor reveals his awareness of the "scanty" resources a country village offered a man of sensitivity.

> . . . Your Royal Highness's kindness in making this addition to the scanty number of gratifications afforded me in this sequestered spot, will never be forgotten; and smoking I am sure is a harmless one if used in moderation. A man who has a pipe at his command, independent of its salutary influence in some instances, has always a soothing companion.
>
> It was with great pleasure that I heard that Your Royal Highness was enjoying so good a state of health. Guard well, Sir, your stomach and your skin, and I am persuaded that you will live in safety from the future attacks of the malady that so often annoys you. Happy shall I be if at any time I can do anything to convince you that I am
>
> > Your Royal Highness's
> > obliged and devoted
> > humble servant
> > Edward Jenner.[69]

One might have assumed that after nearly three weeks in attendance on the King's son, Jenner would have been appointed a Physician Extraordinary, but it was not to be. It is especially strange since when the duke was stricken, he was within nine miles of Cheltenham with its many royal doctors in residence. Yet he had chosen Jenner. As it was, however, I doubt whether the harassed doctor paid much attention at the time. From the son of the King, his sole concern became the son of Edward Jenner, while the autumn dragged bleakly into winter as the deathwatch continued.

Baron, who had finally taken up his post beside Trye at the

Royal Infirmary in Gloucester, visited Chantry Cottage toward the end of the year when both anxious parents were nursing the dying boy. The pattern of his decline was almost identical with Worgan's. First came the typhus with its complete weakening of resistance allowing the lurking seeds of tuberculosis to come to light. Again Baron is a first-hand witness.

His eldest son, Edward, was then lying in the last stages of pulmonary consumption. He had repeated haemorrhages from the lungs, and was evidently approaching his end. Dr. Parry of Bath was in the house. I was introduced into the sickroom and there, for the first time, saw Mrs. Jenner, the anxious and constant attendant on her dying child. Jenner was particularly attached to this young man, and apparently for qualities which in less generous natures would have produced a different effect. He had always been delicate in health, and had, moreover, in some respects, rather a defective understanding. His father felt these deficiencies, and considered them but as stronger claims to his attachment and regard. Some years afterward, he wept when he talked to me of this son, and many times referred to the singular character of his mind with the most touching and affectionate recollection.[70]

In London a similar melancholy occasion was drawing to its end. The painter Hoppner was dying, and, strangely, few people were aware of it. Actually he went before young Edward Jenner, but he had been ailing for some years, and when the end came on January 23, it passed unnoticed. Aside from his son and nephew only six people attended his funeral.[71] To be sure Hoppner was blunt and eccentric, but he was still one of the greatest portrait painters England ever produced and certainly one of Jenner's most celebrated patients. It is strange that Baron makes no mention of him but perhaps it is not so surprising since even the painter's wife did not attend the funeral. His long, terminal sickness seems to have removed him from the ken of men. Understandably, nothing but his son's condition mattered to Jenner in those last trying weeks, and if he was told of Hoppner's death it probably did not register. Even when Sir Lucas Pepys had written to him to come to London for the inauguration of the institute, Jenner had declined and recommended that his friend Moore take the directorship. He would cooperate with them, but for the time his sole concern was with his family. As a matter of fact, the strain was having its effect on him more than he realized. From the autumn of 1809, his activities as a doctor—except to his children and the Duke of Sussex—came to a halt. Edward lingered on, coughing up his lungs, almost through the winter but he never saw the spring. He died on January 29 and his father almost died with him.[72] He was inconsolable. "I feel," he wrote to Hicks, "greatly obliged to anyone who attempts to console me in my present affliction but you, who know so much of the human mind are convinced how vain are those friendly efforts." Later he wrote to Ring: "One would suppose that the mind would become in some measure reconciled to an event, however melancholy its nature, that one knows to be inevitable . . . but I know from sad experience that the edge of sensibility is not thus to be blunted." Nearly two months later he was still prostrate.

February passed in a kind of unreal daze. He kept a long sheet of paper beside him and jotted down an item when it came into his head in order to ultimately send off to his friend Moore. "I do not yet feel myself in that state of composure which will allow me to sit down, begin, and finish a letter to you" There was nothing in Berkeley to take his mind, even temporarily, off his grief. In Berkeley, like Worgan before him, he missed his library. "I cannot refer to your pamphlet; it is among my books in Cheltenham," he told Moore on one occasion. Nevertheless the writing of these long, rambling epistles probably helped to keep him sane during this terrible period. Two months later he still found refuge in this pattern of occupation in lieu of reading. On April 21 he wrote: "I must get to my old plan of the long sheet and filling it up leisurely, or I know not when you may hear from me." There is a poignant postscript at the end of this particular letter. "How is your laughter-loving girl? and that fine boy with the philosophic head?"[73]

While he was rambling on to Moore in these "letters," which touched upon everything that came into his mind, the hours passed somehow, but he was not ready to enter the world again or cope with the tiniest problems of meeting people. Sir Thomas Bernard wrote to him kindly and begged him to visit London, but, even in April, eight weeks after his son's death Jenner was still completely crushed. The gregarious man of the Cheltenham salons wished only to be left alone; time was the only cure. Edward's death, he told Sir Thomas on April 1,

threw me into the state of dejection which makes me unfit to perform my ordinary duties, and I still feel enveloped, as it were, in clouds, so that all objects wear a new and gloomy aspect. You wish me to come to town: you will find me too turpid to perform any useful offices; and I feel confident that even the cheerful company of yourself and those friends into whose society you have so often introduced me would at present do me no service.[74]

If the thought of London was too much for him, so, too, was Cheltenham. He was not ready to go back yet, but he had to get away somewhere. "His symptoms became so distressing," said Baron, "that active means were deemed necessary to obviate them." So Jenner decided to go to Bath with Baron and attempt to recuperate under Parry's care. At the last moment, however, his friend was unable to accompany him so, all alone, he went to seek health and peace of mind at the house of his old schoolfellow. Here he was "cupped and calomeled, salted, etc. etc." but he was still "far from right." He wrote to Baron on June 15 listing all his ominous symptoms, but nevertheless showing more signs of recovery. His mind seems to have lagged behind his body. "I am told to migrate not to think. The first injunction I shall comply with and go to town on Monday for a few days. On my return it is my intention to throw myself upon Cheltenham in a probationary way. Should this be too much for me my retreat is not far distant."[75] But the happy pioneer days were over. This first great family bereavement ushered in a pattern of sorrow and disappointment that dogged him almost continually until his death. The sun was setting.

✍ VII ✍

Domestic Tragedy
and Public Ingratitude
1810

The vaccination campaign had rolled along all through the year 1809 despite the absence of Jenner's hand at the helm. The two events that vitally concerned his interests were the establishment of a local newspaper and resisting an attack on vaccination in Cheltenham itself that might well have had dire effects on the cause had his friends not been there to hold the fort. Ironically, the opening gun of the campaign sounded in the pages of the new paper, which was launched by Pruen, its first editor, and Ruff, the printer. Jenner is reputed to have had a hand in the venture,[1] for which Captain Grey put up part of the money.

The *Cheltenham Chronicle* appeared on May 4, 1809 and was to have a great impact on the vaccination movement. From that date on, a steady stream of news, publicity, and correspondence bolstered Jenner's efforts right up to the day of his death. Most conveniently, the editorial offices were on the corner of St. George's Place and High Street, so that the good doctor had but a few paces to walk when he wished to drop in on Pruen. It is a fact that Jenner particularly liked to have his establishment clustered about him. He was not unlike a comfortable hen sitting on its nest in the middle of the barnyard. Down the lane facing his front door was Rowland Hill's Chapel, which he had watched gradually taking shape through the previous year; close beside him in the other houses of the terrace were his colleagues Newell, Fowler, and Minster; and behind him in Chester Walk was Mrs. Jenner's devoted Dr. Wood.

In a letter to Jenner following the publication of *The History of Cheltenham* in 1803, Dibdin had referred to Pruen, "in his modest mansion of Prestbury." Perhaps that was when the idea of a newspaper first occurred to the quartet: Ruff, Jenner, Pruen, and Dibdin, all of whom during the next year or two published works from Ruff's press. Everyone involved seems to have been a strong Whig, and not surprisingly the paper supported that political position for many years. This same year Lord Berkeley, the most prominent Whig in the county, moved the headquarters of the Berkeley Hunt to Cheltenham, which meant that the family lived here out of season as well as in the summer.[2] As a result the Berkeleys became the "rulers" of Cheltenham for nearly half a century, and since Jenner was the family doctor it is likely that some Berkeley money went into the paper also. This is borne out by the editorial policy of the ensuing years, after the death of the old earl in 1810 and the accession of the bastard Colonel Berkeley as the head of the clan. The *Chronicle* loyally supported the family through its less than decorous activities and predicaments, as did, it should be added, Jenner himself. Despite the fact that the paper only existed during the last fourteen years of his life, it printed more material relating to vaccination and its founder than any other contemporary journal in the world.

In the nature of things the paper of a health resort has a strong slant to medical affairs, and Pruen was well aware of his friend's special field of interest aside from vaccination. It is not surprising, therefore, that in one of the first issues there is a glowing report from Dr. Green, President of the Royal Medical Society of Edinburgh, on the efficacy of the Cheltenham waters in treating dropsy and *diseases of the liver*.[3]

It was tragic that Jenner's domestic problems kept him out of so much that was of vital interest to him. After watching the progress of the new chapel from his front windows for the greater part of a year, he, of all people, was unable to attend the opening. It had been completed the very day poor Worgan died, and when it was inaugurated on August 22, the doctor was tied to the bedside of his doomed son. Nevertheless, it was a grand occasion and most of his friends were present, including a number of people from Oxford and London. It represented yet another temple of vaccine in which Rowland Hill continued the practice of vaccinating people after divine service that he had already instituted at Surrey Chapel and Wotton-under-Edge. Though it is known from the news reports that Jenner was definitely absent from this function, his general movements through the first part of the summer are much harder to follow. He seems to have come home from time to time until the terminal months of his son's illness, and may have been there also when Lord William Bentinck arrived in Cheltenham with his wife. It was the first opportunity he had had to see Jenner since he had personally taken the cowpox virus to India in 1803. A great deal had happened to him since then, mostly of a tragic nature. Despite his zeal in promoting vaccination in the subcontinent, he was blamed for the Mutiny at Velore and dismissed from his governorship of Madras in 1807—the same year, ironically enough, that his father, the Duke of Portland, became Prime Minister of Britain. He was sent to the front in Spain, survived the Battle of Corunna, and the subsequent evacuation of the army, and was at last able to get to Cheltenham on July 12, 1809.[4] Whatever his London commitments Jenner would surely have wished to thank his friend for the money raised in Madras at a time when the Jenner family fortunes were at their lowest ebb. Since the couple stayed in the town until mid-August it is just possible that he found time to see them. The old duke, who was seventy-one years of age, resigned the prime-ministership and died soon afterwards on October 31. He was brother-in-law to Jenner's old patroness, the Duchess of Devonshire, and was, fortunately, succeeded in the premiership by that very enthusiastic vaccination man, Spencer Perceval. Jenner, alas, never lived to see the final vindication of young Bentinck, the colonial administrator who became Governor-General of India in 1833.

The new attack mounted in Cheltenham upon the efficacy of vaccination started out quietly enough in London, but by midsummer had spread to the pages of the local press. Since the intention was manifestly to destroy Jenner on his home ground, it was fortunate that he now had his own newspaper to support him. His record in a community where he had every encouragement and assistance was such that made *sincere* criticism impossible. Nevertheless, his critics did painstaking research in an attempt to discover something resembling failure among the thousands of vaccinations Jenner had performed here since 1798.

Early in the spring a Cheltenham child named Charles Dodeswell came down with smallpox. He recovered and nothing seems to have been said about the case at the time. It later turned out, however, that Jenner himself had attempted to vaccinate the child some two years previously, but without success. The doctor had pleaded to be allowed to make a further attempt, but the parents had refused because the boy had apparently suffered physically from the injection, and he was, accordingly, left unvaccinated. Somehow the anti-vaccination forces heard about the case, and the story was repeated widely with the latter part—the refusal of permission for a further attempt at vaccinating the boy—left out. There is no record of the family's making any kind of protest over the business and nothing in the doctor's diaries or correspondence that even mentions the name Dodeswell. Nonetheless, it soon became well-known in London. It is therefore rather hard on the memory of this family that Dr. Moore was put in the position of having to pillory them for posterity. "It is to be regretted," he wrote, "that when such irregularities occur in the progress of the vaccine it is often difficult to persuade the parents to have the operation repeated. From this obstinacy the life of the child above mentioned was brought into great danger."[5]

As soon as Dr. Jameson heard about the so-called vaccination failure, he reported it to the Royal College of Physicians, of which he was a member. He seems to have sincerely believed that it was, indeed, a bona fide example of the system's inefficacy. He later denied that he was anti-vaccinationist and insisted that his words had been taken out of context. Certainly, what had perhaps been an academic observation to the Royal College of Physicians was given the publicity of a full enquiry and eagerly referred to the National Vaccine Establishment. To make matters worse, Jameson also rashly included two other local cases of as dubious veracity as the Dodeswell boy's—all of which the Royal College was delighted to pass on. Vaccination "failures" in Cheltenham were extremely important. One of the cases to which Jameson referred was reported in full in the *Chronicle* on July 6 with complete explanation given, but by then the vaccine establishment was already engaged in its own exhaustive enquiry. The facts as printed by Pruen were as follows:

> It is said that a case has occurred in this place of a child having had the Small-Pox who had been vaccinated by Dr. Jenner and gone through the regular stages of Cow-Pox.
>
> We have made enquiries into the subject and are able to inform the public, that this is not a fact; the child, it is true, has had the Small-Pox; *but it did not go through the stages of Cow-Pox with regularity*— it appears from the evidence of the servant who took the child to Dr. Jenner that it had the disease very bad, that its arm was a great deal sorer than those of the other children of the family who had it; that she was obliged to rip open its sleeve in consequence of the great degree of inflammation affecting the area, that it was much longer in getting well than the others, and that *Dr. Jenner had it brought to him every day for inspection for about a fortnight and showed considerable anxiety about it.*
>
> It appears, likewise, that contrary to an assertion that has been made, no other person was vaccinated from this child. This is one of those cases, in which the prevalence of herpetic symptoms counteracted the effect of vaccination as it now turns out frequently to have done in Small-Pox inoculation.[6]

It was commonly thought that if vaccine was inserted then *that* was vaccination. The fact that the operation simply did not "take" with some people was ignored, as was the fact that some systems could not receive cowpox without becoming violently ill. Such cases were not, of course, successfully vaccinated and were therefore not protected against smallpox. In certain instances a person who had rejected the serum in this manner could be successfully vaccinated on a subsequent attempt, but perhaps understandably, some people were not too eager to try a second time. Such, however, were the molehills out of which so many doctors attempted to build anti-vaccination mountains. The whisper that Jenner actually used vaccine from this manifestly abnormal child to inoculate others suggests a barbarity on his part that is unworthy of comment.

James Moore made a close examination of all the evidence and wrote a report for the Royal College later in July, by which time gossip was already circulating in Cheltenham. Since Jenner was otherwise occupied, Dr. Newell stepped into the breach and sent the whole text of Moore's report to Pruen at the *Chronicle.* His accompanying letter did not stoop to the defense of his friend; it was merely a case of presenting the facts to the public, so that they may judge for themselves. "As the cases of supposed failure of Vaccine Inoculation which gave rise to the annexed report created a considerable sensation here, last Spring," he told Pruen, "I submit to you the propriety of publishing it in the Cheltenham Chronicle." It duly appeared in the issue of August 17, just about a month after Moore submitted it. In weighing the whole business it might have been more discreet to have ignored Jameson's initial comments, which were most likely inspired by the twinges of jealousy that he continually felt over Jenner's increasing fame. Once released to the Royal College of Physicians, there were all too many men who wished the matter to have the fullest airing. Moore's findings are straightforward enough, but their very existence conceded that an investigation was necessary:

Report of James Moore, Esq. to the Board of the
    National Vaccine Establishment,

Board Room of Nat. Vacc. Est.
Leicester Square,
20th July, 1809

Amidst the numerous authentic reports which are transmitted to the board of the National Vaccine Establishment from all parts of the Empire, describing the great success and extension of the practice of vaccination, accounts have also been received of a very small number of failures.

Most of these failures have occurred at such a distance from town or so long after the event, as to preclude proper investigation, and some of those which were investigated were found to be misrepresented, and the history of the others was destitute of sufficient proof. But in May last a letter was addressed to the Royal College of Physicians, London, by Dr. Jameson of Cheltenham in which he relates three cases where Small Pox occurred, though the patient had been vaccinated by Dr. Jenner some years before. This board having thought to desire me to investigate the cases, the following is the result of my enquiry.

It appears that the first two cases were only examples of that slight variolus affection of the very warty kind which has been termed by some writers Secondary Small Pox. The occasional occurrence of such an eruption, both after the Smallpox and the Vaccine, has often been described and commented on by Dr. Jenner, and other writers. There was nothing, therefore, in these cases to make them be considered as failures.

There was no doubt that Dr. Jameson was very upset at being identified with the anti-vaccination clique. He little thought that the letter to his colleagues in May would have received so much publicity; but when Moore proclaimed to the world that a well-known Cheltenham doctor was questioning the efficacy of Jenner's work, a reply was imperative in the interest of self-respect. Jameson fell back on the excuse that Moore's report was not properly presented. He wrote bitterly to the *Chronicle* on August 21.

I certainly am not, as some persons inferred from Mr. Moore's report inimical to the experiment of vaccination being completely and fairly tried; on the contrary I was a principal agent in introducing the practice into the Finsbury Dispensary in London, and published a series of resolutions in favour of vaccination when Physician to the Charity. But the defective report by Mr. James Moore, Asst. Director to the Board of the Vaccine Establishment impairs the cause it was intended to support. . . .

Perhaps the hapless Jameson was the one who really suffered from the affair. Jenner, with his defense in very good hands, certainly came out unscathed. Being the last attempt to discredit him in his own town until the Cheltenham Vaccination Convention of 1816, it resulted in increasing his prestige among all classes. The last word came in a letter to the *Chronicle* from Worcester on November 16. The correspondent wrote gratefully of the boon of vaccination in his family, and, commenting on a matter close to Jenner's heart, compared the merits of smallpox inoculation with cowpox inoculation. He dismissed the former out of hand as a result of his own experiences, writing: "This may certainly shake our confidence in the immunity afforded by Small-pox inoculation." The letter was from a layman and very important, since at that time many people still believed that smallpox inoculation protected one as effectively as cowpox, but that the latter was to be preferred simply because it was a less odious disease. Jenner, of course, was still trying to drive home the fact that the preventive potential of smallpox inoculation was negligible and the actual injection of the disease was a deliberate spreading of it. The halting of this shocking practice became more and more the obsession of all the vaccination doctors—Trye, Creaser, Moore, Christie, and colleagues—as well as of such powerful allies as Lord Borington, Bernard, and, of course, Lady Crewe. In addition another ally had settled in the town during Jenner's absence in the person of yet one more Physician Extraordinary to the royal family. Henry Boisragon, a rich and fashionable society doctor of thirty-one, appeared in September with his pregnant wife. He was an enthusiastic vaccination man and bid fair to build a large practice among the rich Londoners who patronized the Wells. He would be a perfect counter to the fashionable Riddell cult, which had increasingly flourished during Jenner's long absence.

The *Cheltenham Chronicle,* which had started out so bravely such a short time before, was anything but thriving when it celebrated its first birthday. It had done a notable service to vaccination in its short life, but such literary adventures are very expensive. After about six months it developed serious financial and production troubles. Actually, Ruff was not equipped to handle such an ambitious project from his modest press, and even though he increased the price in the autumn from sixpence to sixpence-halfpenny, the paper continued to lose money. On January 24, in the new year, he transferred the plant to another printer—a Mr. Sharp—who carried on his business in Jordan's Yard off the upper part of High Street, so that when Jenner finally returned home later in the year he no longer had the editor's office at his street corner. Nevertheless, the financial troubles were not reflected in the editorial policy, and Pruen continued the battle as vigorously as ever while his friend was recuperating. Of course, Cheltenham was not England—or even Gloucestershire—and the *Journal,* the long-established paper in the nearby county seat, was under no similar obligation of personal loyalty to Jenner.

Cheltenham and Gloucester are only nine miles apart, but they have always been very separate and independent communities. This applied particularly to their press, and it will be recalled that Charles Trye had a house in Gloucester where, indeed, he spent more time than he did at Leckhampton Court. One might almost call him the vaccination watchdog in the Gloucester camp. A regular writer to the papers, he kept an alert eye on the press of both towns. The *Journal* was friendly enough to Jenner in a general way, but in Gloucester he was not the great figure that he was in Cheltenham. The Gloucester paper would not hesitate to print anything derogatory if it seemed newsworthy, and any disgruntled Cheltenham person who felt that the expression of his spleen would open him to disapprobation in his own community could always air his views in the nearby city. Moreover, it would be likely that none of his neighbors would ever hear about it, still less read it. Pruen, it should be added, was a good newspaperman and would not suppress news or correspondence, but the public feeling in Cheltenham was such that any anti-Jenner sentiments were swiftly answered, if not by the editor then by many an eager defender. This, of course, was not the case in Gloucester, and if anything significant appeared, and Trye saw it, he would pass it on to the *Chronicle*. He wrote under the pseudonym Veritas for both papers up to the time of his death.

So it was, early in the new regime, that he caught an item in the correspondence columns of the *Journal* that he felt should be made known to the Cheltenham public. Apparently a Cheltenham gentleman hoping to keep open, or possibly re-open, the controversy of the previous summer, wrote his allegations to the *Journal* rather than reveal himself among his own townsfolk. It was the old libel about Cheltenham doctors secretly favoring inoculation. Trye wrote to the *Chronicle* on April 5:

I have been led to these reflexions addressed to the Editor of the Gloucester Journal by a Mr. Freeman[7] of this place, in which he states that numerous cases of inoculation took place here in the course of last Spring. This well-meaning liberal-minded gentleman has forgot to inform the public of the extraordinary proofs of the efficacy of the practice he condemns in the very town in which he himself resides where, from the almost universal adoption of it, since its first discovery by Dr. Jenner, the place has been preserved in the most wonderful manner, from that most dreadful of all distempers, the Smallpox. It is well-known that during the last two years the Smallpox has been epidemic in every part of Europe as well as in England; and great numbers have been seized who have not had either the disease before or been submitted to the new inoculation. In the town of Cheltenham, the universal prevalence of the latter has so completely disarmed this scourge of the human race that instances of it have been few and solitary and they would have been still less so but for the inoculations of it, by the opposers of the vaccination, which has disseminated the contagion, and kept it alive much longer among us, than would otherwise have been the case.

Another letter that was printed soon after the new press took over also accented the drive against smallpox inoculation. This time it was from a layman. Mr. W. A. Pruen, Vicar of Fladbury, Worcestershire, cited the experience of his own village in going over to vaccination exclusively. He apparently was an acquaintance of Jenner's, since he said that the system had been explained to him by the doctor himself. During the period from November 1807 to February 1810 he had vaccinated regularly in his parish. "The whole of those I have vaccinated have entirely escaped any infection of the Small pox," he claimed. Over two years without a case was a remarkable record for a lay practitioner during a smallpox epidemic. Mr. Pruen's letter, incidentally, was written on the very day the *Chronicle* announced the death of young Edward Jenner.

All in all, the campaign had taken on a new dimension with the vehicle of the press being locally available for debate and analysis. The logic of the vaccination case in these exchanges always resulted in vindication, and when Jenner was in Bath he was able to discuss the situation, as far as his condition would permit, with Dr. Creaser. In a letter to Baron on his return he had written: "You will see that I have enlisted Creaser in our cause and you will find he will not discredit it." Obviously Jenner did not mean merely the propagation of vaccination, since as Fosbroke tells us, "He [Creaser] introduced vaccination into the West of England, and through life, by many writings and personal exertions adhered to Dr. Jenner with that sincere firmness and fidelity which strongly marked all his attachments and biases."[8] Jenner apparently meant that he had persuaded the loyal ally to come to the Cheltenham fortress to join the constantly increasing band of vaccination doctors. Creaser's son was in poor health and would undoubtedly be happy in the sister spa. Fosbroke, indeed, says that the pair—father and son—moved to Cheltenham on account of the boy's delicate constitution. Creaser had actually reduced his practice in recent years, so it was not too complicated to pull up his roots and settle in a new home.

Fate decreed, however, that Jenner's own return to Cheltenham must once more be delayed. When he came back from London in June and was well on the way to becoming his usual self, his friend Lord Berkeley fell ill and the doctor was called in. It soon became apparent that the old man was on his deathbed, but he nevertheless lingered on for nearly two months, well into August; his death actually left a legacy of worry for Jenner in the serious lawsuit that came with the problem of succession. But for the moment there was a breathing spell. After all the tragic months of death, bitterness, and sorrow, the now reduced Jenner household returned to St. George's Place in September, though even the gentle pleasures of settling once more amid familiar things and faces was marred by yet another passing. On September 1, old Sir Ralph Woodford, former Minister Plenipotentiary to the Court of Denmark, was buried at St. Mary's. Jenner was probably too late to attend, but he would have seen the new grave. They were in some respects kindred spirits who had sought the peace of Cheltenham in their mellow years. Like the doctor, Sir Ralph was extremely fond of children, and on one occasion when the baronet held a children's party at his house, the little ones danced around Jenner and crowned him with flowers.[9] That, alas, was in the days when his own children were tiny—including Edward. There is a memorial to this forgotten but gentle diplomat in St. Mary's Church.

Of all the new developments in the town during his absence, perhaps the advent of Drs. Boisragon and Christie was the most important. Aside from his medical standing, Boisragon was brilliant, rich, and well-connected, with an already established London clientele. He took a large house in Royal Crescent— number eleven—and inevitably attracted a generous portion of the wealthier seasonal patronage. A well-read man, he was also an accomplished musician. Christie, a much simpler type, was fortunate in having as his patron—and devoted friend—Sir Walter

Farquhar. Christie had long been awaiting his release from the East India Company's service, so that he could join Jenner in Cheltenham; he took a house in Cambray near the Theatre Royal. Though the two newcomers were each more than twenty years Jenner's junior, the three soon became close friends.

Creaser, a much older man, maintained a very restricted practice, and eventually only catered to a tiny coterie of people he knew personally. He had come to Cheltenham as a semi-retired intellectual rather than as a practicing doctor. All these men, together with Baron, were concerned with the launching of a Gloucester Vaccination Association, newly organized primarily to find means of stopping smallpox inoculation in the county's capital and to coordinate activities in the whole of the shire.

A list of contributions to the movement printed in the *Chronicle* shows the almost complete spread of Jenner's supporters in the northern part of the county. *All* the Cheltenham doctors contributed except Jameson, the common sum being one guinea—a useful amount in those days—but a few gave more. Both Trye and Boisragon gave two guineas as did Baron; the two thrifty next-door neighbors in St. George's Place, Newell and Fowler, gave the routine one guinea each. This list brings names into our story never previously associated with Jenner: Sir Robert Herries, the banker friend of the late Duchess of Devonshire; Sir B. W. Guise of Elmore Court, who was M.P. for the county; Mr. Darke of Prestbury; Edmund Probyn of Longhope Manor; and a host of others representing everyone of note within twenty miles of the town. The southern part of the county, alas, seems to have been less enthusiastic—especially among the doctors. Bristol was particularly cool.

The Jenners—after the nightmarish year they had just endured—found the town in festive mood with the season having at least a month to go, and they arrived, happily enough, the same day as Mrs. Jordan. Colonel MacMahon was also there, up to his ears in soothing and arbitrating between various ladies who had relationships with the Prince Regent. All the tact of the suave colonel was necessary during this late season at the Wells. He was uncomfortably close to Lady Hertford at Ragley, who still held the principal sway in the Prince of Wales's affections, but Mrs. Fitzherbert, whom many people still considered his real favorite, had taken a house in Cheltenham for the season, and the evergreen Lady Jersey, who had broken up his marriage with the Princess of Wales, had taken a long lease on the house in Cambray where she was to spend the rest of her life.

Mrs. Jordan also took lodgings in Cambray, near Dr. Christie. In a letter to the Duke of Clarence, dated Cheltenham, (Wednesday) September 5, she writes, "We have been very fortunate with respect to lodgings, though dear, they are very comfortable, clean, and quiet, and exactly opposite to the Theatre, which was very crowded last night. It is a very pretty house, well-lighted and perfectly commodious both with regard to the audience and behind the *scenes*. It is a very town [*sic*] and the buildings that are going on are wonderful. There has been four hundred houses built within two years, and whole streets and squares now laid out. It is thought that in a few years it will rival Bath."[10]

It is not surprising that when the Duke of Clarence's mistress came to lodge in Cambray, on Riddell's very doorstep, as it were, it was an opportunity that the alert quack could not resist. Since the appearance of his book, he had openly practiced as a "specialist" in defiance of the disapproval of the official doctors of the town. His first impact on Mrs. Jordan was not very good. "There is a Colonel Riddell here," she told the duke, " a very troublesome man. He has got a beautiful place, and is, I believe, *a quack,* for he teases poor Fanny and myself to death to take his medicine, which we have both declined. We have also declined going to Lady B. who was making great preparations, and who, I fancy, will be very angry, but I cannot help it."[11]

Riddell was at this time living in great state at Cambray Mansion, one of the largest houses in the town, where he entertained the Couttses and the noble families to whom they were related in marriage. Fanny Alsop, who was Mrs. Jordan's daughter by an earlier alliance, had suffered through an unsuccessful marriage herself in 1808, and now travelled about with her mother. It was she who finally succumbed to the Colonel's blandishments, and a week later was one of his "patients." "Fanny has gone through a regular course of Colonel Riddell's 'discipline,' " wrote the actress on the fifteenth, "who has taken a great fancy to her; she is certainly much better. He is a nice old man and has been remarkably civil to us. . . . I have begun the waters the days I don't play, but they make me very sick and uncomfortable all the day."[12] A concluding observation is a little puzzling. "Mrs. Fitzherbert was looking quite handsome last night. I hope the Prince's bed will be well aired for it has not been slept in for a long time. The Thomonds are here and at the Play every night." This referred, incidentally, to the new Lady Thomond, daughter of Jenner's old friend, Dr. Trotter. The allusion to the Prince looks as though people may have anticipated a reconciliation with Mrs. Fitzherbert. As for Mrs. Jordan, she had a delightful three weeks in Cheltenham and was able to leave on September 21 for Liverpool[13] with earnings of three hundred pounds in her pocket.

But as one great lady left the Wells others would arrive—the most important of whom was the beautiful Lady Crewe. Sir Thomas Bernard had been in correspondence with Jenner before the doctor left for Cheltenham and discussed his conversations with her ladyship, who was eager to forward the cause of the new Vaccination Institute and in particular the rising movement to stop smallpox inoculation. She asked him for Jenner's ideas on the most efficacious procedure, before she proceeded to Cheltenham herself, since her name appears on the list of arrivals in mid-September. She apparently decided that it would be better to take up the matter with the doctor first hand.[14]

After being inactive for so long, the bustle and aura of the Cheltenham salons helped Jenner to get back on his feet. Undoubtedly he was now the most important force in the town, and his very social responsibilities could not help but distract him from his personal troubles. The dean of the medical profession, a member of the Board of Commissioners, and a magistrate, he was also to some degree a busy man of letters. After his serious discussions with Lady Crewe, Boisragon, and Christie, the germ of an idea formed in his mind for writing up the Ceylon saga. Jenner's battalions in Cheltenham were stronger than ever as is shown by the spirited manner in which the Jameson-Moore business had been handled in his absence; and there were humbler supporters appearing steadily to bolster the press and the great doctors.

A zealous young parson in the Cotswolds—not so far from Catherine's village—issued a slender volume of poems that added a new and passionate dimension to the advent of vaccination. John Williams, the Curate of Stroud, was a much better poet than Worgan, Drayton, or Snell, but he was buried in the hills and remains almost unknown save for the fact that he was A. E. Housman's grandfather. He was poverty-stricken—almost the prototype of the starving curate—and, inevitably, had a large family. But he was profoundly moved by Jenner's miraculous cure and tried to express in verse what Plumtre had uttered in his sermons. His piety however was tempered by a most unevangelical concern with earthly beauty. Like poor Bloomfield, Williams had a very personal reason for his esteem of Jenner, and his fluid verse is supported by extremely subjective feeling. In his *Sacred Allegories . . . to Which Is Added An Anacreontic: An Ode to the Discovery of Vaccination,* he romantically sees the horror of smallpox as the ugly and evil enemy of love. The simple country maid and her swain are the sufferers:

> A fearful plague whose black envenomed breath
> Loads the pure air with misery and death,
> Dire as the pest that smote Thy servant Job,
> Hath long run riot round this motley globe.
> On beauty's native sweets profanely trod,
> And marred, with cruel joy, the handiworks of GOD.[15]

And, since physical beauty is the stuff of youth and love, smallpox is again the devil. Millions of girls through the ages had been destroyed by the curse that:

> Disunites whom love united
> Makes the fairest maiden slighted;
> Blights the lilies on her brow;
> Makes the swain revoke his vow
> Taints the life-breeze of the grove
> Foe to beauty, foe to love.[16]

But there was also desolation much nearer home. Williams was born in 1779, and had gone through a childhood without the protection of vaccination. "Within a space of three weeks," he wrote, "the author lost two brothers and a sister from that dreadful disease."

> Once, roving wild near my young home it flew,
> And round our walls its wizard circles drew;
> E'en scaled our playground, our fond sports annoyed
> And, of my mother's children, three destroyed.[17]

With the sensitivity of the poet, he deplored the destruction of beauty and protested his bereavement with the bitterness of a brother, but his gratitude to God and to Jenner is the final emotion stirred by the advent of vaccination.

> Which now with philanthropic mind
> He promulgates to all mankind
> That Indian maid or female Rus
> May share the same sweet joys with us
> May the fair, then, give with me
> Thanks, O Jenner, thanks to thee.[18]

Unfortunately Williams's joy at the triumph over smallpox was to be countered by a continuing pattern of tragedy in his own domestic life, but he never ceased to be a devoted and loyal supporter of Jenner. As a country parson he had, perhaps, a different view of the great disfiguring disease. Its aesthetic horror was as terrifying as its social devastation. An intensely religious young man, he confidently looked upon Jenner as the instrument of God, though actually his religious views were markedly different from those of the doctor. He was an extremely narrow, though sincere, Evangelical and deplored the Cheltenham peers' obsession with Catholic emancipation. Actually, many years later, it was one of these peers, Lord Ducie, who presented him with the handsome living of Woodchester after he had struggled along as a curate in Stroud for twenty-eight years. Undoubtedly it was Ducie who, in 1810, showed this little book to Jenner, since we later find the poet in Cheltenham and received by many of the doctor's friends. The ego-building impact of yet another poet's praise notwithstanding, however, the announcement that appeared in the *Cheltenham Chronicle* on November 1, might well have broken a lesser man's heart—even after the ingratitude of royalty such as displayed by the Duke of Sussex once he was cured.

After twelve years of successful application all over the world, after races and nations had been emancipated from the foul disease, when princes and emperors had paid homage to the great emancipator, at last the triumph of vaccination was recognized by the British Crown and the first vaccination doctor was honored. It is hard to imagine just what Jenner's feelings were when he read in the *Chronicle:* "The Prince of Wales has been graciously pleased to appoint Thomas Newell, Esq. of this place Surgeon Extraordinary to His Royal Highness." It would have been kinder to have honored Marshall or Tierney if a bypassing of Jenner had to be performed, but to appoint one of his younger followers who lived almost next door to him in the same street of the same town was unforgivable. It is very doubtful whether the King had any part in this business. His mental condition was seriously deteriorating, and the formation of a regency was only a few weeks away. The utter neglect of Jenner at the Court of St. James from this year on suggests that the Prince of Wales was the motivating force, bearing in mind Jenner's friendship with the unfortunate Princess of Wales.

Jenner, characteristically, reacted to his humiliation with great dignity. Only Catherine would see his tears: the outside world saw nothing. There is not a line in his letters or diaries on Newell's elevation; he simply sighed and turned his mind to Cheltenham affairs. There was much to be done in conjunction with his colleagues for the improvement of the town, and some people were talking of a dispensary. Perhaps Jenner was even thinking about a *Cheltenham* Vaccination Institute, to parallel the one already operating in Gloucester. He must look around and see all that had taken place during his long absence. Certainly his attitude to Newell did not alter in the least. There was too much work to do and all his friends were precious to him—and they also had their burdens.

After much heart-searching, James Moore had finally accepted the directorship of the institute, but not long afterwards that unhappy family was tragically distracted by the death of his brother Charles, who had been ill for some time. Farington, who knew him well, wrote on November 12:

In the newspaper this evening I read that Charles Moore, an auditor of the Public Accounts died on Thursday last. . . . Charles was bred to the law and through the interest of the General (Sir John Moore), obtained a situation under government from Mr. Pitt sufficient to make him independent. About two years ago he was seized with a disorder in the head which gradually reduced him to a state of idiocy. He excelled in humour of a particular kind. His imitation of the oratory of the late Mr. Burke and of Lord Melville were remarkable for the truth of the resemblance both of language and manner. I state this from my own knowledge of him and of this his power.[19]

Undoubtedly the talent for mimicry had a great deal to do with his initial interest in the stage and the Siddonses, which had ended so tragically with his complete mental breakdown in 1808.

After a year of attendance at successive deathbeds in Berkeley, the local scene might have seemed pleasant to Jenner, yet all the improvements Mrs. Jordan had noticed in the town eventually raised a financial problem for the commissioners that came to a head soon after Jenner's return. At a meeting on November 11, it was reluctantly voted to levy a special rate, for this year only, to solve the problem. Jenner and his friends objected strongly to setting such a precedent, and eventually the people of the town escaped the levy by twelve of the commissioners themselves volunteering to advance the necessary funds—some £1,200. Each of these gentlemen provided a hundred pounds at an interest of five percent. In addition to Jenner the ones who contributed were Colonel Riddell, Thomas Gray, Esq., Edward Smith, Francis Wells, Esq., B. Wells, Esq., W. H. Jessop, Esq., T. Gwinnett, Esq., and T. Newmarch, Esq.[20]

Very important among the new developments was the completion of Trye's Cheltenham-Leckhampton tramway, which ran from the new quarries on Leckhampton Hill to link up with the new line to Gloucester in Alstone. Building stone was a valuable commodity during this period of expansion, and the Leckhampton quarries filled a long-felt need in Cheltenham. As an investor in the enterprise Jenner might be said to have played a small part in the physical building of the town. While his civic roots were growing steadily deeper, he was able to appraise the snubs and disappointments of distant London with an objective eye, and once having adjusted to being excluded from the official running of the Vaccine Institute he was quite content to help Moore all he could for the good of the cause. He visited Berkeley in November and wrote to his friend from there suggesting that a good way to subdue the opposition would be to swamp them with masses of evidence from the Berkeley area, where the practice had been going on longer than anywhere else. Jenner's list of suggested research questions and other ideas to help the director in his arduous task make it obvious that any bitterness or even jealousy was completely overshadowed by his earnest anxiety to see the institute succeed in its work. "I shall return again to Cheltenham on Tuesday next," he writes, "where I shall be happy to hear from you, particularly on the subject of my former letter."[21]

In addition to the affairs of the institute he was, of course, extremely interested in Moore's literary activities. Moore was already engaged in writing a life of the brother killed at Corunna, but more important were his works on smallpox and vaccination. In a letter from Cheltenham the week before Christmas, Jenner gives him much more information about source material. He relates the inside story of his controversy with Woodville and explains how that erstwhile "enemy's" kindness to his, Jenner's, children all those years ago had softened his attitude. Then he continues:

Do pray see Paytherus, he will give you a thousand odd anecdotes, and don't forget to ask him for his book on vaccination. He must not omit telling you what once happened at a dinner at Coleman's. . . . I have much more to say to you: indeed, your first letter I do not consider as yet answered; but now I must go to my bed or drop upon my paper. Excuse this sleepy letter.

Truly yours,
Edward Jenner.

Cheltenham, twelve o'clock
Wednesday night, 19th December, 1810.
P.S.   I shall give you some trouble soon in assisting me to liberate a French officer, the brother of Husson (see the list of names in the enclosed paper) who has nearly lost the use of his arm.[22]

The postscript referred to Captain Husson, brother of the great French vaccination pioneer, who had been taken prisoner by the Spaniards at Baylen in July, 1808, and sent to England. Bearing in mind the kindness he had received from Napoleon when interceding for British prisoners of war, Jenner had done all he could to secure the release of this young man the year before. The British government was not as attentive to the pleas of Dr. Jenner as the French had been, however, and after some raising of hopes the prisoner's case was denied. Husson was so distraught that he broke his parole and tried to get across the Channel. He was inevitably caught, and incarcerated like any ordinary criminal in a prison hulk at Chatham. This was the dismal state of affairs when Jenner wrote to Moore. The ships that housed the prisoners at Chatham were normally for civil convicts serving terms shorter than transportation sentences. The sensitive young Frenchman's state of mind can well be imagined. The loss of the use of his arm was probably from dampness or rheumatism. The matter of paroled officers would soon be a problem in Cheltenham, too, where at least four gentleman prisoners from France were due to set up residence.

After Jenner's pleas to enemy sovereigns had liberated British captives, it was inevitable that the traffic would eventually be expected to flow the other way. What people on the Continent did not realize, however, was that the British government held the doctor in far less esteem than did their own. Through the influence of his Cheltenham friends he was able to get such parliamentary action as he needed to keep body and soul together, and, rather laboriously, pursue his vaccination campaign as a public service. But he was not liked by those in power and no *personal* favors or honors came his way. He once remarked to Baron that so small was his interest with those in authority who dispensed favors in Britain that he never succeeded in obtaining an appointment for either of his nephews. He did concede, however, that he had "once got a place for an excise man, but nothing beyond it." The extent of Jenner's influence was made brutally apparent in the case of General Lefevre, the Frenchman captured by Sir John Moore before the battle of Corunna.

Colonel Macleod, an effeminate-looking little man who had, incidentally, been mercilessly lampooned by Mrs. Jordan a couple of months earlier, had himself been a prisoner of war in France some years before. He had received a great deal of kindness from

General Lefevre and was accordingly very concerned when that distinguished soldier was taken prisoner. As the local paper reported at the time, the general had begged his captor to excuse him from the long ocean voyage to England:

When General Lefevre was taken prisoner at the skirmish at Benevente, in Spain, he requested that Sir John Moore would allow him to go to Calais by land, as a passage by sea always impaired his health; and that on his honour as an officer, he would proceed to Dover, and give himself up as a prisoner of war. Sir John Moore replied that he might meet with some danger in crossing the channel, but he would allow him an English frigate, which he knew would go safe to any part of the world without danger and would soon waft him over the bay.[23]

Jenner then was manifestly not the only Cheltenham man to intercede for French prisoners, for at the very time that he was trying to extricate Captain Husson from the Chatham prison hulks, Colonel Macleod was using his great influence in military circles to get his benefactor Lefevre transferred, on parole, to Cheltenham. The tragedy was that Macleod was listened to but Jenner was not.

A year previously, a few days after his son's death, the doctor had been approached by Mr. Corvesart for assistance in locating a young French prisoner alleged to be held at Wincanton in Somerset. "Can you assist me?" Jenner had asked Moore. ". . . I am somewhat at a loss to know where to make my application. I could have easy access to one of the Royal Dukes if this would do."[24] But the three royal dukes who were Jenner's supporters—Clarence, York, and Sussex—apparently availed nothing. The young officer—an ensign named Rigodit—was never found; and then came the Husson case. The doctor was still anxiously waiting for news from the government when General Lefevre arrived in Cheltenham, like a conquering hero, on February 12.

Macleod's friends in high places had done him well. The general's wife had been allowed to join him, and he was accompanied by two other captive generals. To complete his "court" several noncommissioned French soldiers were distributed about the town in Cambray, High Street, and Tewkesbury Road, while the three generals themselves lived in a house on the corner of North Street and High Street—Boots' corner. From the beginning Lefevre was a lion of society. Madam Lefevre was equally popular and the Countess of Buckinghamshire soon competed with the Macleods in lavish entertainments honoring the distinguished French pair.

By contrast, the hardships suffered by the unfortunate Captain Husson were most unjustly laid at Jenner's door by Dr. Husson. The French vaccination pioneer had no way of knowing how little Jenner was appreciated in certain areas of authority and how difficult it was to break the British wall of protocol. Even when the young man was finally released his brother apparently did not associate the event with Jenner's activities that had started so long ago. On April 5 Jenner wrote to Baron, "This day I received a letter from town, informing me that my petition to the Prince had been graciously received." But nothing was done and the young man remained in captivity.

In addition, there were new worries of a domestic nature. Mrs. Jenner's brother, Thomas Kingscote, who also lived in Cheltenham and was sinking under what Baron calls "a painful and protracted disease," was yet another problem for the family to bear. Jenner himself became ill in the spring, though not enough to prevent him from making a brief visit to London in March. He seems to have journeyed back and forth to London frequently during those initial days of the new anti-inoculation campaign, but he always hurried home quickly. He grew to like the capital less and less; he would simply go up and back again when he needed to—no more long sojourns. In April when he was still feeling far from well, another sorrow he had long kept to himself came to its humiliating climax.

The frustration he must have felt when he was unable to return the favors bestowed upon him by his supporters abroad was linked to a fatalistic conviction that, no matter what he did, his own government would never appreciate him. He had treated the royal family without official response, and he had seen one of his younger colleagues appointed Surgeon Extraordinary. On the other hand, all the countries that had adopted his system had rewarded *their* vaccination pioneers handsomely. In 1810 a situation arose that gave Jenner every reason to believe that belated honors might be his. The Indian subcontinent was British, but it was not ruled by the British government, and here vaccination had made extraordinary progress. The merchants who ran the East India Company would be under no obligation to follow the pattern of certain politicians at home whom Jenner's bluntness had possibly ruffled. All through the tragic year of 1810 talk had been prevalent about the company's gratification at the elimination of smallpox from its territories. At first Jenner must have been puzzled when, despite the recognition and rewards he received from the people of India, no word came to him from official sources. So the months went by and he meekly waited as he always did. There is no mention of the business by any of his contemporaries so he undoubtedly kept the matter to himself. But sooner or later the most patient worm must turn. Jenner had been content to see Christie's fame as the conqueror of smallpox in Ceylon resound over England. It was all in the interest of the cause and Ceylon was but a small country of the Far East. The cleansing of India was the greater feat, and that, one would assume, was indisputably Jenner's victory. But the fates in the form of the East India Company were not so sure.

The labored efforts to get vaccine to Madras through Bentinck and others had been both slow and difficult, but fortunately De Carro had been able to get samples of his supply of Jennerian vaccine from Constantinople by short stages to Bombay in good condition. Jenner was, of course, delighted. He was not concerned with the transmitting details as long as the precious serum arrived, and he had always looked upon the Austrian doctor as one of his most valuable disciples. Indeed, during the pioneer years the two men had been extremely close, and Jenner had actually sent his friend a silver snuffbox in appreciation of his work. Consequently, when the directors of the East India Company sent De Carro a substantial grant of money for his part in eradicating smallpox from the company's territories, Jenner saw it as a general recognition of the movement, and waited to hear from them himself. But they had made their award for the cleansing of India, and a much higher authority would shortly reward the work in Ceylon. Despite the grateful thanks Jenner had received from Wellesley, Wellington, Bentinck, Russell, and many other company servants, not a word in support came from the nabobs.

Despite his feeling for De Carro, this was too much. He went to the banker Sir Francis Baring, who was a director of the company, and, more important, intimately related to several of Jenner's friends. His son George had married Sir John D'Oyly's younger daughter Harriet, and it will be recalled that the older girl, Maynard D'Oyly, had married Farquhar's son, who was then in the East India Company's service. Possibly the latter man was Jenner's go-between. The old banker was sympathetic and would probably have interceded had he not died on September 12, 1810.

Once more, as in the Newell case, Jenner maintained a dignified restraint and mentioned the humiliation he suffered to none of his friends. In the six months following Sir Francis's death he sought out one director after another but to no avail. Nothing, in fact, would be known about this affair had it not been for the discovery in 1971 of a letter hidden in the frame behind an engraving of Jenner. The letter, kindly put at my disposal, was written to a lady whom Jenner hoped might speak on his behalf to Sir Hugh Inglis. He had apparently already discussed the business with her.

Dear Madam,
That I may not load your memory with the detail I laid before you a short time since, respecting the circumstances I wished you to do me the favour of making known to Sir Hugh Inglis I beg leave to trouble you with it in writing.

As soon as I became perfectly satisfied that the vaccination discovery was in every respect complete I began to turn my views to India and made several efforts to introduce the new practice there by sending the matter to Madras with ample instructions to the medical men at the different Presidencies. However, from the length of the voyage or want of practice among those into whose hands it fell it was ineffectual.

My friend and pupil Dr. De Carro of Vienna soon after availed himself of an opportunity of sending it to Constantinople and by renewing it at different stations as it pass'd on it at length reached Bombay in a state of perfection. Dr. De Carro's meritorious services claimed the attention of the East India Company and they were noticed by a pecuniary present. This event gave me peculiar pleasure as no-one among my numerous followers has labor'd more to spread vaccination over the globe, or has been more successful than this gentleman.

Now my dear Madam to my point. How it came to pass that the *second* person concerned in this important business should have been honor'd with attention and not the first? For I must observe the Doctor had the matter from me and from this source it moved onward. The advantages derived from the universal adoption of vaccination throughout the Company's settlements in India are represented to me as immense. Millions have already been saved from an untimely grave who would have been sent there by the ravages of the Smallpox. But this need scarcely to be mentioned to Sir Hugh Inglis as he must already be well acquainted with the Fact. My application must appear to come rather late, but this may be explained. I have many times mentioned it to more than one of the Directors, particularly to the late Sir F. Baring who assured me he thought I had a claim on their attention.

As I mentioned to you in our conversation on the subject it is not the munificence of the Honble Company I presume to solicit but some mark (should I be thought to be deserving of it) of their notice. For how very odd it must appear a century or two hence to see the name of Dr. De Carro recorded in their books as the source of that benefit which India has derived from the Vaccine Discovery and not that of . . . Madam

> Your obliged
> &obed^t. humble serv^t.
> Edward Jenner.

St. George's Place,
April 8th, 1811.[25]

Nothing appears to have come of the letter that reveals a poignant sorrow imperfectly concealed by a businesslike style.

Following this De Carro seems to have faded out of Jenner's life. There were no recriminations but the relationship drifted. There was a brief word in a letter to Moore the following February. Commenting on a Spanish newspaper story, Jenner says rather bitterly: ". . . it is on vaccination they so lavishly pour forth their praises, and not on me. I have not received any late report either from Dr. De Carro, or Professor Odier, at Geneva." What is remarkable about this unprecedented example of official ingratitude is that the doctor never let the company's behavior influence his feelings for Christie, who was also basking in public attention. In fact, even while he was pathetically and secretly trying to obtain recognition for his services to India, he was preparing to present the story of the Ceylon campaign to the public despite a hundred other pressing matters demanding his attention. The ever cheerful and hopeful pioneer was not so sanguine anymore, however. Perhaps had not Catherine been going through a period of better health and obviously enjoying her return to a peaceful domestic life after the ordeal of bereavement, he would have given up the struggle.

Young Worgan and Edward had occupied some two years in their lingering departures from this world while it was becoming more and more apparent that the doctor would never get the recognition he had earned. Society had to acknowledge the realities of vaccination, but it did not have to celebrate its discoverer. Jenner was paid money, albeit grudgingly, so that he might carry on his labors in the public interest, but no honor of any kind from the state went with it. It might be well at this point to analyze the circumstances around Jenner as he entered his sixty-third year.

Vaccination had swept the world despite the almost continuous state of war between the great powers. Abroad Jenner's name was everywhere: streets bore his name, children were named after him, and festivals were held in his honor. But in Britain it was vaccination that was esteemed—with certain reservations—and a vaccination pioneer, Thomas Newell, was granted the royal patronage, presumably to cover the state's obligation to the movement. When Jenner nursed the King's son through a dangerous illness—and indeed probably saved his life—he received no such official recognition: he was instead given an excellent water pipe. Not, however, by the grateful royal father but from the thankful patient himself.

The decline of Jenner's standing with the Prince of Wales seems to have commenced after the invitation to the command performance at the Theatre Royal in 1807. By this time, fortunately, the doctor's backing in the House of Lords was too strong to break, but thereafter this support from the highest in the land could not bring him *official* distinctions. For him no royal appointment, no order of chivalry, no office under the crown; indeed, no further financial grants. What happened between that Chel-

tenham theater party and the first snubbing after Sussex's illness
was the friendship between the Princess of Wales and Jenner.
His visits to Blackheath with her friends Angerstein and Lawrence might have ruffled the Prince's vanity and made him see
disloyalty in a man he no doubt felt had benefitted from his
earlier patronage. But unfortunately the problem was much
wider than this.

Jenner was *not* idolized in England the way he was abroad. His
solid coterie of nobles in the Cheltenham salons and his wide
circle of friends among the medical intelligentsia in no way reflected the attitude of the thousands of general practitioners and
the public throughout the kingdom. Save for his business trips
to London and a visit to Scotland his activities were practically
confined to his native county for the entire span of his professional life. Even in Gloucestershire his ideas were suspect, outside
of Cheltenham, right up to the time of his death. With the exception of Edinburgh, none of the great provincial cities of the
country knew him, and no mobs milled in the streets begging his
attention as they did in St. George's Place. His lecture engagements were remarkably sparse for a man of such importance, and
the number of papers he read before the learned societies during
his entire career was negligible. In effect, he had a population to
cope with that was suspicious of his ideas and helped along in its
ignorance by a cynical phalanx of doctors who saw disruption and
loss of revenue in his interference. Added to this were the monumental voices of the Lord Chancellor and the Lord Chief Justice
of England passively blessed by the pettish irritation of the Prince
Regent himself. To be sure, many learned associations—those
under such personal friends as Astley Cooper, Saunders, or Bradley—accepted him, but both the Royal Colleges denied him
membership. Even the National Vaccine Establishment itself was
given to another. If this situation could exist when he had so
much backing in the highest realms of society one cannot help
wondering what would have been the fate of his life's work without it. Since Charles James Fox, he had known every Prime Minister *personally;* yet his associations were not sufficient to bring
him the recognition he deserved—nor did the situation ever
change.

⤷ VIII ⤶

The Perfidy of Princes

1811-1812

Perhaps no project of Jenner's had ever been so buffeted and delayed as his plan to publish Christie's Ceylon narrative. Aside from the heartache of the East India Company affair, in this year of 1811 he was beset by every kind of obstacle. There was the matter of the Berkeley Succession trial and also the Grosvenor business, both of which took weeks and months of time he could ill afford, but the book remained his principal concern.

Certain things had developed since his return to Cheltenham that made the publication project viable. The fact that the *Chronicle* once more fell upon evil times actually worked to his advantage. Thomas Pruen, who continued to lose money, finally gave up the struggle and sold the paper on January 17, 1811. The purchaser was a Mr. J. K. Griffith, head of a printing firm that was fast outstripping Ruff in his particular field. Pruen was loyal and dependable in his support of vaccination, but he was an enthusiastic amateur and had neither the money nor the knowledge to run a newspaper. Griffith, on the other hand, already had the largest printing plant in the town at Portland Yard and was one of a large family of experts (including his mother). But most important of all, he was also a friend of the Jenners' and had a crusader's zeal to stamp out smallpox inoculation. It is significant to note that Jenner's interest in Christie's book developed during the time the Griffiths were negotiating to buy the *Chronicle* from Pruen, toward the end of 1810, and properly publicized, such a venture could strike a formidable blow against smallpox inoculation. For Jenner the word "inoculation" could well be left out. The fight, in terms of newspaper policy, was against the deliberate

spread of smallpox—a crime of the worst order that had no logical
excuse when the mild form of cowpox could be injected as an
effective preventive. Christie's fortuitous arrival in Cheltenham
presented a new and potentially powerful weapon in the cause.
Once the younger doctor was settled in his new home in Cambray
Street with his wife and two children, the organization of the campaign was started in earnest. Dr. Coley lived only two doors away
and was rapidly becoming sufficiently prominent in the movement
as to be second only to Jenner himself. And Jenner's plan was a
book on the eradication of smallpox from the island of Ceylon
solely as a result of the complete substitution of vaccination for
smallpox inoculation. It would be prima facie evidence of the
most irrefutable kind.

Christie, however, had to be persuaded. When he had left the
island in February 1810, he had assumed that the battle for recognition of the practice was over. The campaign for the future
would be the providing of vaccine and vaccinators to spread the
blessing throughout an eager and accepting population. During
the months at sea on his voyage home, he had seen nothing to
interfere with this assumption. At every point between India and
Europe, vaccination, in a world at war, was eagerly embraced. It
was clear that throughout the years in his voluminous correspondence with Farquhar, Elgin, and even Jenner, the bitter
resistance of certain powerful medical forces in Britain had not
been made clear. When he arrived at Cheltenham in September,
however, he was very disillusioned. "I had considered the question
at rest;" he wrote, "the more so as in an extensive communication
and correspondence with the Medical men in different parts of
India, *I never heard of one* who had the smallest doubt as to the
preservative efficacy of Cowpox, or the propriety of the general
system of vaccination there adopted."[1]

But he was not long in learning the state of affairs in Britain.
Perhaps Cheltenham gave a rosy picture of the situation, but Jenner himself was soon able to make the younger man aware of the
need for every extra pen that could be marshalled in the cause. The
fight must now be pressed with renewed hope since among Jenner's
greatest virtues were his doggedness and almost superhuman patience. He apparently never tired of having to answer the same

attacks year after year, and his answers were the same year after year. His enemies did not vary their approach very much: cowpox inoculation, according to his detractors, did not secure the patient against smallpox, a claim proven by the many cases of smallpox contracted after vaccination. Jenner monotonously replied that the protection was complete, and the operation never failed if the correct procedure was followed. In the happy year of 1804—when he first heard from Christie about the Ceylon triumph, when he received his first grant money and had bought his house—Jenner had written to Lord Berkeley: ". . . a great number, perhaps a majority of those who inoculate, are not sufficiently acquainted with the nature of the disease to enable them to discriminate with due accuracy between the perfect and imperfect postule. This is a lesson not very difficult to learn, but unless it is learnt, to inoculate the cowpox is folly and presumption."[2] Six years later, when at the bedside of his dying son he wrote to Moore relative to the same problem: "I have taken a world of pains to correct this abuse (inexpert operation) but still, to my knowledge, it is going on, and particularly among the faculty in town."[3] And so he went on until the day of his death: vaccination was the certain preventive for smallpox *if properly performed*.

The fact that these obvious truths had to be monotonously driven home year in and year out despite the manifest universal evidence eventually convinced Christie that England was not Ceylon, and that the battle still had to be won. He was particularly concerned about the hazard to children implicit in the tactics of the opposition and he had good reason. "A son of my own who had a vesicle, regular in form, but premature, the oreola having commenced on the seventh day, has since been inoculated six times without effect."[4] In fact, the summary of his preface suggests that this was the reason why he finally agreed to relate the story of the Ceylon experience. If it "shall induce one parent to secure his offspring from the contagion of smallpox by means of vaccination I shall be satisfied that my time has not been misemployed."

Through the bleak winter of 1810–11, still rather numbed by the bereavements he had suffered, Jenner went over the vast array of materials the young doctor had brought with him from Ceylon.

What a record they represented: a glorious and unopposed progress of the system until a tropical and "backward" Asiatic country was completely *free* of smallpox while civilized England hesitated to cleanse herself. There was no question but what this story had to be released to the world as soon as possible. Christie tells how he was "particularly urged by the great author of the discovery, Dr. Jenner, that an essential service might be done to the community by a description of the circumstances attending the introduction of vaccination into Ceylon in August 1802." Nor was Jenner alone in his importuning; many other medical acquaintances added their pleas, and finally Christie, who had stated that he had no intention "of ever writing on the subject again," was persuaded to cooperate. So it was all arranged. Jenner's friend Griffith would publish the book and it could be ready that very year.

Once the project was launched Christie's reluctance vanished, and from the published result, it seems clear that Jenner assisted him in the actual writing. It was finished by July 1, 1811, the date of its dedication to Sir Walter Farquhar, which referred to "the deep sense of gratitude I feel for the great obligations you have conferred on me, by directing my studies in youth; and affording me your uniform support and protection in more mature age." Perhaps it would have been more fitting for the author to have dedicated it to the much passed-over Jenner who discovered the system about which it was written, had suggested and helped in the production of the book, and whose friend Griffith had published it. But one passage in the preface made up for everything in Jenner's eyes. Christie hoped "that the expulsion of smallpox from so large an island as Ceylon may excite considerable attention in Great Britain, and that the means pursued by the government there for *Prohibiting variolus inoculation,* and encouraging vaccination, may be thought worthy of the attention of the British Legislature."[5]

The book had an extremely long title, which may be briefly stated as follows: *An Account of the Ravages Committed in Ceylon by Smallpox . . . With a Statement of . . . the Introduction, Progress and Success of Vaccination Inoculation in that Island. Printed by J. & B. Griffith, Portland Passage, Cheltenham, 1811.*

Jenner was delighted. Nothing had ever appeared before of such devastating proof of his doctrine. He wrote to Moore the following year, ". . . pray do not let Dr. Christie's be forgotten. Among all the good ones, *there is nothing to surpass this.*" Certainly the support for forbidding smallpox inoculation was increased by the work. Legislative action, indeed, did follow in 1812 with Lord Borington's first bill in the Upper House.

With the honors which were showered upon Christie following the appearance of his book one might say that it was yet again the case of the protégé's being rewarded instead of the master, but fortunately Jenner's disposition was not such as to allow bitterness to impair his relationship with an ally. It was as important to maintain the support of Christie as it had been to hold that of Newell after the humiliation of 1810.

The launching of the book from Griffith's office and the new initiative in the *Chronicle*'s policy suggested to Jenner that there might well be a case for setting up a vaccination institute in Cheltenham. Certainly London was getting increasingly discouraging. The Sussex, Newell, and East India Company rebuffs, coupled with his exclusion by the National Vaccine Institute and the Royal College of Physicians, made it clear that there was little future for him in the ruling medical establishment. On the other hand, the anti-smallpox inoculation movement instituted in the county seat at Gloucester the previous year was mainly the work of Cheltenham doctors and had been very well supported. To concentrate the main body of vaccination research in the vicinity of his own home would really be making official what had long been the unmistakable de facto trend. Perhaps Jenner's bitter reaction to the East India Company's snubbing was the decisive factor, since exactly three weeks after his letter to Sir Hugh Inglis's friend, the following announcement appeared in the *Chronicle:* "Dr. Jenner has nobly manifested his zeal in the cause of humanity by having most liberally offered to give a piece of ground to erect a vaccine institute in this town."[6] Presumably the building plot offered was to be taken from his large garden on the opposite side of St. George's Place next to Rowland Hill's little burial ground.

Griffith followed up this item in successive issues with the latest and most impressive vaccination news he could find from all parts of the world. A week after Jenner's offer he printed a glowing tribute from Dr. Barrey, the eminent French physician, entitled "Vaccine and Its Effects." After expatiating on the value of the discovery and its impact on civilization, he pointed out that it was acclaimed by all the leading doctors of Europe. "Even war and disease united," he proclaimed, "cannot accomplish so much misery as the vaccine will produce of benefit to mankind." A few weeks later it was announced—once more from France—that "young Napoleon was vaccinated on the ninth (of May)."

This almost defiant spurt of journalistic activity from Cheltenham was rudely halted in midstream when Jenner was peremptorily called to London by the Earl of Grosvenor, whose third son Robert was dying of smallpox. Unfortunately it was on record that the doctor himself had vaccinated the child in May 1801, but in fact the mother had interfered through overanxiety and had not permitted the regular procedure to be followed. Jenner wrote at the time, "I vaccinated this young gentleman in a puny state of health at about a month old. Lady Grosvenor was timid and prevailed upon me to deviate from my usual mode of practice; and to make one puncture only; and the postule it excited was unfortunately deranged in its progress by being rubbed by the nurse. The smallpox which followed went through its course in a shorter period than usual and scarcely left any mark." None of this, however, was made known at the time.

Extraordinarily enough, even though the boy was stricken on May 26, 1811, his two royal doctors—Jenner's friends, Sir Henry Halford and Sir Walter Farquhar—did not recognize the disease as smallpox for some days, being undoubtedly misled by the assumption that there had been a successful vaccination ten years before. Under normal circumstances, therefore, having received no appropriate treatment, the boy should have been dead when Jenner arrived. Belatedly, on June 1, the smallpox diagnosis was made by Farquhar, and was of such a serious nature that he gave little hope for the child's recovery. Nevertheless, they were confused "that the latter stages of the disease were passed through more rapidly in this case than usual; and it may be a question whether this extraordinary circumstance as well as the ultimate recovery of Master Grosvenor, were not influenced by previous vaccination."[7]

It took a week to inform Jenner and get him to London, so that when he visited the patient on June 8, in the company of Farquhar, the child was already on the way to recovery. Fortunately, the earl's other children, though exposed to the contagion from their brother, were unaffected. A subsequent inoculation with smallpox was equally without effect, even though they also had been vaccinated as far back as 1801. Nevertheless, this case played into the hands of the enemy as an example in the highest possible rank of society in which vaccination had provided no protection against smallpox. The National Vaccine Establishment put out a special report on the case, and Jenner explained the complete background. The 1801 vaccination had not properly taken, therefore the immunizing effect of cowpox had not applied. The real tragedy of the situation, however, was that despite young Grosvenor's recovery, many people rushed to have their children inoculated with smallpox. It was the Dodeswell episode all over again. No matter what pains Jenner took to prove his case the enemy exaggerated the tiniest hitch into another "failure." As a footnote to this occurrence the principal actor, little Robert Grosvenor, lived until 1893, when he died as Lord Ebury on November 18, well within the memory of many people living today. Yet he was one of the first to be vaccinated by Jenner.

But by far the worst ordeal of this turbulent spring was Jenner's attendance, at intervals between March and midsummer, at one of the most famous trials ever staged in the House of Lords. As the family doctor and lifelong friend of Lady Berkeley's, he was required to testify at the hearing on the Berkeley succession. The late Earl of Berkeley was alleged to have forged the entry in the parish register at Berkeley showing him to have married the countess in 1785 instead of 1796 and making his four sons legitimate, including the eldest. The case was lost and the Lords proclaimed, on July 1, that the new Earl of Berkeley was Morton Berkeley, who was born after the recognized marriage in 1796. Counsel for the Crown, Sir Thomas Plumer,[8] was brilliant and ruthless in winning a case that everyone felt would end in favor of the eldest son. "The Solicitor-General has gained great credit by his ability and perseverance in proving the forgery of a pretended *former* marriage of the late Lord Berkeley," wrote Farington.

Jenner was called upon to testify at length on two occasions,

though he was obliged to be on hand most of the time in case one
of the learned Lords required him to clarify some point in the
medical evidence. The point that the Lords, who opposed Her
Ladyship's claim, sought to make was that it was generally understood by the Berkeleys' friends that there was no marriage before
March 16, 1796,[9] but the eldest son, born before this marriage,
insisted that his parents had been married in Berkeley church on
the thirtieth of March, 1785. In the course of the investigation,
Jenner was asked, on March 8, 1811, whether Mrs. Jenner had
ever called upon Lady Berkeley at the Castle before the 1796
marriage. He was obliged to admit that she had not. The pious
Catherine knew nothing of any earlier marriage and could not
bring herself to call socially upon a lady who was living in sin.
Paytherus, Caleb Parry, Sir Isaac Heard, Gwinnett, and Gardner,
among others, were subjected to exhaustive questioning in order
to establish a common admission of Her Ladyship's irregular
status. A great deal of importance was laid upon her first pregnancy after the 1796 marriage. It was alleged that Lord Berkeley
was very concerned about producing an heir, a concern, if established, that would show that he did not consider his existing sons
legitimate. Jenner was questioned along these lines on June 18.
"During that pregnancy did you never hear Lord Berkeley express
his anxiety that it might be a son in order to have an heir to his
title?"

To which the doctor replied stolidly, "O never."[10]

"Were you at Berkeley Castle at the Beginning of the year
1797?" he was asked.

"Yes, I was," he replied.

"In what part?"

"I believe I was there the whole year. . . . It was my permanent residence, save for one or two excursions."[11]

At another point in his evidence Jenner admitted that he had
been responsible for the medical care of the eldest son ever since
his birth; his testimony revealed that whatever Catherine's qualms
might have been, Jenner himself had waited upon Lady Berkeley
and her children, wedlock or no wedlock, from the very beginning. He had been her doctor for twenty-six years. Nor was his
role of doctor the only aspect of the Lord's interrogations. He was

obviously accepted as one of the closest and oldest friends of the family and was even asked to identify signatures. All the panoply of a modern Scotland Yard came into play during this long hearing. Not only were handwriting experts called in but also authorities on paper. Jenner was closely questioned as to the authenticity of the signatures of the late Lord Berkeley himself, and of the alleged performer of the 1785 ceremony, Rev. Augustus Thomas Hupsman, vicar of Berkeley, who was long since in his grave. The doctor was particularly pressed about the matter of open and closed loops in the late peer's handwriting and about the way certain letters were formed. His replies indicated a knowledge of the subject that undoubtably strengthened the probability of forgery as did those of the late vicar's wife.

All in all, it was a tragic business, and the principal sufferer was the unfortunate Lady Berkeley. What had started on February 11 as "The case of William Fitzharding Berkeley, Earl of Berkeley, on his petition to the King, to be summoned to Parliament, for the earldom of Berkeley," became a long, drawn-out investigation, in the most merciless and clinical detail, of the countess's morality. Indeed, nothing could be more indicative of the fact that the real appellant in the business was Lady Berkeley than the great document that issued from the trial: the "Address to the Right Honourable Peers of the United Kingdom of Great Britain and Ireland, from Mary, Countess of Berkeley"[12] ran to 212 pages and put the real issues into proper perspective.

Despite the verdict of the Lords, the Cheltenham press was very sympathetic to Lady Berkeley. In fact the whole family, including Morton who became the new earl as a result of the trial, was indignant. It seemed to be Jenner's fate to have to testify on the side of the prosecution. The Reed murder case would have had a terrifying impact on him had "his" side won, and, in this case, as the Berkeleys' family doctor, he was called upon to give evidence that could only help to prove the illegitimacy of the early issue of the liaison. Few people believed the claim of an earlier marriage; their siding with the family was impelled purely by the affection with which Her Ladyship was generally held. It seemed outrageous that she should be submitted to this humiliation after more than twenty-five years of domestic bliss in a household dominated by her kindness and care, and Jenner was particularly concerned about her ability to stand the strain. After the evidence of a particularly damning witness, he wrote from Cheltenham in the middle of the trial, "I grieve to think how long and unnecessarily this distressing business is procrastinated; but I trust your ladyship's health will be supported under it." He wanted it to be very clear that whatever admissions the keen interrogation of Sir Thomas Plumer elicited from him, his sympathy and loyalty were entirely with Her Ladyship.

Nor was the support for the cause confined to her Gloucestershire friends. To his credit the Prince Regent himself was extremely concerned. He sent her a letter of encouragement on March 4 and soon afterwards visited her so as to let society know exactly where his sympathies lay. Fortunately there was no question of a criminal prosecution, since the forger of the earlier marriage record, Lord Berkeley, was dead. Nonetheless, the strain of the six months' trial was a terrible ordeal for the widow. She had never anticipated the opposition and final humiliation at the bar of the Lords. Her counsel, Sergeant Best—later Baron Wynford, Deputy Speaker of the House of Commons—was one of the most able men in the country, and had anticipated that the case would be disposed of in a few days. But now, in July, as Farington put it, "he looks his disappointment."[13]

After he had given his evidence, Jenner had remained in London until the trial was over, staying as usual at Fladong's Hotel in Oxford Street whence he could return to Cheltenham at a minute's notice if Catherine needed him. He wrote enthusiastically to Worthington of having dinner with Humphrey Davy, who had just received an honorary doctorate from Dublin. But it was not pure science they talked about, it was that somewhat twentieth-century aspect of medical research, snake venom. On June 26 Jenner wrote:

Yesterday I dined with Professor Davy. I wish you had been with us. His mind is all in a blaze. He seems to be one of those rare productions which nature allows us to see once in a score of years. We touched on hydrophobia. He started an ingenious idea, that of counteracting the effects of one morbid poison with another. What think you of a viper? not its broth, but its fang, as soon as the first symptom of disease appears from *canination*. If this should succeed we domicilate vipers as we have leeches. But from this hint I should be disposed to try, under such an event, vaccination; as it can almost always be made to act quickly on the system, whether a person has previously felt its influence or not, or that of the smallpox.[14]

The following year Davy was knighted—and also took as his laboratory assistant a twenty-year-old youth named Michael Faraday.

When the trial was nearing its end, Lady Berkeley turned to the man to whom Jenner had introduced her twelve years before—Sir Isaac Heard. She pleaded with him to help her with regard to the registration and baptism of her eldest son, whose legitimacy she was fighting for. She wrote on June 20 from an address at Spring Gardens,[15] but there was nothing the old man could do to help her. Actually his position as Garter King of Arms had no bearing on deciding whether an entry in the Berkeley church register was a forgery, but the poor distraught woman vaguely saw him as an authority on family history and was willing to seek aid wherever she could. By this time the thinking of a harassed woman under such emotional pressures would not be too logical.

But Jenner still seemed fated to continue, on official occasions, in the role of an unwilling prosecutor, and if the major performance of this nature took place in the House of Lords it was not, unhappily, the only one this year. When he returned home after the trial he hoped to pick up the threads of his professional and domestic life in his usual manner. He was worried about young Husson on the one hand and eager to resume activity about a Vaccine Institute in St. George's Place on the other. Then there was the matter of promoting Christie's book, and of course the ever present shadow of smallpox inoculation. But there were also the irritations that came from time to time relative to his office as a town commissioner. On a much smaller scale, he was again required to play a reluctant part in official business against a personal friend. Rowland Hill's chapel was one of the new centers for vaccination, and though Jenner had been unable to attend its opening and the consequent celebration, he *was* present to inflict what he himself must have considered a grossly unreasonable financial levy upon it. By some misunderstanding, Hill had listed himself as sole proprietor of the institution, but there were, in fact, twelve trustees. Under the law of the time this apparently made him liable for taxation, even though the edifice was a place of worship. The poor man had provided most of the money for the building, and now he would have to pay for his magnanimity. On July 25 the chapel was accordingly declared taxable for the poor rate.[16] The Overseers of the Poor—which meant the vestry—were the immediate authority for this, but the ultimate rulers of the town were, of course, the commissioners. Unquestionably, Jenner would have been bitterly opposed to this anomaly, but he was in the minority and had to witness the board sanction a tax on a place that, every Sunday, vaccinated the poor gratuitously. Unhappily it was the law of the land and not any kind of persecution, but that was small comfort. Likewise, the murder trial in Gloucester and the Lords' tribunal had also been the law of the land.

A chronological record of this year is quite impossible. Jenner was continually required to leave tasks half done and return when he could, but all was not tragedy and heartache. There were periods when he and Catherine could enjoy certain singular aspects of life together, and this summer, fortunately, continued to find her in relatively good health. Music was an important part of his life and it was a part that was very well catered to in his particular geographical location in the town. There were not only the concerts in Mr. Ruff's rooms on the corner but also those at the Fleece Inn. Then there was that celebrated pianoforte artist, Mrs. Cooper, who lived only a few doors away from him, definitely within hearing distance of Catherine's sitting room as was, of course, St. Mary's Church where the great oratorios took place.

All of which brings us to another of Jenner's protégés in a somewhat different category from Christie's—"poor Thomas Cam," a rustic composer of some native ability. "Though compelled to labour at an humble trade," writes Baron, "and little indebted to education . . . (he) contrived, while living in a secluded hamlet, to acquire such a knowledge of the theory of music as to be able to compose pieces of music of considerable length and adapted to a great variety of instruments, some of which he had never seen or heard."[17] Cam was not a young man, however, like Christie or

Fosbroke. He had plodded through the years denied the experience of music as a result of penury, but content to hear it in his mind. A phenomenon of this nature never failed to stir the doctor who might have wondered: What would be the reaction of such a personality if he heard the greatest orchestral music and, perhaps, the greatest singer in the world?

Approaching the end of his days, Charles Trye—who was a great patron of music and a Steward of the Gloucester Music Meeting (later known as the Three Choirs Festival)[18]—contrived to get Catalani[19] to sing for the benefit of his beloved Gloucester Infirmary. As a matter of fact, the festival in 1811 was very much a project of the Jenner coterie. Daniel Lysons, Trye's brother-in-law, was the director and also its historian, and even the ubiquitous Mr. Entwistle, a patient of Jenner's, played the violin. Indeed, the great Catalani herself was something of a figure in the medical world. She performed as a money raiser for hospitals, though she was not always appreciated. After many of her concerts she would linger in the city or town concerned and seek some worthwhile cause to support with her services before she left.

It must have been to this concert that Jenner took Thomas Cam. "There he witnessed an orchestra more varied and complete than any he had ever before contemplated. He listened with extraordinary satisfaction; and when Jenner asked him if he was not astonished at the strange concord of sweet sounds issuing from a number of instruments new to him, 'Oh!', said he, 'I knowed how it would all be.' " Samuel Lysons was rather more fortunate after the concert. He took dinner with Madame Catalani and her husband and told Farington all about it. "He said she was very humane and extremely disposed to do acts of kindness, and is always ready to sing, when in health, for public charities."[20] Needless to say, her charitable spirit was well received in Gloucestershire. Lysons's brother, Daniel, and Trye decided that any generous offerings by the great singer would be more than welcomed by the Gloucester Infirmary. It is pleasant to think that in the closing days of his life Charles Brandon Trye should be closely associated with one as beautiful and talented as the Catalani, but so it was.

When the festival was over, Madame Catalani spent a couple of days looking around Gloucester before leaving for Cheltenham, where she intended to live for a while. "During a visit made by Madame Catalani to the County Prison," writes Daniel Lysons, "she proposed under the most evident impulse of benevolent feelings that a concert should be given for the release of poor debtors, during her intended residence in Cheltenham, offering the gratuitous exertions of her great talents on the occasion. Her kind proposal was instantly accepted; and the Stewards of the late Meeting undertook to be Directors of the Concert. . . . One of the Stewards [Trye?] . . . proposed that a share of the profits should be appropriated to that excellent charity, the County Infirmary."[21] She had already moved to Cheltenham when the Stewards had held their meeting, but she expressed her willingness to come over to Gloucester so that the concert could be held in the immensity of the cathedral. With a thousand people buying tickets at five shillings each (Gloucester could not demand Cheltenham prices), the Cathedral was packed, and a total of £264 was raised. All expenses were defrayed by the promoters of the concert and the poor debtors' liabilities only amounted to £71-3-4. When £62-15-8 had been set aside for future relief, the entire balance, some £130, went to the infirmary. Not, perhaps, just what Madame Catalani had anticipated when she visited the prison, but she was very happy, nevertheless, when she returrned to Cheltenham.

Mr. Watson of the Theatre Royal, an old friend of the singer's, had paid her a thousand guineas for a week's performance in Birmingham, two years before in 1809, and, by all accounts, her run at Cheltenham must have cost him even more. It is known that she performed there for over two weeks, and the seats for one performance of the *Messiah* at the Parish Church were ten and sixpence each—a huge sum for those days. In addition, there were *a hundred other musicians*—a mighty event indeed—and for Jenner this Cheltenham appearance was, as it were, a command performance. Sitting in his little back room overlooking the churchyard, he could listen to the transcendental rhapsodies of the great soprano not so many yards from his chair, with Catherine, who did not go out by night, sitting beside him.

Thomas Cam, moved but not awed by it all, lived to see some

of his compositions in print. "I am told by good judges," said Baron, "that, considering his opportunities, they are very astonishing." I cannot find evidence of their ever being performed, but it is not unlikely that Jenner and Boisragon tried them out on one of their musical occasions.

It was while Catalani was in Cheltenham that Jenner lost one of his most valuable contacts with the royal family. The Duke of Clarence broke with Mrs. Jordan while she was playing at the Theatre Royal. At the age of fifty she would present no more babies for vaccination. She arrived on what was to be her farewell visit on September 17. She was not feeling well and was already worried over her relationship with the duke, who was beset by creditors and was secretly debating the possibilities of a wealthy marriage. From Cheltenham, on Tuesday, September 17, she wrote: "I have been so unwell that I cannot keep anything on my stomach, a most cruel sensation produced frequently by agitation but which I never experienced before and trust in God I never shall again." After a couple of days, however, she was better—at least physically:

Madame Catalani is here. She left her card with a very civil invitation to her concerts. I in return wrote her a *civil* answer, concluding with saying that I never went into public when from home—so there our acquaintance ends.—so much the better. . . . Many people have left cards here that I do not know—those I do know I have made Thomas return.[22]

To make matters worse, the autumn set in like a premature winter. Even the loyal Cheltenham people did not wish to leave the warmth of their comfortable salons to visit the theater. "The badness of the weather is thinning this place very fast," she wrote on the twenty-eighth and the thirtieth. "This day has turned out shocking and if it continues so tomorrow my pocket will pay for it, for a wet night here ruins the Theatre." But the next day it did indeed continue so. "This place is thinning fast and another few days of bad weather will make it miserable."[23]

Mrs. Jordan left Cheltenham forever on October 2, 1811. It is said that while she was actually playing a letter arrived from the duke ending their twenty-year liaison, and it may be so. One observation of hers on September 24 reveals an unbroken will fighting a broken heart. ". . . I play tonight, Play and Farce, and fear I shall do it with very bad grace. Many people have taken notice and have said, 'Mrs. Jordan does not appear in spirits,' but it is impossible at time to force them."[24] She was a gallant woman, and it should never be forgotten that her splendid brood of ten royal children, even though borne on the nether side of the blanket, was the first entire royal family to be inoculated with Jenner's vaccine. He owed her a great deal. Perhaps history should remember her more for this rather than for being a great actress and a future king's mistress.

On October 11, just under three weeks after Madame Catalani's concert at the cathedral, Charles Brandon Trye died at his Gloucester house, Friar's Orchard. He had been ill for several months with severe pains in the head. He told his brother-in-law, Lysons, early in the year that "he felt sensations in his head which he was sure had a fatal tendency."[25] In fact he composed an epitaph for his memorial plaque in Leckhampton Church and picked out the spot where he wished to be buried in the church of St. Mary Le Crypt in Gloucester. He had spent so many dedicated years at the Royal Infirmary that his heart was there rather than at his birthplace in Leckhampton.

The final attack had come on Thursday, October 3, and Jenner was summoned from Cheltenham. Baron was already in attendance when he got to the house, but it was apparent that there could be no recovery. Baron said later in describing the occasion: "I allude to this occurrence here, because it brought me for some days into close and constant professional attendance with Dr. Jenner." It rather looks as though the two men had had little association before this. Trye was very stoical and even "gave various minute directions concerning his affairs with the utmost calmness." It was, at first, thought that he had cholera, but this was soon seen to be incorrect. Jenner never gave up the fight to save the life of his earliest medical friend; as Baron put it, "his services were unremitting." They battled on all through Friday and Saturday, with little or no sleep, but on Sunday there was a turn for the worse. The patient, who in his innermost thoughts was something of a saint and ascetic, received Holy Communion and died very early the following morning. It is no reflection on Jenner's devoted friendship that he was most concerned to find out what had killed his friend, and after four days of an exhausting day and night struggle against death, the two doctors performed a postmortem. They discovered that the tissue of one side of the brain was in a deteriorated condition. Poor Trye must have suffered for many years.[26]

He died a rich man, of course. He left his eldest son an estate which brought him an income of £2,400 per annum, while the medical practice made about £1,200. This latter was actually very small for a man of his renown, since he seldom took any fees from poor people, who constituted the bulk of the population in any community. His philosophy caused him "to give his assistance to the lowest ranks of people with as much readiness as to the highest regardless of any emolument," as Lysons put it. He told Farington the way the property was divided amongst the eight children. In the eldest son's bequest there was the living of Leckhampton, Leckhampton Court, and the estate that included several villages. "To his younger children," says Farington, "he left £28,000, which, when divided will allow to each four thousand."[27]

One of the things that came out some time after Trye's death when his executors had gone through all his private papers was the fact of his deep religious convictions. He was, indeed, something of a priest-doctor as mentioned earlier, but in his humility he kept this aspect of his life very secret. Jenner, who was a good man but quite unostentatious and admittedly no theologian, was strangely moved by his friend's piety during those last days of his life. In fact, this thought must have played upon Jenner's mind even more than the loss of a friend or even the professional aspects of the case. It was a week after Trye's death, when the funeral was over and everything seemed to have settled down, that Jenner wrote to Daniel Lysons, who had taken charge at Friar's Orchard.

My dear Sir,
In the Prayer Book which stood in Mr. Trye's room there was a prayer in Mr. Trye's handwriting, and which I took to be his own composition. If you would have the goodness to favour me with a Copy of it, I should feel greatly obliged to you.

Remember me kindly to the family and believe me,
                Most truly yours,
                Edward Jenner.
Cheltenham
15th October, 1811.[28]

There is no record of a reply to this short letter, nor do we know
if Jenner ever received the prayer, but it is remarkable that, of
all the likely mementos or keepsakes in the familiar household,
this prayer should have been so important to the appellant.

On September 27, Jenner had received a long, rambling letter
from the poet Coleridge—one of the famous literary figures who
Fosbroke lists as being friends of the doctor's. With Parry, Coleridge's old fellow student in Germany, now residing in Cheltenham, it is quite likely that the poet visited the town occasionally,
particularly since he appears to have known Thomas Pruen also.
At all events, this letter was, in the main, a suggestion that vaccination might well be the theme for an epic poem. But what is more
surprising than anything is the revelation that, at least on the
poet's side, Jenner and Coleridge were the closest possible friends!
He refers to the great work that he was too lethargic to do himself,
but which "has been effected in my own lifetime by men whom I
have seen and many of whom I have called my friends; inshort,
that I have known and *personally* loved. Clarkson, Davy, Dr. An-
drew Bell, and Jenner." And he signs the letter, "Your respectful
friend and servant, S. T. Coleridge." In a postscript he adds, "Be
pleased to remember me to Mr. Pruen when you see him."

At the outset the poet refers to Jenner's discovery as being a
counterpoise from the All-Preserver "to the crushing weight of
this unexampled war." He goes on to ask when the idea first
came to Jenner, and who was the best authority on the subject.
Then the letter's character changes after about six hundred words,
and Coleridge quite unabashedly occupies the final four hundred
words in seeking medical advice for a lady friend of his who suffered from toothache.

She has many decayed back teeth; so many as to put extraction almost
out of the question. . . . I am convinced that the locality of the pain
is in great measure accidental; that it is what I have heard called a
nervous rheumatic affection of the stomach or other parts of her inside.

She is single, about six-and-twenty, has excellent health and spirits in all other respects and bears this affliction with more than even feminine patience. . . . Her last attack was in November last when she was confined to her bed more than a month by it, and reduced to a skeleton. Yesterday she had a return, and I am sadly afraid of another fit of it. Should you remember any case in point in the course of your practice, and be able to suggest any mode of treatment, I will not say that I should be most thankful, but only that you will make a truly estimable family both grateful and happy.[29]

There is no record of Jenner's answer to this letter. What we do know is that no great vaccination poem was ever written by Coleridge. Perhaps the letter was simply a plea for free medical treatment, which would at least show that some degree of intimacy existed between poet and doctor.

The year ended with a rather more tangible honor than the letter from Coleridge. In December, Jenner was made a member of the French Institute, or rather, that is when the news reached England; the decision was made in Paris on May 30. It is interesting to note that Farington certainly heard the good news before Jenner himself. He went to dinner with Lysons at the Royal Society Club on the night of December 5. They ran into Sir Joseph Banks there, and he said that he had "just received of the Institute Society, in Paris, the official documents which constitute Dr. Jenner, author of the *Vaccine Discovery*, a member of the "Institute." Farington asked him whether he was able to keep up a regular correspondence and communication with the institute.

He said it was a matter of great uncertainty, depending upon the caprice of Buonaparte. Sometimes he has been in the humour to allow the communication to be easy, and at other times when he has appeared to be out of humour with the Institute it has been stopped. Sir Joseph added, "I have been a year and a half together without receiving any communication, and having had it signified to me that receiving letters from me might be dangerous, I have foreborne from writing."[30]

He had sent the diploma to Cheltenham the day before, on December 4, which means that if it had been put on the very first coach that was leaving, which was doubtful, it would have reached Jenner the following day. However, the post office arrangements in the town under the easygoing Entwistle often caused letters to be left overnight or even a day or two in the office. So Jenner certainly could not have known of the high honor conferred upon him earlier than the fifth, and in all probability it was the sixth or seventh, particularly given the wintry road conditions. Banks pointed out in his covering letter that the National Institute had defied the Emperor's edict to change the name to Imperial Institute, which he rather illogically saw as evidence that the members "are as little satisfied with the barbarous mode of warfare adopted by their chief as we English can be." As a matter of fact Jenner's diploma had the abbreviation "IMP." inserted in small letters after the word "INSTITUT." It was a nice Christmas present, however, imperial or national.

All too often the free labor offered by many of the vaccination pioneers was revealed only in their obituary notices. Trye and Jenner seem to have been completely indifferent to the accumulation of wealth, and Baillie, who never charged the poor, became a rich man solely from the enormous amount of work he did. In the case of Lettsom, however, there was an even more philanthropic approach. Thomas Pettigrew[31] relates that "necessitous authors and clergymen of all denominations and their families were attended by Dr. Lettsom gratuitously, *and often assisted by pecuniary donations.*"[32] It was also to Pettigrew that Jenner confided the fact that initially Lettsom was opposed to vaccination. Like John Fosbroke, who was six years his junior, Pettigrew was extremely precocious. He had been admitted to the Medical Society of London in 1808, when only seventeen years of age, and was to become secretary to the Royal Humane Society at twenty-two. He began to appear in Jenner's circle after the death of Trye. Also a friend of Coleridge's, he was very close to Lettsom, whose biography he wrote, and seems to have had a special quality that impressed the elderly doctors and scholars. That extraordinary old man, Dr. Thomas Cogan—physician, philosopher, novelist, archeologist, clergyman, translator, and founder of the Royal Humane Society, and who was fifty-five years Pettigrew's senior—was a striking example of this.[33] Having successively followed the ministry of the Congregational, Presbyterian, and Unitarian faiths, a large part of his last years was occupied by his even greater faith in the genius of Pettigrew. This patronage ultimately led to the highest honors from several members of the royal family while the young man was still in his twenties. He had the ability, also apparent in Christie, of being able to climb over the heads of his sponsors without incurring any resentment. To Pettigrew, Jenner was one of the greatest names in medicine, and he always remained a loyal and humble supporter, even when he was chosen above Jenner to vaccinate in the royal family.

Not but what Jenner was firmly established in the highest circles of his own particular world. It was all a matter of degree. There were the inevitable functions a member of the Board of Commissioners and a magistrate was expected to attend, and on November 14, we find him among the two hundred people present at Mr. Herve's lecture in aid of the National Benevolent Institution. For a wonder Jenner was the only notable Cheltenham doctor present—Lady Castle Stewart, Lady Hunlock, Lady Meredith, and one or two other titled people shared the platform with him.[34] It well illustrates the position he had now reached, at least in the society of the town. A far cry, indeed, from the journeyman surgeon who rode through the mud of the Berkeley lanes for twenty years.

But even transparently honest people like Jenner can become the victims of their own good nature. He always thought with his heart before his head, and never seems to have learned the unwisdom of it to his dying day. Only four days after Mr. Herve's lecture an entry in Farington's diary revealed how thin was the line between respectability and social disaster. It would seem that Jenner's manifest loyalty to Lady Berkeley, despite the course of the late trial, could have been a very risky business for him. His contention had always been that she was a mother defending her son's inheritance, and if there were any discrepancies or contradictions in her testimony it was due to the stress under which she was functioning. He had forced himself to believe that the systematic forgeries, perjuries, and conspiracies involved had all been on the part of the late peer now safely in his grave. And it is probable that the obvious respect and trust that he showed for her at the trial had some impact in the popular assessment of her guilt or innocence. His social reputation was so unspotted that it would, in a sense, make a deeper impression than that of the Prince Regent and other loyal but scarcely unsullied aristocrats. On November 18, however, Farington recorded how Lysons had visited him and told him of the real situation—in what secret contempt Lady Berkeley had been held by her legal advisers. "Sergeant Best, her council [sic] now says that he never before met with so great a Lyar as Her Ladyship. She told him her Mother was dead at the time she was living in Lincolnshire and to Her Knowledge."[35] One would assume that the perjury had been for the purpose of preventing her mother being called upon to testify. Lady Berkeley was not, as Jenner saw her—a confused woman attempting to remember things long past; she was a systematic schemer intentionally trying to deceive the court. Poor Jenner would have been horrified. Fortunately, neither Farington nor Lysons ever told him or—more important—Catherine, of the barrister's rather unprofessional revelations. As it was Jenner was just about on his feet again after the nightmarish year of 1810.

Activity in Cheltenham definitely accelerated as the impact of Christie's book was felt in ever widening circles. The drive and tenacity of the local doctors impressed at least one Cheltenham peer to decide on presenting a bill in Parliament. It was ironic that the gentleman in question, Lord Borington, should come from the very family that had supported Lady Mary Wortley Montague on her introduction of smallpox inoculation into England. Now he would reverse the position and fight for its extinction. A man of impeccable reputation, but perhaps more enthusiastic than able, he was undoubtedly moved, in great part, by the Boringtons' long record of combatting smallpox. But his zeal carried him swiftly rather than efficiently, and he had a bill for the eradication of the practice drawn up with little preparatory work and no consultation with the experts—including Jenner himself. The folly of this was soon to be apparent.

The new year opened promisingly enough, however, and the uncertainties and vicissitudes of the Vaccine Institute in particular took an encouraging turn for the better when Jenner's old friend, Sir Francis Milman, was made director in February 1812. A great deal had happened since the early years of vaccination and honors had been heaped upon this dignified elder statesman of medicine.

He had received a baronetcy in 1800 and was appointed physician to George III in 1806. Now at the age of sixty-six he deigned to become, in effect, the national leader of the vaccination movement. A man above politics and aloof from the bickering of jealous doctors he was the ideal—almost unattainable—choice. In addition to his impressive career as a doctor and a scholar, he was of vast importance in the medical establishment—particularly the Royal College of Surgeons where there was so much overt jealousy of vaccination progress. Jenner was delighted. "I rejoice at seeing so distinguished a person as Sir Francis Milman at the head of vaccine affairs," he said to Moore.

We wanted firmness and decision, and I now see that we shall have it. I beg you to present my best compliments to him, and to say, that when I go to town I shall have the honour of waiting upon him, and hope he will indulge me in a full conversation on the subject, particularly that part of it which relates to the conduct of the first board, the cause of my seceding, etc., etc.[36]

With it all, however, the problems of the institute were by no means over.

Also in February, Daniel Lysons finished his labor of love—a life of Charles Brandon Trye.[37] It is a pathetic little effort really; only thirty pages of large print with a reproduction of Rossi's sculpture as a frontispiece. But the real significance of this event lies in the public interest roused upon its appearance. To be sure, Lysons sent out presentation copies to all he felt would be interested, but the replies he received from nonmedical literary personalities show with what esteem this pious but retiring doctor was held. Perhaps local figures like Bransby Cooper and Richard Raikes[38] are understandable, but who would have expected Hannah More, Mrs. Piozzi, or even Anne Hunter—all in the evening of their days—to feel so strongly and to write the most moving tributes.[39]

The comments are redolent of the eighteenth century and a literary world so very far removed from Regency England. Mrs. Piozzi was the confidante of Dr. Johnson; Mrs. Hunter the friend of Haydn; and Hannah More—what a galaxy of memories there! David Garrick, Reynolds, Burke, and countless others long in their graves were the people of *her* world. Yet Jenner was much

older than Trye, and the voices of these three old ladies remind
us that the vaccination tract came out in Jenner's fiftieth year,
and that he too was essentially a man of the eighteenth century.

Perhaps a Ph.D. student many years from now will labor
through all the court records and write an account of Jenner's
life as a magistrate. The cross-section of Regency England that
continually passed before his eyes undoubtedly aided him both
as doctor and man. The cases that came up in Cheltenham in
those days are only barely suggested by the occasional clues we
get through consideration of more pertinent matters, but more
of this later. In addition there are the names that occur in his
own writings—a fleeting mention and then gone forever—and
we are left to wonder who such and such person was. Jenner's
poems are full of allusions to people we can never identify at
this distance of time—"Death and Mr. Peach," "Harmless Will,"
"The Cook at Newcastle," "Alexander," and so on, but we *can*
identify a name here and there. Who, for instance, was Jemmy
Wood? Jenner wrote a poem to him that is now in the Hellman
Collection in New York.[40] Wood was, as a matter of fact, a well-
known Cheltenham eccentric in his day and was one of Pitt's
partners in the Cheltenham and Gloucester Bank. (We have
noticed Jemmy Wood's bridge when St. George's Place ended in
the fields below Fauconberg House.) At one time he owned a
large part of the town—or the land on which it was eventually
built—though he actually lived in Gloucester. Jenner's interest
in him was based on his notoriety as a miser; his parsimony was
so extreme that it might well have been the subject of a medical
thesis. Jemmy Wood was once described as "perhaps the richest
commoner in His Majesty's dominions," and yet he dressed like
a tramp and would pick up a piece of coal in the street and take
it home for his fire. The folklore relating to him is extensive,
and to his contemporaries he must have been an unending
source of wonder. On the other hand his partner, Joseph Pitt, was
a much more rational being. He sat with Jenner on the magistrates' bench and supported the vaccination movement with the
rest of the town fathers. The two men would also have come
together at the meetings of the Town Commissioners, so I suppose they knew each other quite well. It will be recalled that

Jenner's house, or possibly the land on which it was built, had once been partly in Pitt's possession. He was an important figure in Regency society though nothing has ever been written on him.

The war was the one thing that dominated everyone's mind throughout this crucial year, and Jenner must have bitterly pondered over the exertions of the most unenergetic Prince Regent in succoring Macleod's protégé, Lefevre, while ignoring the doctor's pleas for young Husson. As in the Newell case, it was surely too local to be coincidental. Lefevre was sought out for the prince's clemency while living as an actual neighbor to the impotent Jenner, and despite the bitterness of the Peninsular campaign, the local affection for the general and his lady seems to have continued unaffected under the royal smile. In fact, when rumors went round that the general was to be exchanged for the Earl of Beverley, there was actual dismay in certain quarters. The Prince seized upon this moment to show the royal favoritism, as related in the *Chronicle:*

General Lefevre had an excellent watch when he was taken which he valued highly, and such was the attention shown to him that his watch, after three years bestowed in research and enquiry among the dragoons engaged in the skirmish, and afterwards in guarding the prisoner, was at length by the exertions of the Earl of Moira and the Prince Regent, recovered last summer and sent down to him in this town, by the hands of Major Carnac, private secretary to Sir H. Wellesley.

And while men were fighting and dying in the Peninsula, Cheltenham men and women continued their unbounded hospitality to this heroic figure from the enemy camp. Then came the news that put even the war out of the public mind—at least for a few days. The mail coach arrived from London on the morning of May 11 bearing the news that Spencer Perceval, the Prime Minister, had been assassinated the previous afternoon in a corridor of the House of Commons. Goding, the industrious town historian, implies that Mrs. Perceval was not in residence in Cheltenham at the time. "In 1812," he says, "*after* the dreadful catastrophe, Mrs. Perceval and her widowed family repaired to the town." On the other hand, in the chronological table attached to Goding's work, "culled partly from the newspapers of the day," it is stated categorically: "At the time of the murder of her husband . . . Mrs. Perceval and her orphan family occupied a cottage in Constitution Place."[41] There is evidence that she had not been very happy about her husband's appointment in the first place and might well have preferred to stay away from it all in Cheltenham. As usual, it is Farington who informs us with a curious anecdote relative to the Percevals. When Perceval was first offered the premiership and his wife was informed,

she came into the room and conjured him not to accept it. The gentleman deputed said "the good of his country requires it"—on which she shed tears and replied "then my children will be sacrificed;" meaning, it is supposed, that his constitution could not stand the fatigues of office and parliamentary duties, and that she and her family should lose him.

The tragedy of poor Mrs. Perceval was naturally the main topic of conversation in the town for the next day or two, and one assumes that since General and Madame Lefevre had become so much a part of the social activity of the place, they shared the correct sentiments and expressed the proper condolences. Then came the complete disillusionment—appropriately enough from the town crier, swinging his bell in the High Street and the alleys. "General Lefevre has escaped!" The issue of the *Chronicle* for May 14 put it more forcefully: "The French General Lefevre Desnouettes, has absconded from his parole in this town."[42] The public indignation at what was considered the basest treachery was as severe as had been the recent adulation. The government, for its part, ordered the remaining prisoners to be removed from the sylvan haven of Cheltenham to the bleaker surroundings of the Welsh mountains at Abergavenny.

From the battles in the Peninsula, the "war" at home came rudely to the forefront when the long-awaited Vaccination Bill in the House of Lords was finally presented. But so many things were mishandled. Had Lord Borington the ruthlessness of people like Lord Eldon or Lord Ellenborough, smallpox inoculation might have been destroyed many years before it was, and thousands of lives saved in the process. While the peer was undoubtedly one of Jenner's most loyal supporters in Parliament, he was easy game before ridicule or contempt. He brought two bills before the House of Lords to fight the cause of vaccination and curb inoculation but quailed before his opponents on both occasions. Despite the distinguished vaccinationists among the Prince Regent's doctors, His Royal Highness also patronized one of the most vitriolic anti-Jenner men in the country—John Birch,[43] who was a rabid smallpox inoculator and had a great influence over his master. By 1812, the halting of inoculation had become far more important to Jenner than the spread of vaccination itself, but this terrible and senseless practice was still allowed to challenge the progress of the last sixteen years. It was a tragedy that, of all the brilliant orators in the Lords, the well-meaning but faltering Borington insisted upon presenting the bill to stop inoculation.

On the surface Borington's proposal looked like a sound enough arrangement. Since his second marriage, to Frances Talbot in 1809, he had remade his life and become one of the most lavish hosts in the kingdom. His wife was a perfect partner in his pattern of living and was as brilliant a woman in her knowledge and appreciation of the arts as the greats such as the Duchess of Devonshire or Lady Crewe. The blow to Borington's morale suffered at the hands of the frivolous daughter of Lord Westmorland was apparently completely forgotten. In addition, unlike Lords Sherborne, Berkeley, or Ducie, he was, at least officially, a supporter of the government. Surely it would be more practical for him to present the bill than one of the forthright Whig members.

The writer, Cyrus Redding,[44] who himself spent a great deal of time at Cheltenham in Borington's day, gives us a good description of the peer at just about the time he drew up his bill. "At the age of forty he was a well-proportioned man with regular and handsome features, pallid complexion and sedate physiognomy."[45] We are told, further, that he spoke French and Italian fluently and had considerable taste in the fine arts. But with it all the vaccination debate became a farce—not even reaching a vote. The intention of the bill was "To prevent the spread of smallpox by supplying provisions for vaccination." Eldon, the Lord Chancellor, had his own way of dealing with it. As the debate proceeded points of difference kept coming up, and the innocent Borington tried to compromise with them rather than repudiate them. The result was that eventually he had made so many qualifications that the bill was unintelligible. The Lord Chancellor waited until the hapless man was utterly confused and embarrassed, and then suggested that the bill be withdrawn since there seemed to be more alterations than bill. It was a complete victory for the anti-Jenner forces that could have been avoided had a more astute person been in charge. The only compensation was that Borington was just as determined as ever to go on fighting, and remained, for what he was worth, one of Jenner's loyalest supporters. He would try again.

Birch, inevitably, continued his smallpox inoculation as avidly as ever, and while there is no comment from Jenner himself on the matter of the Borington bill at the time, we do have, later in the year, his view of Birch. "What a sad wicked fellow is that Birch," he wrote to Moore. "Had I the power to exercise vaccination as I liked, in one fortnight this dismal work of death should entirely cease."[46] He also spoke bitterly of Lord Ellenborough, a man whose petty vanity submerged the debt of gratitude he owed to Jenner's discovery. (Ellenborough's own children had been protected against smallpox by vaccination.)

It was yet another disappointment, but by this time the idea of government action was growing ever more remote. On August 6, when Lettsom and his wife arrived,[47] there was a great deal to be discussed, in particular a future program that did not depend on politics. Despite the firm hand of Sir Francis Milman, all had not been progressing too well at the institute. Business seemed to have gone completely dead when Jenner wrote to Moore from Berkeley on June 20.

It is a long time since I heard from you and longer still, I fear, since you heard from me. What has become of the Annual Vaccine Report? Have the hurley-burleys of the state annihilated it? If it exists pray let me see it. If the South America and Havannah reports, with which I furnished the Board, are not noticed, those who sent them to me would think themselves not attended to with due respect. Poor Sacco and the seeds! This is a bad story and I am in a scrape. Sir Francis, perhaps, did not apply to Sir Joseph; or if he did, a request of mine was thought but little of.[48]

His hopes from the accession of Sir Francis had apparently been shattered as on so many previous occasions.

It was in the course of this summer that the poet Byron decided to come to Cheltenham—possibly to get away from the attentions of Lady Caroline Lamb, but more likely to pay court to Lady Oxford. He already knew most of the vaccination peers, and both his boyhood doctor, Baillie, and his Cheltenham medical advisor, Boisragon, were close friends of Jenner. To be sure, Elgin was *persona non grata* as a result of the removal of the Parthenon marbles, and was the butt of the poet's ire in "The Curse of Minerva," but perhaps that was more than balanced by the deep friendship that existed between the poet and Lord Holland, one of Jenner's oldest supporters. After Holland returned from Spain in 1803 he became a regular seasonal visitor to Cheltenham, virtually picking up where his uncle Charles James Fox had left off. It is likely, indeed, that he continued the lease of Vernon House, which was in the middle of the area at the top of the High Street where most of his set lived. Baron does not even mention Byron, but this is in keeping with his silence on practically all Jenner's friendships with people of loose morals. It is certain that Catherine would not have permitted the poet beyond the front door, but a remark made by young Fosbroke, who was fifteen years old at the time, suggests that the doctor was rather more compassionate to Byron than most of his fellows. It will be recalled that this was the year that the poet sold his home, Newstead Abbey. "What is the unbefriended man of genius," asked Jenner, "but a wanderer without a home who sits down by the waters and weeps? He came with all the good in his soul, held out the right hand of friendship to the sufferer and took down the harp from the willow."[49] When he was feeling somewhat depressed later in the season Byron almost paraphrased these lines in a letter to Lord Holland.[50] In addition, not only were Colonel Berkeley, Lysons, Campbell, Lawrence, and Thomas Moore *close* friends of both the doctor and the poet, but the influx of visitors this summer included as usual the Berrys, the Hollands, the Jerseys, the Lansdowns, and Lord Donoughmore, at all of whose salons Jenner would certainly have run into Byron.

Despite the fact that the poet had been taken to Baillie by his mother when he was a boy, he was not interested in that eminent doctor when he came to Cheltenham. He preferred to be under the care of Boisragon whom he had probably met in London. He was not a good patient and did not always follow his medico's advice. Byron did not stay with any of the great ones while he was in Cheltenham. He took his own quarters at 430, High Street, almost adjoining Barratts' Mill beside the River Chelt. Lady Oxford's cottage, where the Duchess of Devonshire had lived, was almost within sight near the Cambray meadows, while Charles James Fox's Vernon House was on the other side of Byron's garden wall. Lord and Lady Jersey may have stayed with Lord Jersey's mother, the dowager, who lived nearby. Thus the whole Byron coterie was lodged together around Barratts' Mill and the willow trees of the Chelt. The younger Lady Jersey, it will be remembered, was the sister of Lord Borington's runaway wife. The Milbankes were in the town as usual, together with Lady Milbourne, Lady Caroline Lamb's mother-in-law, who is generally assumed to have been the matchmaker of the Byron-Milbanke union. Her niece Anne Isabella Milbanke, was the soul of modesty and decorum, and it may have seemed a good way to break up Caroline's notorious affair with the poet while at the same time securing a distinguished marriage for the more respectable girl.

Dear as all this social-literary activity would have been to Jenner's heart, it seemed that tragedy was never far away from the family hearth. The brilliance of the seasons following young Edward's death were not always to be enjoyed by Jenner because of some new domestic problem. This particular season of 1812 found him absent for several months owing to the illness of his last surviving sister who lingered on through the late summer under his anxious care in Berkeley. He left the Lettsoms sipping the Cheltenham waters while he watched beside yet another deathbed, but as usual, he made the best of his melancholy lot. If he had no one to talk to in the country, there was, at least, plenty to observe. He wrote to Moore on August 9:

Certain it is I have no society here but clods; but out of these clods I contrive to make something. The produce of their fields has been a plentiful source of enjoyment to me. This year there has been more of liver disease among sheep, cows, oxen, hogs and some other animals than I ever remember. I long since discovered that the ordinary source of scirrhus is the hyatid, when passed on to its secondary stage; but there was another sort of scirrhus which puzzled me till now, and I make this out to originate into diseased bile ducts. Some of these I find dilated to the size of a child's finger, and passing in this state almost to the extreme edges of the liver; their internal coats highly inflamed, like a croupy trachea and throwing out mucus and coagulable lymph. Others which have weathered the inflammatory stage, thickly encrusted over with stony matter. Here, then, is a little apology for seclusion in this sequestered corner of our island.[51]

He manifestly did not wish his friend to think that he was wasting his time.

When, some two months later, his sister succumbed he was both grieved and, in a way, relieved. She had suffered for over a year. "The event I have long been expecting has at length taken place," he wrote on October 11 to the same correspondent. "I have lost my only sister, and the last of my family of that class. So that I am now insulated in that way—the only one left of ten —I could not come to town while she lay on her deathbed; but now I shall come and try to cheer myself by mixing with my friends for a week or two." Then follows a very interesting allusion to the war that had been declared against Great Britain by the United States on June 18:

The inclosed I received from Waterhouse at Boston. There is something so striking in it with regard to the politics in America, and so unlike what we are taught to believe at home, that I have inclosed it for you, thinking it might be of some value in the hands of some of your political friends. I know you are well-acquainted with my Lord Lauderdale, and many others. It may be sent to a newspaper if you think it may be useful; in that case no names must be mentioned. Dr. Waterhouse is a man of correct habits. For the seven first years of vaccination I corresponded with him regularly. He upbraids me justly for late irregularities.[52]

I can trace no letter from Waterhouse at this time—if, indeed, it was a letter to which Jenner referred. It may have been a pamphlet or document of value presumably to Lauderdale,[53] or one of his supporters, rather than to the government. Whatever it was Waterhouse had sent must have left Boston *after* the outbreak of war since some four months had elapsed. Lauderdale had once been a powerful figure in politics and was a friend of Charles James Fox's, but after 1807 had been in opposition to the government. It would be interesting to know what material Waterhouse had sent that would have been of significance to a leading Whig politician and to the press. With the warning that "no names must be mentioned," (presumably the names of Jenner and Waterhouse), there is a slight cloak-and-dagger atmosphere here. Coincidentally old Dr. Anthony Fothergill had returned to England from Philadelphia a short time earlier when war had seemed inevitable, though, strangely enough, when we recall the venerable doctor's association with Cheltenham, his name is not even mentioned in any of the Jenner records. He would certainly have known a great deal about the progress of vaccination in America. He died in London at the age of eighty-one the following year, 1813.

During the weary deathwatch at Berkeley through September and October, Colonel Berkeley, Byron, Grimaldi and the theatrical crowd were bobbing back and forth between the castle and Cheltenham. Byron, despite his many other involvements—emotional as well as business—actually accomplished a great deal of literary work during those last months of 1812, and Jenner himself actually addressed some verses to the poet's friend and great comedian, Grimaldi.[54] He probably wrote them after the death of his sister left him free to resume his role in society.

The high water mark of the much extended 1812 season came with the great rally of the National Benevolent Institution Fund at the Assembly Rooms on November 16, when Jenner was definitely back in circulation. The Trustees for Cheltenham and Gloucester were Jenner, Christie, Parry, Newell, and Boisragon of Cheltenham, and Baron of Gloucester. The main feature of the function was a lecture by Mr. Peter Herve, the founder. It was specifically stated that "no money would be accepted." Apparently the point was to persuade a substantial number of prominent people to pledge specific amounts. A further interesting event followed on the twenty-first, when a number of public-spirited actors and actresses under the patronage of Lord and Lady Gormaston gave their services free at the Theatre Royal. The play was *Lover's Vows*, and the professional actors were assisted by enthusiastic amateurs. The prices ranged from a shilling and sixpence to four shillings, and an encouraging note, considering the time of the year, was the announcement "Good fires will be kept to warm the theatre."[55] It was the first time that Jenner had been involved in the organization of stage activities, and one can only wonder how Catherine felt about it.

The local newspaper gives us a continuing summary in detail of the day-to-day life of the doctor among his neighbors at this time. The disasters, mishaps, and civic concerns were typical of the provincial society. Most alarming, at least for Catherine and the children, was the fire in the drawing room of Mr. Butts, the grocer, only a few doors away, even though it was put out before any serious harm was done. A much more tragic occurrence was described in the *Chronicle* two weeks later. Mr. Lambert, who kept the livery stable adjoining Jenner's garden, lost his son under the most terrible circumstances.

Tuesday, as Thomas Lambert, son of Mr. Robert Lambert, of St. George's Place, apprenticed to a surgeon at Dudley, was returning home from visiting a patient, the night being dark, he missed his way and was in consequence precipitated to the bottom of a coal-pit and dashed to atoms.[56]

He was the third promising young man from this thoroughfare to die prematurely in as many years. He would undoubtedly have known the two boys from the Jenner household and might even have been influenced in his ambition for a medical career by his distinguished next-door neighbor.

In the more mundane realms, Mr. Morhall made an excellent report on the conditions in St. George's Place, though they were not entirely related to Jenner's sewer problems.

The return streets—St. George's Place, Winchcombe Street, etc., are rarely entered (by the scavengers) and never for the purpose of moving ashes and rubbish from the dwelling houses. Though the act specifically requires the same to be moved every Tuesday and Saturday. . . . The road in St. George's Place, being too low, the water lodges in a continual pool after the rain and this added to the heaps of dirt makes a filthy road to the Crescent, etc.

If this was the situation in a thoroughfare that had at least a rudimentary main drain, the condition in most areas must have been shocking. Fortunately, that part which related to the delinquency of the dustmen could be remedied—and it was. From the day Jenner joined the Board of Commissioners, in fact, there was a marked improvement in the upkeep of his own thoroughfare where the camber had long been a problem. Jenner was not entirely without power, and his zeal was not devoted solely to earthshaking medical decisions. He was undoubtedly very happy when his voice was listened to in civic affairs. As a local administrator he was, of course, involved in the whole spectrum of urban life—much of it sordid and far removed from the glitter of the fashionable salon. This side of his daily routine was probably in a great part responsible for his tolerant views on what is loosely called "morality." The respectable merchants of the upper end of the High Street were highly incensed when the local vice descended below the level of the nobility, unnoticed, apparently, by the police. "Complaints of residents that a disorderly house is being kept to which the constables are indifferent," was noted in the press, "a twenty-pound penalty is threatened against them." The house in question was in St. James's Street but nothing, it seems, was done about it. The plebians will ever imitate their betters, and it is doubtful whether the town commissioners were unduly concerned. But these were the things that formed a permanent if minor part of Jenner's life and perhaps make him all the more real to us; particularly when we place them in juxtaposition to the impact his real work was making in the farthest corners of the earth.

The season ended pleasantly enough with great news out of Russia—news that might perhaps compensate for some of the sorrows Jenner had endured. Dr. Alexander Crichton,[57] the Scottish Physician-in-Ordinary to the Czar, sent him a long report on the growth of vaccination in the Russian Empire where, it was said, every seventh child used to die of smallpox. In eight years, from 1804 to 1812, 1,235,597 children had been vaccinated and therefore, observed Crichton, "vaccination has saved the lives of this empire of 176,514 children; and in an empire like this where the population is a great deal too scanty in proportion to its extent, such saving of human life is of great importance. Many generations must pass away before Russia will have any occasion to dread Mr. Malthus's predictions."[58] Contemplating the labored progress of his work in Britain, Jenner must have sighed over the advantages of Russia's dictatorial government. The Emperor merely commanded—in language that was simple and to the point—that vaccination be universally accepted, and it was. "Three years is allowed for vaccinating the whole empire, after which period there must not be found man, woman or child, the newly born excepted, who have not been vaccinated." The report does mention a tiny sect who for purely religious reasons did not accept the practice, but they were so insignificant that the government came to "the wise resolution of leaving this dispute to time."[59]

The tenor of the letter suggests that Crichton and Jenner might possibly have met before the former settled at the court of St. Petersburg in 1804. The fact that Russia and England had been at war during a part of this period again indicates the esteem in which the British doctor was held. "The re-establishment of peace between England and Russia being happily concluded," he writes:

I embrace an early opportunity to sending you a letter on the state of vaccination in this empire as I am convinced that the encouragement it meets with from the government, its gradual extension and success, cannot fail to be interesting to you. . . . *Having been, as you well know,* one of your earliest advocates in England, and having never wavered in my opinion concerning its great advantages, you need not doubt that I do all in my power to encourage and support vaccination in Russia . . .

He concludes with the suggestion that his information might be worth publishing: "I have thought that this short account of the state of vaccination in Russia would be acceptable to. Bradley, if you deem it sufficiently interesting for his Journal." Unfortunately, Bradley, who had retired from the Westminster Hospital in 1811, died the following year.

◈ IX ◈

The Death of Catherine
1812-1815

While Jenner's idea of a Cheltenham Vaccine Institute built on his own land did not materialize, within the year a much more ambitious scheme did. Perhaps the increasing pace of the variola-inoculation feud and the uncertainty of Catherine's state of health made him shrink back at the last minute from something that would have been solely his responsibility; but the seed had been sown and the Cheltenham Dispensary was born. One might almost say that it was Jenner's scheme under another director since one of its two joint purposes was the promotion of vaccination; but actually it was established and run by the younger doctors of the town, led by Jenner's protégé, Charles Parry. It was Parry, according to young Fosbroke, who "suggested the first proposals and the first code of regulations,"[1] and had it not been for this fact one might have justifiably assumed that Jenner was cool to the idea. Parry, however, was as close to him as his own son and the feeling was more than reciprocated, so that the three vaccination elders—Jenner, Creaser, and Baillie—left the arrangements to their younger brethren and Jameson. Except for the latter, no one involved was out of his forties, and some were in their twenties. I suppose the real situation was that Parry's action at the head of all the younger vaccination men greatly appealed to Jenner. It may well have seemed churlish to the older man to move into a group where he would have to become the leader, and, as it were, steal the limelight from his young friend. Jameson, though one of the older local practitioners, was not nearly as prominent, and would work with the others as a kind of background figure. Jenner did support the society financially, however, for the rest of his life.

Another point of extreme interest is that about this time Jenner purchased number seven St. George's Place adjoining his own house.[2] This gave him a vast Cheltenham headquarters of some thirty rooms, "with outbuildings and cottages" in addition to his land on the opposite side of the street. It was a worthy center for the world vaccination crusade and certainly provided plenty of room for an initial base of the new organization. (There is also a tradition that Jenner subsequently acquired the entire terrace, but I have not been able to find concrete evidence of this.)[3]

Fosbroke, who at the age of sixteen would have been keenly aware of all that was going on, recalls:

From the younger medical men the public would thus be made to receive the benefits of plastic minds filled with the more improved views of modern science in surgery and medicine, and unsophisticated with habits and prejudices in practice long formed and stubbornly adhered to.[4]

Nevertheless, it was unusual to see a local medical project launched which included Jameson but not Jenner.

Informal meetings had been held before Christmas, 1812, but the first official gathering took place on March 6 with the Rector of Cheltenham, Rev. Foulkes, in the chair. The committee formed consisted of the following volunteers: Parry, Jameson, Boisragon, Minster, Newell, Wood, Lucas, Seager, and Fowler; and the name chosen was the Cheltenham Dispensary for Administering to the Sick Poor Advice and Medicine Gratis; and for Promoting of Vaccination.[5] A further meeting was arranged for the ninth, when the four doctors to serve for the coming year would be chosen by lot, and all the organization details would be worked out. The Irish peer, Lord Ashtown (whose father-in-law was a distinguished medical scholar[6]), presided, and the four men selected were Jameson, Parry, Newell, and Seager. A tariff of charges was made out for the donors. For two guineas a year the subscriber could have four patients continuously on the books. A prorata principle applied to larger and smaller donations.

On St. Patrick's Day (March 17), there was a great ball and

dinner at the George Inn with the wealthy Irish peers there in force. Again Lord Ashtown presided, and the *Chronicle* reported that "several of our *distinguished* medical characters were present."[7] The ball apparently went off satisfactorily, for the following day the dispensary advertised for its first paid employee; moreover, the ubiquitous Mr. Morhall joined the committee. A notice appeared in the *Chronicle* inviting applications for the post of resident assistant at the Cheltenham Dispensary. The salary was seventy pounds per annum plus an allowance for lodging and fuel. Not a very tempting offer in that community of wealthy, fashionable doctors, but typical of the time. Anyone interested, who was of good character, was invited to write to Mr. Wood, surgeon. At least part of the new institution's wages problem was solved on the following Sunday when a collection for the dispensary at the Catholic Chapel raised £11.9.8d.[8]

To one Irish family in Cheltenham, however, the feast of St. Patrick brought tragedy. John Boles Watson, who had managed the successive Theatre Royals since 1774, died at the age of sixty-five:[9] "the gout . . . terminated his existence by an attack on his vitals." Of the happy quintet at Kelly's cottage in the cornfields, all those years ago in 1796, only Kelly and Jenner were left; Mrs. Crouch and Lord Howth had passed on soon after the turn of the century. Watson was highly esteemed all over the western and midland counties. In his time he had brought every prominent international figure in the world of the stage and music to entertain the great in Cheltenham.

Perhaps it was an indication of the days to come as far as the town's destiny was concerned. When the Cheltenham Dispensary was born, the theater began to die: when Watson was laid to rest in the old churchyard, on March 22, the golden age of the Cheltenham theater passed with him.

Undoubtedly, Jenner's leaving the matter of the dispensary to the younger men had a lot to do with the local commitments that were encroaching on his vaccination work. Strange though it may seem, he was faced with considerable opposition in his determination to get a main sewer laid down the length of the High Street. A correspondent in the *Chronicle* on March 4, though less articulate than the doctor, nevertheless thanks him for his stand. Writing in the third person he states, "Fortunately he was assisted by the learned Dr. J.—whose letter answered the writer's purpose in drawing forth shrewd practical and intelligent illustrations of an undertaking of so much importance to the already sufficiently burdened inhabitants of Cheltenham."[10] Unfortunately his "sewers for Cheltenham" campaign was not as successful as the vaccination one. The sewer was never built in his lifetime, though the preliminary work he completed bore fruit soon after his death.

Jenner was also very concerned about the progress of James Moore's book on the history of smallpox. Young Edward Davies, his niece Anne's son, visited Moore in London just before Christmas and was allowed to read some of the manuscript. He gave a glowing account to his great-uncle, which Jenner repeated back to Moore. "Mr. Moore read to me a very considerable part of his intended publication. The style, in my opinion, is admirable; nervous, concise, gentlemanly and severe without descending to scurrility. It is also so amusing as to render it interesting to every class of reader." Jenner enclosed the report he had just received in the mail from the Deputy Inspector of Hospitals at the Cape of Good Hope. It described "the annihilation of the smallpox which appeared there in one of its most horrible forms, by vaccination." Jenner went on:

There may be no necessity for my sending it, as I find the National Vaccine Establishment is in possession of a similar document or at least the purport of the communication made to me. However, as mine may go into more detail, I beg you will present it to the Board, together with the Russian Report. But I must again entreat you to request Dr. Harvey to see that they may be restored to me on demand for I hold these things as sacred deposits and they will pass from me as heirlooms. . . . I wish Sir F. Millman would recollect that upwards of seven hundred reports in favour of vaccination lie buried among the archives of the College of Physicians.

Poor Jenner; he always seemed to be on the outside looking in. One often gets the impression that his help and knowledge was received impatiently by the pompous officialdom that usurped his rightful throne. In conclusion he pleads, "Let me hear often while these important movements of the Board are going forward."[11]

The war, of course, made communications much slower, particularly from overseas, and, as one more worry, Moore himself was half expecting to be sent abroad on some kind of active service. In fact, the war did actually swirl around the feet of Catherine's medical advisor, Mr. Wood, when he was called to be Surgeon to the Cheltenham Yeomanry Cavalry, in succession to old Dr. Minster (father of Thomas), of Stow-on-the-Wold. Everyone was very eager to be somehow involved in the fighting, and there seems to have been little or no cynicism. When the recruiting detachment for the Seventy-second Regiment of Foot came to the town and surrounding villages there were numerous enlistments, even though the Seventy-second was not even a local regiment. So many of the young men wished to become part of the companies of "dashing heroes." The reality of the Peninsular holocaust was brought right into the Cheltenham High Street on April 8. A poor girl collapsed in front of Sheldon's Hotel sick and half-starved with her infant in her arms. Good Samaritans appeared from all directions. Charles Parry was called and had her taken to a house and put to bed, while two good ladies—Mrs. Travell and Mrs. Postans—took tender care of her. When she was able to speak they learned that she was the widow of a lad killed in the war and was trying to make her way on foot to her village in Essex (over a hundred miles away), carrying her little girl in her arms. Since she was penniless and desolate, the good ladies fed her and provided clothes for her and her little one. Finally, when the gentle Dr. Parry had her well again, a collection was made, and she was given a sum of money, and as the *Chronicle* put it, she was soon "on her way home to Essex."[12]

On May 6 the dispensary opened for business. The date coincided with a veritable flood of Irish peers—Catholic and Protestant. Lord Kenmare and Castlerosse and Sir George Gould, the disappointed delegates from yet another abortive London conference on Catholic relief, were joined in the week of the sixth to the thirteenth by the Marquess and Marchioness of Donegal, the Bishop of Dromore, Lord Belfast, Lord Gormaston, Lord Charlemont, and Lord Adair. The dispensary benefited considerably by their visitation, but this promising opening of the new season was dampened by the appearance of smallpox in one of the alleys off the High Street. For Jenner, however, it turned out to be a further vindication. He writes:

Though the situation was exposed and numbers of children who had been vaccinated were within reach of infection, yet none of them took the disease. However, it happened that a young fellow who had been inoculated some years ago for the smallpox, at Upton, was not so fortunate. He became infected and had this distemper with some degree of severity. His case, by the way, which illustrates the truth of my observation respecting the cause that proves an impediment, in either inoculation, to that constitutional change that nature demands as a safeguard against future infections. This young man at the time of his being inoculated had Tinia Capitis and for some years after.[13]

Undoubtedly had it not been for Jenner there would have been an epidemic of smallpox in midsummer, the worst possible time of the year.

Yet with every striking vindication there seemed to be a rebuff. The Royal College of Physicians was, for reasons beyond understanding, still reluctant to admit him to its ranks. When one realizes the size of the organization and the fact that there were members in every town and city of the kingdom, it is incredible that a man of Jenner's international stature should still be denied admission *fifteen* years after the publication of the vaccination discovery. In Cheltenham, however, Jenner was something in the nature of an international potentate. Couriers and messages came from all over the world, and the famous doctors came from all over the country. Nor was the sister kingdom to the north flagging in her interest. Late in the season, old Dr. William Wright, in his seventy-ninth year, made the arduous journey from Edinburgh to Cheltenham.[14] As President of the Edinburgh Royal College of Physicians he had presided over Jenner's election to that body in 1806, and like his English colleague, was both doctor and naturalist. Griffith fittingly celebrated Wright's arrival by printing the great news out of Scotland: Glasgow—traditionally one of the most plagued cities in the kingdom—had been completely cleansed of smallpox through vaccination. During the past year there had been but twenty-four deaths in a population of 100,000—certainly something to talk about.[15]

In the middle of these pleasant occasions, Thomas Bradley, who was at death's door, begged Jenner to accept the president's chair in an effort to revive the almost forgotten Royal Jennerian Society, but the doctor was obliged to refuse and poor Bradley went to his grave three weeks later. The frustrations of attempting to deal with the whims of the London doctors over the years had purged Jenner of any idea that he could work *with* them. He now preferred to stay at home and help from without. And with what time he had left over from his vaccination practice, there was plenty to do on the Board of Commissioners. As both legislator and magistrate Jenner saw a very full cross-section of provincial life. Indeed much of it was under his very nose. There was the case of the pregnant lady in Cheltenham Chapel, where he spent so much of his leisure time listening to Rowland Hill's sermons. The *Chronicle* reported:

We have received a serious complaint against some unknown miscreant who, on Monday evening, threw a brick-bat into the meeting-house in St. George's Place and forcibly struck a female who is in a state of pregnancy. We cannot too loudly condemn such a wanton inroad on the religious ceremony of any sect, however at variance with the private opinion or public practice of any individual, and sincerely hope that discovery and adequate punishment will ever follow [the] offence.

There were no repercussions so we must assume that the lady recovered and that the assailant went free. Nor was this all. The same correspondent started a series of letters and journalistic debate on the activities of "an unhappy maniac" who roamed the High Street unattended and upset the local females. There was some doubt, at first, as to whether the magistrates had any authority to interfere with him, but after several weeks' discussion it was decided that they had.

The stiffness between Jenner and the Royal College of Physicians is put into strong relief when one observes the official recognition that came the way of other vaccination pioneers. Matthew Tierney, an admirer of Jenner's when little more than a boy, and still a young man in 1813, had every conceivable favor heaped upon him. He was the Prince Regent's doctor at Brighton, and it was only a matter of time before he would receive the accolade of knighthood. But the bitterest pill of all for the most patient Jenner must have been the appointment of Physician Extraordinary to the Prince Regent, which in 1813 went to Christie. The young doctor, who had waited in Ceylon for eight years in daily anticipation of coming to England to work beside Jenner, had finally set up in Cheltenham, written his book with the help and encouragement of his master, and then received the recognition that was denied Jenner! But Jenner was still far too engrossed in his Cheltenham activities to take much notice, and Christie was too valuable an ally for the misplacing of honors to separate them. Perhaps Jenner's day would come. "You see I was not quite in so great a hurry as my friend Christie to show myself at Carlton House," he wrote bravely to Moore on December 6. "I shall be there in good time you may depend on it, and then hear your history of the rise, progress and downfall of a monster still more horrible than Buonaparte."[16] Presumably he was referring to smallpox inoculation and anticipating the action in Parliament.

Unhappily, as was often the case, Wright's visit was not representative of the entire situation north of the border, and some later news from Scotland did admittedly upset Jenner. A Dr. Watt of Glasgow—possibly Robert Watt, who was made Physician to Glasgow Infirmary the following year—wrote a very devious pamphlet entitled *An Inquiry into the Relative Mortality of the Principal Diseases of Children*. It was supposed to relate to measles, but it was actually an argument against vaccination. By stretching his arguments, Watt endeavored to show that the epidemic of measles among Glasgow children had come during a period of almost universal vaccination, ergo: the smallpox that had been eradicated was indeed the "preparative" that made measles more mild. Reporting on Watt's pamphlet, Jenner said: "In short, he says, or seems to say, that we have gained nothing by the introduction of cowpox; for that the measles and smallpox have now changed places with regard to their fatal tendency. Is not this shocking?" Fortunately Jenner had all the facilities with him in Cheltenham to make an exhaustive survey and was able to prove by the evidence here in his own fortress that this relationship between the two diseases was nonexistent. He continued:

Here is a new and unexpected twig shot forth for the sinking anti-vaccinationist to cling to. But mark me—should this absurdity of Mr. Watt take possession of the minds of the people, I am already prepared with the means of destroying its effects, having instituted an inquiry through this populous town [Cheltenham] and the circumjacent villages, where, on the smallest computation, 20,000 must have been vaccinated in the course of the last twelve years by myself and others. Now it appears that during this period there have been no such occurrence as fatal epidemic measles. You would oblige me by making this communication to the Board, with my respectful compliments.[17]

Soon afterwards Jenner was reassured by a doctor from a large industrial area similar to Glasgow that Watt's contention did not have any basis in reality. There seemed to be no limit to the wild theories that were desperately advanced to discredit the triumphs of vaccination.

How much Jenner would have enjoyed Moore's visiting him in Cheltenham and seeing for himself a society ruled by Jenner alone and an oasis of disease-free contentment in an England still bedevilled by smallpox! Jenner had written to Moore in October:

Dear Friend,

I have had so much intercourse with you lately by means of London visitors, that my being a letter in your debt almost escaped my recollection. You have doubtless seen Charles Murray since his return from Cheltenham. I had two days of his company, and we pretty well talked over London matters. It was not then known that your late excellent president was tottering on his vaccine throne from which I find that he has since fallen. This is very tantalizing, as he was in possession of that stock of knowledge which rendered him fit for his government. I am a little acquainted with your new chieftain but I want to know your sentiments of him. I have always considered him as a very worthy man, of manners extremely gentle. . . . I long to see the progress you have made in your book. Is it possible to bring it here? You may be in Piccadilly at seven in the evening, and your arrival in Cheltenham be announced by the horn of the mail-coach at ten the next morning. I am sorry you have not succeeded in infecting a cow. . . .

Did I ever inform you of the curious results of vaccinating carters? These people from their youth up have the care of horses used for ploughing and cornlands. Great numbers of them in the course of my practice have come to me from the hills to be vaccinated; but the average number which resisted has been one half. On enquiry many of them have recollected having sores on their hands and fingers from dressing horses affected with sore heels; and being so ill as to be disabled from following their work; and on several of their hands, I have found a cicatrice as perfect and as characteristically marked as if it had arisen from my own vaccination. How goes smallpox among you? I am almost afraid to ask; and afraid, too, to enquire about Lord Borington's intended bill. There has certainly been ample time for its preparation. I think it a little strange that he should never have made any communication to me on the subject; the more so, as I am acquainted with his lordship, having vaccinated his eldest child.

I have some reason to think that all *etiquetical* impediments to my becoming a member of your Board will soon be removed. . . .

You begin to yawn over my long letter, and so do I for it is almost twelve o'clock; so adieu my dear friend, and believe me ever truly your,

Edward Jenner.

Cheltenham, October 27th, 1813.[18]

On the whole, a very cheerful letter—full of hope and determination to persevere, though Lord Borington's second bill for the prohibition of smallpox inoculation would not come up until well into the following year. The letter also reveals the fact that Jenner had not been making the routine visits to London of late. Moore's letters kept him informed quite adequately. The several mountains could always come to Mohammed if they needed to—and a large number of them did, including a pioneer "psychologist," the celebrated Dr. John Mackie,[19] author of *Sketch of a New Theory on Man;* he arrived in town on July 22. Perhaps he met Griffith, because in the current issue of the paper the editor printed a very modern-sounding psychological item: "A German moralist has put an analysis of German women in thirty-two parts: vanity 4, love of rule 4, sexual passion 4, fickleness 4, timidity 2, inocency and superstition 4." Regrettably, he does not give us the name of the analyst.[20] Such things were apparently of interest to the patrons of a fashionable Spa in 1813. This use of "sexual" in the above context is surely unusual for the time; the common term of that day would have been "carnal."

The dispensary was able to report an excellent initial half-year of operations on October 7. Only 4 out of 272 patients had died, and 86 had been completely cured of various illnesses. Griffith found the occasion a good one on which to make an observation on vaccination, which was, of course, given gratis at the dispensary. There was, he pointed out, no excuse for anyone's not being treated—particularly after vaccination's endorsement by the first medical men in Europe.

Christie was rewarded for his year's work when his wife presented him with a son on September 24. But as is often the case the autumn was also a period of some sadness. The great house at Hardwick was put up for sale by Lord Hardwick on September 9. Since being removed as Viceroy of Ireland, he had spent less and less time in the district, and this was the final break. Georgiana Cottage had also been sold earlier in the summer. On June 10, Byron had gone off to Italy with the Oxfords, and a month later the cottage of so many memories was empty and awaiting a purchaser. But if old faces left new ones continued to arrive.

One of Jenner's earliest allies, Lord Somerville, arrived with his entire family on October 14 and stayed well into the winter as more and more people made the town their winter quarters. The *Chronicle* noted in particular the Irish families that were setting up establishments. That delightful firebrand, Lady Lucy Foley, had been in and out of the town all through the autumn months, and still preaching Irish home rule while her gallant husband, the Admiral, was busy fighting his wife's spiritual allies the French. Lady Charlemont, Mary Berry's latest friend, gave the most lavish parties in the town during the winter, and Mary herself, now fifty, was still a lion of society sought after by all the social leaders.

Of more importance, of course, was the continuing influx of dons from Oxford, mostly in medicine—and attracted, I suppose, by Jenner. The University authorities decided just before Christmas to give him an honorary Doctor of Medicine degree. When he heard the news he reacted more enthusiastically than he usually did on receiving honors. He was the only Jenner in several generations who, for financial reasons, had not been able to go to Oxford, but where poverty had frustrated him vaccination had rewarded him. There was more than one path to a university degree. He dearly hoped his friend Moore would share his experience:

The University of Oxford on Friday last, conferred on me the degree of Doctor of Medicine, by diploma, without a single *non placet*. This is the more honourable, as I understand that they consider this gift so precious that it is not bestowed twice in a century. Some early day next week (Tuesday, most likely) I intend going to Oxford to accept this boon, and staying one clear day. Now, my friend, what may you? Do you feel bold enough to face me there? It would be a high gratification most certainly; and I would envolop you in a frank, for you have no business to jaunt about and spend your money.

Perhaps anticipating Moore's refusal to come (he had unavailingly invited him to Cheltenham not so long before), Jenner pointed out the possibility of some help from the great library facilities the university offered.

By the way, would not some of the sages there aid your research in conducting you over the Bodleian Library? There are several coaches go from town every morning. I have a thousand things to say to you. Pray enquire of Dr. Harvey whether I may not knock boldly at the door of the College of Physicians and gain admittance; and desire him to explain the nature of the ceremony that would take place. . . . If you can come to Oxford write soon.[21]

He sent this letter off from Cheltenham on the sixth, but whether Moore was unable to come or for what reason we know not—it was more than a week before Jenner was finally able to arrange his trip with a friend who lived closer at hand.

According to Baron, the university had been considering this move ever since 1798 when the *Inquiry* came out but had cautiously waited until the system of vaccination had proved itself. Baron, in this instance, becomes a very valuable source, for it was he who accompanied Jenner to Oxford for the ceremony. The young Gloucester doctor was always so grateful when he had the opportunity to take part in anything related to the great man.

He invited me to accompany him to Oxford to receive the diploma; and I did so with much satisfaction. We left Cheltenham on the morning of Tuesday the fourteenth of December 1813, and arrived at Oxford in the evening. He was playful and ingenious as usual, during the progress of our journey, but at times a little depressed by anxiety for his son Robert, who had just returned from school with a cough. He said that he so much resembled his son who died, that he could not but feel alarm. Next morning he was waited on by Sir Christopher Pegge and Dr. Kidd[22] the professors of Anatomy and Chemistry. They presented the diploma with becoming expressions of respect, and remarked that it was an honour that had not been conferred on any man for nearly seventy years before. Jenner behaved with much simplicity and dignity. "It is remarkable," said he, "that I should have been the only one of a long line of ancestors and relations who was not educated at Oxford. They were determined to turn me into the meadows, instead of allowing me to flourish in the groves of Academus. It is better, perhaps, as it is," he then observed, "especially as I have arrived at your highest honours, without complying with your ordinary rules of discipline." He then reluctantly put on his gown and cap, because, he said, the thing was unusual to him, and he could not help thinking he should be an object of remark in the eyes of others—forgetting for the instant that he was at Oxford and not at Cheltenham.[23]

Jenner's hope, as he had expressed to Moore, that the honor conferred by Oxford might influence the Royal College of Physicians was quite without basis. By now, practically all the learned societies in the world had recognized Jenner's importance. In fact the Royal College was the only distinguished international body that refused to join in the common policy. The Oxford ceremony was accordingly ignored by the Royal College officials and Jenner returned to Cheltenham and his own affairs.

With Christmas in the offing he found time to attend to a matter that had been in his mind for some time. By now there was a brilliant array of doctors settled about him—and many of whom had literary ability. Men like Parry, Baron, Boisragon, and Christie, who were scholars as well as doctors, presented a splendid nucleus for a literary organization, and during the Christmas holidays Jenner invited a few of them around to St. George's Place, where plans were made for the establishment of such a society. Baron, writing twenty-five years later, seems to have thought that the time was not ripe. Pointing out that while, in 1838, "the establishment of literary and scientific institutions in our provincial towns forms a striking feature in the character of the present time," he suggests that in 1813 (possibly because of the war) the mood was much different. "He (Jenner) even outran the spirit of the age, in attempts to cultivate this goodly tree. In this spirit he endeavoured to establish a Literary and Philosophical institution in Cheltenham. Several preliminary meetings were held at his house, No. 8 St. George's Place, in the end of the preceding year."[24] Baron was present at some of these meetings, of course, and they must have been spoken of in the town, because the press reported on January 19: "We are happy to announce the prospect of the speedy establishment of a Philosophical and Literary Society in this place, and it is also rumoured in fashionable circles that an annual musical festival will shortly be established at this watering place." This was more than two weeks before the first official preliminary meeting, but things were undoubtedly held up by a serious change in the weather, and Jenner was marooned in his house by successive blizzards. An old lady collapsed in the snow in front of Bedford Buildings, on the corner of St. George's Place and Chester Walk, and was only saved from death by being quickly taken indoors and treated by a householder. The streets were, indeed, so blocked by snow that travel on foot or by carriage was extremely difficult. Poor Mr. Morhall, as Town Surveyor, was under constant pressure from the discomfited citizens and had little time for anything but the weather emergency. By February, however, conditions improved and an inaugural meeting was finally held at the Assembly Rooms on the fourth; Jenner was formally elected President of the Cheltenham Literary and Philosophical Society and Morhall was made Secretary. A week later on February 10, the first regular gathering was held. The *Gazette* reported that "about thirty members are already elected and Dr. Jenner is appointed president for the year. The first periodical meeting was held on Thursday evening at which a paper was read by Dr. Baron and received with considerable approbation."[25] In his account, written after a quarter of a century, Baron inaccurately recalls that, beside himself, Parry and

Boisragon read papers. He was also confused as to the fate of the institution itself. After "his [Jenner's] retirement to Berkeley," he goes on, "it soon fell to the ground." To be sure it underwent a decline for a spell given the all-consuming sorrow of the doctor's last years, but there were other members still available. Two years after Jenner's death Boisragon reorganized the society, and it had a very active life until 1861.[26] In 1836 it moved into a splendid new building of classical design located in the Promenade where from time to time internationally known scholars gave lectures.

The Christmas and New Year of 1813–14 had been Cheltenham's first as an established winter resort, and the social activity despite the weather had been equal to the height of the summer season. It is significant that Jenner chose December to hold the gatherings at his house prior to launching his society, but his modest hospitality was nothing compared with the routs, suppers, and balls that were held in other people's private houses. Mrs. Dowdall, the lady of a Dr. Dowdall who had arrived in the town in July and was undoubtedly very rich, gave a ball and supper at her house in Bedford Buildings on January 27. But even the wealthy doctors were outdone by the "fashionables." On the fourteenth Captain Richardson gave a ball and supper to "upwards of two hundred fashionables." On the sixteenth Mr. Barrington gave a concert and supper to a numerous party at his lodgings in the Crescent, and on the twenty-first Miss Seaton gave a ball and supper to nearly two hundred. The spaciousness of these new Regency houses is revealed by the company they were able to accommodate, and one might assume that Jenner enjoyed a great part of the hospitality around him. Certainly the new, crowded winter season offered unlimited scope for his own gatherings, which became very much a part of the town's social life.

Morhall also played an important role in making St. George's Place as attractive as possible. He actually had an old house removed from the corner of Chester Walk and Well Walk, which had rather blocked the view from Jenner's rear windows, and planned to erect a pleasant "lighted archway" at that entrance to the churchyard; but for some reason his plan never materialized. Of course there were some problems that he was unable to solve. Some humorless correspondents were extremely concerned about the little boys who went swimming in a pond at the far end of St. George's Place where it met the fields about Bayshill. In order to dry themselves after their ablutions, they apparently ran about in a state of nature. Nothing was ever done about it, as far as research shows, and the crimes went unpunished. Save for the weather and Catherine's uncertain condition, winter ended on a very satisfactory note. Jenner had made his own world among his own friends. There would be only one more venture to London.

Indeed, with the launching of the Literary and Philosophical Society his interest seemed so far removed from the metropolis that when the Royal College of Physicians categorically and finally refused to admit him, Jenner was not as upset as one might have expected. As a matter of fact, his friends were far more indignant than he. Baillie, we are told, "spoke his sentiments with unusual animation and warmth." Jenner would have been much happier if no one had *urged* his admission. If the college wished to honor him, as Oxford had done, all well and good, but he wanted no one to plead for him. On March 15, when he had been president of his own society for just over a month, he wrote with delightful independence to Dr. Cooke.[27]

You saw by my reply to your first letter that I was not ambitious of becoming a Fellow of the College of Physicians; your second has completely put an end to every feeling of the sort, and I hasten to request you to put a stop to the progress of anything that may be preparing for my approach to Warwick Lane. In my youth I went through the ordinary course of a classical education, obtained a tolerable proficiency in the Latin language, and got a decent smattering of Greek; but the greater part of it has long since transmigrated into heads better suited to its cultivation. At my time of life to set about brushing up would be irksome to me beyond measure; I would not do it for a diadem. That indeed would be a bauble. I would not do it for John Hunter's museum: and that, you will allow, is no trifle. How fortunate I have been in receiving your kind communication! If the thing had gone on it would have been embarrassing to both parties——[28]

So much for the Royal College. Their excuse for refusing him, incidentally, had been his apparent unwillingness to take a language test—or rather, their assumption that he would be unwilling.

There was one cause to which Jenner considered himself committed, however, despite his increasing withdrawal into his Cheltenham shell. Jenner's zeal for releasing prisoners of war seems to have continued unabated right up to the end. His final coup was the son of no less a person than Sir Francis Milman, though the London papers got very confused in their reporting of the affair, much to the amusement of Griffith, who reported as follows in the *Chronicle* for April 14:

Captain Milman, son of Sir Francis Milman, Bart. just arrived from Verdun where he was sometime a prisoner, owed his liberation to the influence of Dr. Jenner, now in Paris, who was in such high esteem with Buonaparte, on account of the success of vaccination in that capital that he was informed that the French Emperor would readily grant him any favour he might request. The doctor in consequence solicited the exchange of Captain Milman, which was immediately granted. We copied the above paragraph from a London print and it possesses everything to recommend it but the truth; the celebrated character in question being at present in this town.

There is little doubt that Napoleon released the young soldier at Jenner's behest, but the doctor was never in personal contact with the Emperor, nor, indeed, was he ever outside the British Isles. Sir Francis and Lady Milman came to Cheltenham some six weeks later, but by then Jenner was not home.[29] He had left for London at the end of April.

There were several reasons for the journey to the capital. Lord Borington's bill would be coming up in the Lords very soon, and while the doctor was not too sanguine after so many rebuffs, he was so vitally concerned about the dangers of smallpox inoculation, he wished to be present himself. In addition, with the closing of the war there would be many foreign potentates in London with whom he had been in correspondence and whom he now hoped he might meet. Catherine was not very happy about his going, but she was very safe in the hands of the dependable Mr. Wood, who apparently handled the practice in the absence of his colleague. Baron states that this gentleman was "one of Dr. Jenner's oldest and most attached friends, and attended to *all* his affairs during his absence from Cheltenham,"[30] but that is the sole sentence he gives to this apparently very important character in his entire two volumes.

Upon arrival Jenner found the capital swarming with his friends, and the Cheltenham clan was very active. Lysons was in poor health but as full of gossip as ever, particularly about the foreign royalties Jenner hoped to meet. He told Farington that the Emperor of Austria, he was informed, "was of limited mental capacity." Of the Duchess of Oldenburgh, on the other hand, one heard the most glowing reports. The lady's reputation seems to have impressed Jenner greatly and as a consequence it was she to whom he first addressed himself when he was able.[31] Lawrence felt there was more character in the face of the King of Prussia than in that of the Emperor, and he was specially concerned with such things since he was officially commissioned to paint all the allied royalties. (This year was the most successful of his career and marked him as the leading portrait painter of Europe.) Even the aged Warren Hastings was in town and was introduced to most of the great personages. Jenner's friend, Sir John Sinclair, accompanied Hastings to the Thanksgiving Service at St. Paul's Cathedral. But in this whirl of activity, it was exclusively the foreign royalty who sought Jenner's company.

Jenner took the ailing Lysons under his care in conjunction with Baillie soon after his arrival, even though engaging in practice had been the last thought in his mind when he left Cheltenham. In the long entry for May 15, Farington gives such a detailed account that one must assume that he had discussed his friend's condition with both the doctors.

Lysons I called on this afternoon. He looked ill. His face a bad colour and thin. His eyes yellow and heavy, with a light spot at the point of vision. He spoke as desirous to make the best of his state, but he said he had not got the better of his essential complaint; that he went to bed at half-past-ten and usually slept seven hours, and when he rose at half-past-six or seven o'clock his pulse was at eighty, but afterwards any exercise or exertion it still rose to ninety or more, and what he called "a sinking of the heart" accompanied it. Dr. Jenner recommended him to eat roast meat in preference to *boiled meat,* as it contained more nourishment, and he advised him to dine of *meat* and bread only, forbearing from *vegetables,* as by that means he would take in a larger proportion of really nourishing food. It was strongly recommended to him by Dr. Baillie and Dr. Jenner to forbear from application to study, as rest for his mind was highly necessary; but, said he, "what can I do? I cannot sit wholly idle?" I told him that his known activity and industry made the advice of his physicians prudent, but that I apprehended that if he would limit his application so far as to make it rather an *amusement,* it might be beneficial to him. Before I left him I manifestly saw that he was considerably weakened in his bodily state, for contrary to his usual ardent manner, his conversation sunk into short answers to what I said. On the whole I felt convinced that his constitution was labouring under great difficulty. He said he continued to take the blue pill every night, containing five grains of mercury so prepared as to moderate its effect. He was prohibited the use of wine or malt liquor.[32]

For some reason, despite the fact that he was looking forward to a possible meeting with the great ones of the earth and hoped that they would benefit his cause, Jenner found London more unpalatable than ever. In addition he was probably lonely. "Though I can't get away," he wrote to Baron on May 18, "yet I am quite sick of the life I lead here, and certain I am that your presence would relieve me. The mighty potentates will be here soon, and I suppose I shall see some of them. The Duchess of Oldenburgh is a more interesting being than I ever met in a station so elevated." He was also worried about his wife, though the scrap of the letter given by Baron is somewhat unclear. "Poor Mrs. Jenner has suffered severely during my absence. So ill was she that I held myself in readiness daily to go down on the arrival of the post. My last accounts *have been very pleasant.* Judge what a life of disquietude I have."[33] Besides these reassuring accounts, Jenner was encouraged to stay in London by the continued concern with his work shown by the duchess. Altogether he met her several times and was profoundly impressed. He must have visited her again a week or so after this letter was written, for the *Cheltenham Chronicle* relates on June 2 that Jenner "had the honour of a long audience." His subsequent meeting with the Emperor of All the Russias is given in "very nearly" Jenner's own words by Baron.

I was very graciously received, and was probably the first man to contradict the autocrat. He said, "Dr. Jenner, your feelings must be delightful. The consciousness of having so much benefited your race must be a never-failing source of pleasure, and I am happy to think that you have received the thanks, the applause and the gratitude of the world." I replied to His Majesty that my feelings were such as he described, and I had received the thanks and the applause but not the gratitude of the world. His face flushed. He said no more, by my daring seemed to give displeasure. In a short time, however, he forgot it, and gave me a trait of character which showed great goodness of heart and knowledge of human nature. My enquiries respecting lymphatic diseases, and tubercles, and pulmonary consumption had reached the ears of the Grand Duchess. She was present and requested me to detail to her brother, the Emperor, what I had formerly said to Her Imperial Highness. In the course of my remarks I became embarrassed. She observed this and so did the Emperor. "Dr. Jenner," said she, "you do not tell my brother what you have to say so accurately as you told me." I excused myself by saying I was not accustomed to speak in such a presence. His Majesty grasped me by the hand, and held me for some time, not quitting me until my confidence was restored by this warm-hearted and kind expression of his consideration.

It will be remembered that the Prussian royal family had been the first foreign house to be vaccinated when Jenner had sent his vaccine to the Princess Royal in 1799. He was consequently very grateful when he received an intimation that the King of Prussia would grant him an audience. The system had been put into effect more thoroughly in that country than any other with the result that smallpox had been completely eliminated. Jenner later met Marshall Blucher and some of the lesser Prussian generals. There was no question but what all the allied statesmen were eager to meet so great a benefactor, and a number of his friends suggested a scheme whereby a delegation should be formed to approach the allied sovereigns on his behalf, so that a fitting recognition might be made of his work. Count Orloff, the Russian Ambassador, however, felt that this was too restrained. He insisted that Jenner had every right to approach their majesties himself, direct. Undoubtedly, on the evidence of the past actions of foreign royalty in both war and peace, the gesture would have borne fruit, but because Jenner was Jenner, nothing happened. He was far too diffident to even consider such a move and the whole idea was forgotten. The London visit, at the time of mutual exchanges of international victory honors, secured no official recognition for Jenner. Not a decoration, not an order, not a gift from the assembled mighty to him "who by his discovery had saved our own fleets and armies from the pestilential ravages of smallpox, and had rendered not less important services to the people than to the military force of every potentate in Europe." It is perhaps a pity that Wellington, Hutchinson, and Admiral Berkeley were not the arbiters in the allocation of rewards for the victory. To be sure the victorious rulers of the German and Russian allies had thanked Jenner—but not the Prince Regent of his own country.

Nor was the second well-intentioned move of Lord Borington any more successful than the first. Again Jenner was betrayed by ingratitude in high places. Both the Lord Chancellor and the Lord Chief Justice opposed the bill. Jenner was particularly bitter about the latter, Lord Ellenborough, who should have known better but who was probably smarting from a social rebuff he had received from the doctor a short time previously. They had both been present at a drawing room in St. James's when Ellenborough had made a comment on vaccination of a very stupid nature, probably not realizing that Jenner was within earshot. The doctor's reaction was as scathing as it was indignant, and his lordship was silenced by a rhetoric that was outside his province. "It is all very well," said Jenner, "to attain to a certain rank, but there is one beyond, where mind and nature cease and a man becomes a thing of imaginary dignity, of form, rules, starch and ruffles."[34]

Baron records an anecdote of a similar nature.

"When occasion required, he [Jenner] could well sustain the dignity of his name and station. In the drawing room at St. James' he chanced to overhear a noble lord, who was in high office, mentioning his name and repeating the idle calumny which had been propagated concerning his own want of confidence in vaccination, in consequence of his acting as has already been stated in the case of his son Robert. He, with the greatest promptitude and decision, refuted the charge and abashed the reporter. His person was not known to the noble lord, but with entire composure he advanced to his lordship, and looking fully in his face, calmly observed, "I am Dr. Jenner."[35]

The objectionable reference was to the late Dr. Cother's careless behavior in Cheltenham in 1798, but it survived for many
years in the drawing rooms of the enemy. Undoubtedly Jenner's
ready anger and blunt speech when the vital principles for which
he stood were involved contributed a great deal to the lack of
appreciation in many high places. Both the Eldon and Ellenborough families were in the Cheltenham orbit. In fact, both
eventually settled there—the Eldons at Stowell Park and the
Ellenboroughs at Southam de la Bere. Lord Eldon achieved tremendous prestige when he became Lord Chancellor of England
in 1801, and Ellenborough became Lord Chief Justice the following year. Neither man was popular with the people and neither was a rake, as were most of the Cheltenham peers. Jenner
knew Ellenborough but not Eldon, who may have been the subject
of Baron's anecdote.

Jenner enjoyed the company of the learned and enlightened
nobility from the royal family downwards, but he was completely
intolerant—even arrogant—where rank and wealth demanded
respect otherwise unmerited. Young John Fosbroke, who certainly knew him in his last few years better than anyone else,
described him thus: "Where reason was subdued by personal
pride, and aristocratical distinction and artificial superiority put
forward to level and reject supereminence according to intellect
and nature, there the swelling contempt of his soul burst forth
in unrepressed indignation."[36] But all this, splendid as it was, did
not make for getting a bill through the House of Lords. Jenner
may have unwittingly offended many a noble lord by his scarcely
concealed contempt for fools—and there were hundreds of peers
outside his personal circle. Even so Borington started out in a
much more promising manner than in 1812. The bill was presented to the House on July 1 and entitled: "For Regulating the
Practice of Smallpox Inoculation and Checking the Diffusion
of That Disease." Baron's report of the presentation indicates
that, this time, it was all-inclusive.

His lordship on introducing it to the House, took occasion to observe
that the principle on which it was founded had often been acted upon
and recognized by the legislature. He showed that all civilized communities, individuals were restrained from exercising unlimited

dominion over their persons or property; and that many statutes had been passed for preventing the spreading of contagious diseases. He particularly dwelt upon those which had been enacted in order to stay the progress of the plague . . . that similar provisions ought to be put into force against the plague of smallpox. He therefore recommended that regulations should be adopted in all cases where this disease existed, either in consequence of inoculation or casual infection.[37]

The very completeness of his case perhaps hurt him on this occasion, however. The noble lords could not confuse him with amendments and suggested alterations, but they could claim that the bill was unnecessary. His best approach would have been simply *a bill to end inoculation with smallpox* and nothing more. But he was up against the two greatest legal minds in England, among others, and once it came to a debate he was outclassed. Lord Ellenborough practically implied that the bill was frivolous.

What was unforgivable in the Lord Chief Justice was the fact that he himself had taken advantage of vaccination to safeguard his own family. In the familiar House of Lords, however, the great lawyer had an easy prey in the rather nervous Borington and was merciless. Ellenborough claimed that the elimination of smallpox inoculation could not be covered by legislation; common law could well deal with any actions that deliberately forwarded the spread of smallpox. He openly ridiculed some of Borington's points. Of vaccination he was tolerant:

No doubt it was of some use, but he did not concur in all the praise bestowed upon it in this bill; but if the noble lord considered it a complete preventive of smallpox, he differed with him in opinion. At the same time he had shown his respect for the discovery, for he had had eight children vaccinated. He believed in its efficacy to a certain extent: it might prevent the disorder for eight or nine years, and was desirable in a large city like this, where there was a large family of Children.[38]

Despite the care with which the substance of his bill had been drawn up, Lord Borington was demolished by the opposition. After a few remarks by another Gloucestershire peer, Lord Redesdale, the bill was withdrawn on the grounds that the position was already covered in common law.

Though Jenner had not really expected an act to be passed, Lord Ellenborough's behavior shocked him deeply. For a man of that stature to use the privilege of the Upper House to damn with faint praise a system he himself was glad to utilize, and which deep in his heart he must have known to be right, violated every decent principle. Coming from a person of such august station the remarks were doubly injurious. Baron reported:

I have seldom seen Jenner more disturbed than he was by this occurrence, and not certainly because he had any fears that the unsupported assertion of his lordship would prove correct but because it unhappily accorded with popular prejudices, and when uttered by such a person, in such an assembly, was calculated to do unspeakable mischief.[39]

Of course all his friends were as disgusted as Jenner was, but it was not clear how the influence of so exalted an orator as Ellenborough could be countered among the masses. The reaction of hordes of ignorant parents must have a dire effect upon their children.

In the anxiety and resentment of the moment the loyal Baron prepared a pamphlet pointing out how the peer's observations were completely negated by the prima facie evidence of the past years, but finding the publication process unduly slow, and noting Jenner's final disgust at the whole business, he let the matter drop. The doctor's one concern now was to get back to Catherine in Cheltenham as soon as he possibly could. The contrast between his gracious reception at the hands of the foreign royalty and his failure in the Parliament of his own country must have been very much on his mind during the long coach ride home that July night.

Nonetheless, as Baron put in, "all these things passed away and we find Jenner again . . . in the midst of his domestic circle at Cheltenham." To be sure, it was a chaotic and troubled household, but at least he was wanted. Probably the first thing Catherine showed him was the current issue of the *Chronicle* in which Griffith had printed an impressive news item for his friend's return.

July 21st. As an additional honour to the already imperishable name of Jenner, we observe that his Holiness the Pope, in order to arrest the progress of that pestilential curse, the smallpox, which had broken out in a populous part of Rome recommended vaccination as "a precious discovery which ought to be a new motive for human gratitude to Omnipotence!"[40]

One can hope that this recognition put the treatment by Eldon and Ellenborough in its correct perspective.

The immediate domestic situation facing Jenner was very serious indeed—thankful though he was to shake off the disappointments of London. He worked frantically to bring his brood back to health. When he had time he wrote to Baron:

You know how actively I have been employed here since my return from town, and the impossible miseries I have endured from domestic affliction. The three servants are still in bed, I think convalescent; but there is no marked termination of the fever, except in Frank who suffers only from hunger, as nothing seems to satisfy him. Mrs. Jenner is rather better; but there is another on the sick-list—alas! myself. I was seized on Sunday with cholera and sad work it has made with me. Within these four hours things have changed for the better, or I could not have answered your letter by return of post.[41]

As was so typically the case, his letter of many complaints ended on an optimistic note. He was grateful for every mark of appreciation, and the comments of the Pope were not the only welcome words that heartened him. In October a moving letter came from Brunn in Moravia written in the most picturesque English and addressed to "The Rt. Hon. Physician, Edward Jenner, Discoverer of the Cowpock, the Greatest Benefactor of Mankind," and signed by "Med. Doctor Rincolini, Physician, and Claviger, first surgeon and vacciner [sic] of Vaccine Institute at Brunn." It reported the deep feelings of the people of Moravia for the great doctor's work and described the monument they had erected to his memory on the occasion of his birthday,

—a constant monument with thine breast-piece in the 65th year of thine age, erected even in the same time as the great English nation by her constancy and intrepidity, rendered the liberty of the whole Europe. . . . Accept generously, great man, that feeble sign of veneration and gratitude and Heaven may concerve your life to the most remote time.

A drawing of the "monument" was enclosed. Baron was visiting St. George's Place when the letter arrived, and he said that it gave his friend "unqualified gratification." He was not sure that it was ever answered, though in all probability it was, since Jenner felt it deeply enough to write a poem to celebrate the occasion entitled "Cheltenham to Brunn."[42]

Old Dr. Saunders had arrived at the Wells on May 11, but we do not know whether he was still there when Jenner came home. Another interesting visitor was the historian John Lingard, who had arrived a week later.[43] He had already been working for three years on his monumental *History of England,* which he completed in 1830, and, presumably, had come to visit his friend, that great Benedictine scholar, John Augustine Birdsall who settled in Cheltenham in 1810.[44] With the rise of anti-clericalism on the Continent, many Catholic orders turned their eyes to more tolerant Britain. Father Birdsall, who possessed a large private fortune, was probably the most learned English Benedictine of his day, and in later years became president of the order. It is an index of the importance of Cheltenham to the great Catholic families that he was sent to this relatively small town to establish a mission rather than to one of the large centers. Perhaps Lord Holland was partly responsible; he was no papist, but a man who had spent many years in Spain and had indeed played a role in the negotiations between His Catholic Majesty's court in Madrid and Jenner at the time of the Balmis voyage. Father Birdsall built his chapel in Somerset Place, perhaps two hundred yards from Jenner's house, and the two men sat on various committees together during the next ten years. Since the visiting historian would almost certainly have lodged with his friend, Jenner may well have met him. Birdsall was a sought after conversationalist and wit, and one of the most influential men in the Catholic establishment of England.

Gregarious man that he was, Jenner unquestionably enjoyed seeing the ever changing stream of folks who passed—or entered —his door during twenty-five years at St. George's Place.[45] But the time available for studying the lists of arrivals for new and interesting visitors was definitely limited, and all too often after an extended absence his almost perfect control of the smallpox scene slipped a little. No matter how efficiently the vaccination protection functioned within the town, there was no way—short of refusing treatment—of controlling infected patients who were brought in from outside. One very sad incident had taken place during Jenner's absence. A little boy of two and a half, John Clark, "the son of a respectable tradesman" had died of smallpox. The child, who lived in Russell's Passage, off Lower High Street, had caught the disease in Evesham and had been rushed home to be tended by the dispensary doctors. They worked tirelessly to save him but it was in vain. A number of children who lived in or near the house, but who had been vaccinated, came through unscathed.[46] Of course, the *Chronicle* urged all who were not so protected to go to the clinic right away. At that point, a death from smallpox in Cheltenham was a very rare and serious matter.

The visit of the allied sovereigns to London on the conclusion of the war had stolen the summer crowds from all the fashionable resorts. For a short period in June, Cheltenham was virtually deserted—at least, that is, by the "fashionables." Once the London "stage" had completed its performance, the opposite obtained. The flood of celebrities that poured into the town was without precedent. Griffith estimated that a "majority" of the House of Lords was present in July—most of them with their families. In the fortnight following Jenner's return on the fourteenth, nine generals and three admirals joined the throng, and more crowds of distinguished visitors continued right up to Christmas. The dawning of peace after nearly twenty years of war drove people a little mad. The balls and dinners of the wealthy were more than matched by the rank and file. The very night that Jenner got home an ox was roasted in Rose and Crown Passage, and forty people feasted and made merry. The following day Mr. Richards, landlord of the King's Head in the High Street, broached a hogshead of beer for all to enjoy. But the biggest celebration of all was arranged by the nobility and gentry who each gave six guineas so that the whole town could feast and celebrate in Well Walk—right behind Jenner's house. Just how poor Catherine survived this period of raucous nights is hard to imagine, but perhaps her patient soul understood and accepted the spontaneous bedlam that celebrated the end of almost twenty years of con-

tinuous warfare. Jenner, tending his household of invalids, might
have stolen a minute now and then to gaze down upon the revel-
lers from his windows.

Inevitably this period of happy hysteria had its blacker side.
Vandalism after copious drinking was rampant, and there was a
shocking wave of lamp smashing as well as—or to facilitate—general lawlessness. Some hundred and fifty street lights were destroyed, and the *Chronicle* observed that, on a pro rata basis, the
culprits could serve as much as twelve years in prison when
caught! Though a magistrate, it is doubtful whether Jenner
sat on any of the hearings surrounding these activities of the week
or so after he came home.

It was almost a month after his return before the family was
back on its feet and Jenner was free to resume his seat on the
magistrates' bench—and a changed, chaotic society he found
around him with the households of his own friends often involved. The very proper and Reverend Mr. Farryman had a most
upsetting experience. During the confusion of the celebrations
his housemaid, Ann Williams, must have been left a great deal
to herself; she and her male companion, named Buffon, had stolen
a number of household items including some sheets, which she
was in the process of making into shirts when arrested. Both prisoners were committed to the Assizes at Gloucester. In a somewhat
lighter vein there was a case which, quite improperly, benefitted
the local medical establishment. Two ladies of pleasure, Miss
Kendall and Miss Higgs, were apprehended and lodged in the
lockup overnight. They were charged with riotous conduct and
with obtaining two guineas from a gentleman on false pretenses!
(Apparently the bench did not accept that the services they
offered were legitimate merchandise.) Having spent the night in
jail, their sole punishment was that they hand over the two
guineas to the dispensary.[47] It was a most improper procedure,
but it did help the cause of medicine—and does, perhaps, indicate
the influence of the doctors in the town's affairs.

A case that came before Jenner and the magistrates' bench
a few weeks later was a far cry from the usual misdemeanors.
Miss Sarah Humphris, a brothel keeper in Grove Street, had a
bitter quarrel with her paramour over another woman and in

a fit of anger, drank vitriol. She apparently had not intended suicide because in her agony she kept repeating to the doctor that she would never have used vitriol had she known the pain it would cause. But her internal burns were such that the corpse was in a shocking condition when she succumbed. From the evidence of her comments and her rational speech during her last hours the magistrates had to declare her to have been of sound mind. She was, therefore, legally a suicide. Fortunately there was sufficient humanity on the bench to waive the usual barbarous ritual of driving a stake through the body, but the poor soul could not be buried in consecrated ground. She was tipped into a rough grave at the crossroads leading into Swindon Village. The body had so offensively decomposed by this time that they not only filled the coffin with quicklime but the grave also. The *Chronicle* explains that this particular spot was chosen because it was a favorite rendezvous of prostitutes plying their trade. According to Goding it was the last such case on record. "Sarah Humphris. a felo-de-se buried in the cross-road leading to Swindon, the last instance of a cross-road burial in the parish."[48]

As the season waned Jenner's friends continued to follow him to Cheltenham. Lord Egremont appeared on the scene at the end of September as breezy as ever despite his sixty-three years. It was the peer's first visit since the establishment of Jenner's Literary and Philosophical Society and there was much to discuss. Meanwhile, the *Chronicle* continued to pour out superlatives from all over the globe, keeping up the tempo of enthusiasm. "In Sweden," announced Griffith on October 13, "Dr. Jenner ranks as one of the greatest benefactors of the human race and vaccination is performed in all children nine days only from their birth. The court, the clergy and the medical profession have zealously concurred and consequently the smallpox is considered as extirpated from the country." Nor was this all. On the same page was the report of a woman named Vantudello who had been prosecuted in London for "exposing in the public walks a child infected with smallpox."[49] The story proceeds to the effect that such action should draw people into appreciating the work of the National Vaccine Institute. The reasoning is not too clear, but the writer does go on to inform us that this was the first prosecution on record for such an offense. Perhaps it showed that there was some basis in Lord Ellenborough's contention that the law, as it stood, had authority to curb the culpable spreading of disease. Never has a modern chamber of commerce worked harder in promoting the fame of a local celebrity than Griffith did for Jenner.

Though the great world struggle with Napoleon was over, the unpopular conflict in America still dragged on, bringing periodic desolation to local homes. In this month of autumn colors, two tragic items were reported. A very popular young Cheltenham man—Captain James Brook Irwin—was killed in the assault on Fort Erie. "The heroic Captain . . . of the 103rd regiment . . . leaves an amiable widow and two children." And just over two weeks later, on the twenty-seventh, a poem appeared to the memory of that gallant Irishman, General Ross, victor of Washington, killed in action at Baltimore. War was still very much with the Cheltenham people, though under a surface of often superficial gaiety. Jenner in particular had a much more gentle recollection of the name Fort Erie, but now the very field of his Canadian triumphs was drenched in blood.

Riddell and Boisragon seemed to be set on outdoing each other in the lavishness of their entertaining. Boisragon had given a magnificent concert to a hundred "fashionables" when Lord Egremont arrived, at which two celebrated artists performed— Madame Marconi and a Mr. Magrath. But Riddell replied with a superb banquet to Lady Buckinghamshire when he returned to Cambray on November 10. This grand old lady of Cheltenham society had apparently recovered from her "betrayal" by the Lefevres and was as active as ever. When Colonel Berkeley took over the Theatre Royal for his amateur theatricals this week, she and the aging Lady Jersey were right in the thick of it. Lady Buckinghamshire, of course, could be gently distracted away from her disillusionment, but for Jenner the Lefevre incident was a tragedy in its effect on government policy. No further action was ever taken to locate young Husson, and his father—a power in French medicine—turned bitterly on the English doctor, even to the extent of disputing his discovery of vaccination.[50]

But the somewhat hectic autumn passed, and when Egremont

was joined by Worthington who came for a long visit late in November, things at St. George's Place were back to normal. Worthington's arrival about coincided with a letter amusing in its flamboyance and dated Munich, November, 1814; under present conditions it would have taken two or three weeks to reach Cheltenham. It was from Dr. Von Soemmering of Bavaria and accompanied by that country's Diploma of the Royal Academy of Sciences "as due acknowledgement of the superiority of that salutiferous genius by whose infinite merit mankind stands delivered for ever from the most hideous and dreadful of all diseases. . . . Bavaria can boast of being the country in which your glorious discovery not only found the highest applause, but which from the very first beginning till the present day continued regularly and steadfastly its universal introduction." This routine introductory praise, gratifying in itself, was followed by something that was particularly heartening to Jenner, fighting his eternal battle against the school that maintained inoculation by cowpox was little different from the injection of smallpox.

Our meritorious and most famous physician in Germany in regard to smallpox, Dr. Ch. L. Hoffman, Physician of the late Elector of Mainz, a lynx-eyed man, though more than eighty years old, regarding attentively the first cowpox shown to him, energetically exclaimed, "This pox surely will secure against the smallpox, being indeed nothing else but a real and true genuine smallpox of the mildest sort; and you all know that ten thousand poxes give no more security than a single one." He used to tell me confidently as a result of his long experience, "Believe me, my friend, there exists a certain form or a particular sort of smallpox, so mild, so regular, and of so short a duration,—in short of such benignity,—that the patient whatever regimen he follows, this sort of smallpox by no means will kill him; nay, even in any way hurt him."

The letter concludes in a manner even more flattering than any Jenner had previously received: "May the blessings of so many millions whose lives you saved or whose deformities you prevented, contribute to exhilarate the days of their benefactor. I am dear sir, With the profoundest veneration, Your obedient and humble servant, Dr. S.Th. Von Soemmering."[51]

Inevitably, after every little breath of encouragement, there

came the melancholy balance in the other direction, and after
a brief rally when Jenner returned from London, Catherine's
health continued to deteriorate, so that she was almost permanently confined to her room through the autumn and winter,
with Jenner as her nurse as well as her doctor. It was cold though
not as snowbound as the previous winter, and the town was
crowded, with the line of demarcation, socially speaking, between
summer and winter seasons becoming harder and harder to de-
fine. The year concluded with Jenner's outrageous old landlord's
feeling the edge of the satirist's pen. The *Chronicle* carried a
poem commenting on a recent eulogy of one of Riddell's beauty
potions. The author, who slyly signed herself simply "A
Woman," openly laughed at the self-professed doctor:

> On Riddell if thy powders give health
> We're too generous not to confess
> That we prize them far higher than wealth
> Which sickness can never suppress.[52]

By contrast, through all the years of his very full civic life Jenner was never lampooned, still less, threatened. Whatever elements he and his fellow commissioners offended in their running
of the town no overt act as far as I can gather was ever taken
against them. The same could not be said for innocent Mr. Morhall, the executive who so efficiently carried out their orders. One
dark night in February some ruffians broke into his house in
Milsom Street, terrified his wife and child, and did a great deal
of damage before leaving. Then they marched up the High Street
smashing street lights as they went—some thirty-two in all.
When Mr. Morhall returned home he found his wife in a state
of collapse and most of his windows broken: a sad comment on
law and order in a fashionable spa. As a result of this incident
the anxious Jenner and a group of prominent citizens formed a
society for the prosecuting of felons,[53] suggesting that the existing police system was not considered very effective. There is
something very contemporary about all this, but Jenner was still
not discouraged. The die was finally cast as far as he was concerned. There would be no more long absences from Catherine,
no more anxious seeking of help in the capital. He would handle

his crusade from home, and concentrate his activity in the ever growing society at the Wells, both as doctor and civic leader.

An early manifestation of this new direction occurred on September 13, 1814, when he was appointed Vice-President of the Cheltenham Auxiliary Bible Society. Up to this time he had never shown any active interest in religious affairs despite his wide family associations with the clergy of the Established Church; but the deep sorrows he had suffered during the past few years and the increasing concern for his wife's life could well have made him turn more to contemplative concerns. On the other hand, it may have been pressure of a different kind as well, since the man who put his name up at the meeting in the Town Hall was the poet, John Williams. Williams was still very poor and now had nine children to support. He had the evangelical zeal of his faith to sustain him, and he somehow found time to help establish the Bible Society in the sinful town of Cheltenham. Only one other of the local doctors attended, Jameson, and he was elected a member of the committee. It was a rare occasion indeed for these two medical men to be exclusively associated with each other in any public activity, and the unusual character of the committee makes it even stranger to find Jenner there at all, Catherine notwithstanding. A side of Jameson's personality is shown, however, that emphasizes his occasional aloofness from the fashionable and somewhat easygoing doctors of Cheltenham. The meeting was concerned about the pagan state of Regency society, and the organizers decided to seek out the public rather than wait to be approached. Early in November six little groups of three or four perambulated the walks and streets stopping residents and visitors, "soliciting donations and explaining their motives."[54] Jenner appears to have taken no part in this, however. His attitude to the Deity was an extremely humble one, and he seems to have been troubled by no intellectual curiosity of a theological nature. Baron mentions at least one fragment of a prayer written under affliction and which reflects the simplest accepting faith. In it Jenner prays "that I may never lose sight of Thy divine mercies; and thus by my faith and practice, when it may please Thee to send my body to the grave, may my imperishable soul be received into Thy habitations of eternal glory."

The inscription he put in a Bible he gave to young Parry's little girl also reflects his simplicity: "To Augusta Berty Parry, with the best wishes and affection of her God-father, Edward Jenner; who most devoutly hopes, as this is the greatest book that ever was written, she will give it not only the first place in her library, but convince those who love her dearly, that it occupies the first place in her heart."[55] None of this suggests the aggressive evangelism that resulted in Dr. Jameson's committee accosting the sinners in the streets of Cheltenham. Meanwhile, poor John Williams returned to his curacy and continued his life of sorrow. All his children died before him including young John, who passed away at the age of twenty-four during his final year at Guy's Hospital.

Without making the slightest reflection on Jenner's sincerity in attending the above function, it should be noted that there was another man on the platform whom he found at least as interesting as the poet Williams. "The meeting was addressed," we are told, "by eleven resident members of the Established Church, seven Dissenting Ministers, and by two members of the Society of Friends, one of whom was the celebrated Dr. Pope, Physician to George the Third." This amiable gentleman had long maintained—vainly—that he could cure the old king's mental condition, but he had also been concerned in the tragic illness and death of the monarch's daughter, Princess Amelia, in 1810. His treatment for her extreme, all-encompassing case of erysipelas was apparently continual bleeding, and eventually the worried family insisted upon bringing in Dr. Saunders and Dr. Baillie, but by then it was too late to save the girl's life. Pope had a tender and most engaging bedside manner and maintained the patient's confidence right up to the end. Tragically, she resented the intrusion of the other and more expert doctors—particularly Baillie, whom she considered abrupt and unsympathetic—and by her resistance to their presence probably sacrified her only hope of recovery. But when he appeared on the platform with Jenner, the Quaker doctor was still looked upon as one of the great practitioners of the land.[56]

Certainly Catherine must have been very pleased with this public effort on her husband's part to assist in propagating the

Gospel, and as she grew increasingly weak during the sunless winter months he subordinated everything else in his life to her care. "The tenderness and delicacy with which Jenner superintended the arrangements of everything that could be thought of for her comfort, the administration of her medicine and the preparation of her food (which a difficulty in deglutition rendered necessary) all indicated the warmest attachment and the kindest feelings." The strain of the constant attention was to a certain extent relieved by the advent of young John Fosbroke, who appeared increasingly on the scene about this time and became an invaluable junior partner to the much harassed doctor. Only eighteen years of age, he was the constant companion of Jenner for the rest of the older man's life, and being a competent writer he was also able to help in most of the later literary work. Whether or not he served an official apprenticeship with Jenner is not certain, but on the evidence it would seem likely. He went up to Edinburgh to obtain his M.D. in 1820, and in 1826, referred to "ten years practice" in Cheltenham. Since he was thus in the town through five years of medical preparation from 1815 to 1820, it is hard to believe that he could have been under any other mentor.

But if professional wrangling and vaccination research could be shelved for the moment, Jenner's more urgent medical cases could not be neglected. Another of his patients was gradually coming to the end of her travail not a hundred yards from his front door. Mrs. Entwistle had been ailing for the past year, and the constant bickering with her daughter, mainly because of the shiftless character of Mr. Entwistle, did not help matters. The situation got so bad that Harriot preferred not to come home any more, though she dutifully kept up the flow of money for such comforts as her mother expected, and the same money undoubtedly paid Dr. Jenner's bills. Old Mr. Coutts's wife died on January 14, and six weeks later one of those "real-life" fairy tales came true. The *Chronicle* reported, rather briefly considering the circumstances, "On Wednesday the 2nd of March was married at St. Pancras Church, Middlesex, Thomas Coutts, Esq. to Miss Harriot Mellon. The charitable disposition of this lady entitles her to the good wishes of all. She is the daughter of Mrs. En-

twistle of this town and is now the mother-in-law of the Dowager
Countess of Guilford."[57] And, they might have added, the richest woman in the land. To be sure, she was now thirty-eight
years old and far too buxom to take the younger roles that were
her stock-in-trade on the stage. (In fact it was Michael Kelly's
daughter who had gradually taken over a number of these parts,
though she never attained the celebrity of the older actress.) As
might have been expected, the news of the marriage did a great
deal to restore Mrs. Entwistle's health, and she did rally to a certain extent in the spring. The new Mrs. Coutts saw that she had
every conceivable care, but the improvement was short-lived.
Also, it would seem, there was again some coolness between
mother and daughter. At the end of March Mr. Entwistle wrote
to Harriot:

> Cheltenham,
> Good Friday, 1815.
>
> My dear Mrs. Coutts,
>
> Your mother was much better yesterday. . . . I wish I could say
> she was so well to-day—she appears heartbroke that she shall never
> see you again—Pray write to her. Dr. Jenner has just been to her and
> speaks very favourable of her, but my fears and doubts are not re-
> moved. May heaven bless you! She has been two days disappointed at
> you not writing.
>
> Sir Richard Clayton from Wigan, a person I have not seen for thirty
> years, called on me today to pay his respects.
>
> > I am my dear Mrs. Coutts,
> > Yours most affectionately,
> > T. Entwistle.
>
> I did get her to eat about half an ounce of boiled mutton to-day and
> take a glass of wine.[58]

It is amusing to note that in a letter manifestly written to inform Harriot of her mother's condition, the pompous Entwistle
has to remind the wealthy Mrs. Coutts that he too knows distinguished people. Clayton, an essayist of some prominence in
his day, was recorder of Wigan.

The new status of Harriot Mellon, now the controller of untold wealth, inevitably caused speculation in the town as to the
future of her parents. It was hard to believe that they would con-

tinue to run the post office, or, indeed, indulge in any labor at all. Jenner, always ready to help, had in mind a very worthy candidate for the position of post mistress. Possibly in his attendance on Mrs. Entwistle some remark had been dropped by her husband as to his pending retirement. Jenner's letter to a friend in London relative to this is interesting, as it shows his continuing concern for his friends in humbler walks of life. It is addressed to Sir Francis Freeling, Secretary of the Post Office, London, and himself a Gloucestershire man.[59]

Dear Sir,

Will you pardon the great liberty I take, on a supposition that a recent event in the family of Mr. Entwistle will occasion his retiring from our Post Office, in recommending to your attention Mrs. Eliz. Roberts as a fit person for his successor? She is very active and intelligent, and has for a series of years conducted herself with strict propriety as a superintendant of one of our public libraries. I have the honour to be, Sir, your obed[t]. & faithful, humble servant,

Edward Jenner.[60]

It was some two weeks before Jenner received a reply from Sir Francis. Since neither letter has before been printed, I give them in full. From the opening sentence, it is apparent that the two men knew each other fairly well.

G.P.O. 14th April, 1815.

My dear Sir,

Be assured that my delay in writing to you has not proceeded from any diminution of my personal and unaffected esteem and respect for your character, but from circumstances attached to the object of your application.

The Patronage of the Country Post Offices has lately passed from the hands of the Postmaster General into those of the Lords of the Treasury and hence had proceeded my inability to reply to your letter. I did mention the circumstances to Lord Chichester and I am certain his inclination towards your application was as strong as my own,—I have not however the power of saying more at this moment.

We have not yet heard of any intention on Mr. Entwistle's part to resign his office.

Believe me, etc.

F. Freeling.

Jenner lost his patient exactly a month later and Mr. Entwistle did, indeed, retire, but we do not know whether the doctor's efforts on Mrs. Roberts's behalf bore fruit or not. In these last months with Catherine, however, Jenner dedicated himself increasingly to helping his and her own people. It was his reputation for giving free medical treatment to the poor as well as vaccination that made him one of the most revered men in the town and beyond. To many simple people the gift of vaccination —at any price—placed him in the position of something akin to a priest. Because of its heartfelt sentiments, I believe the following letter, which appeared in the *Chronicle,* might be printed here, as evidence of the way his own poor felt.

Thursday, Feb. 2nd, 1815.
To the Editor of Chelt. Chron:
Sir,
    Impressed with gratitude to God, and the author of that mild substitute for Smallpox—*Vaccination,* I take my pen though I never ventured to address the public before, but I cannot restrain the feelings of a mother, who is not experiencing the benefits and comforts of this modern discovery. A dear infant now at my breast, sleeping in peace, notwithstanding it is at this moment, under the full influence of the vaccine on the eighth day, I am led to express thus publicly my feelings of gratitude, from observing, which I do with astonishment and regret, the neighbourhood in which I live, once again visited by the horrible and loathsome of all disorders, the Small-Pox. I am stimulated by sensations I cannot resist, to call upon every mother whose eye this may meet, who has been induced by her own unnecessary fears or by the ignorance and prejudice of self-interested advisers, not to adopt this safe and harmless preventive. Can you consent to be instrumental in keeping the other dreadful disease in activity? Suffering your own dear children to escape the most afflicting consequences of *this Plague* (for which I shall ever consider it, since I witnessed its distressing though, thank God not fatal effects on my first child) are you sure that you may be the cause of many innocents receiving the infection you are the means of disseminating, how can you answer to a poorer neighbour, before God, should she charge you with being the murderer of her child.—Should you hear the afflicted mother say, "but for you I might have kept still a darling and only child alive, who is now lost forever to me, a spectacle of horror and disgust"; I shudder at the very thought. Rouse yourselves then, you mothers who

either have experienced or can easily conceive what it is to lose the infant of your bosom, suffer not prejudice to operate with you, think of the goodness of God in permitting such a discovery, in giving us so unexpected a blessing reward the labours and kindness of him who made this mild process his study and who has been pleased by God with completing success to his labours—give him all that is in your power, the grateful adoption of his discovery in your own families, and those of your poor cottagers; your self approving hearts will well reward you in return.

Yours (as I must be whilst I am)
A Mother[61]

Jenner also found natural allies in those newcomers to the town whose interest in vaccination matched a concern with gengeneral peace in 1814. On July 13 the *Chronicle* observed: "Sir Arthur Faulkner[62] worked with the doctor and his friends to alleviate the growing problem of poverty that had followed the general peace in 1814. On July 13 the *Chronicle* observed: "Sir A. Faulkner's recently submitted plan for the ameliorating of the condition of the poor in this town, not being—from its philanthropic tendency—sufficiently known, we shall next week endeavour to give sufficient educidative observations as will make the scheme more generally understood and appreciated." The paper accordingly followed this up by printing a long account, in the issue of July 20, of the learned knight's proposals. Lest Faulkner be unaware of the philanthropists already active, Griffith pointed out the generous contributions already forthcoming from the clergy and the medical profession—"among some of the most forward J. C. Mathieson and Dr. Jenner hold distinguished prominence."

Mathieson, who appears more and more on the charity scene, had another interest in common with Jenner, namely, music. On April 15 he organized with Boisragon the first meeting of the Cheltenham Harmonic Society at Ruff's Regent Concert Room. A Major Fermor was in the chair while Lord Tara and "50 nobility and gentlemen selected a committee and arranged a dinner." There were representatives from the Worcester and Gloucester choirs, and Woodward played the pianoforte. (The Woodward family, incidentally, was a prominent musical family

in Cheltenham for several generations, almost up to the present.)
Boisragon held concerts at his house in the Crescent for many
years. We are reminded that Jenner himself still included song
writing among his many activities by his remark to young Fosbroke that "the music group of the drawing-room heard the
solo of a self-composed medley."[63] Perhaps there were, indeed,
musical evenings at St. George's Place to cheer the housebound
Catherine during these last months.

On the whole, Jenner's circle was a talented group. Aside from
the wide range of professional poets, artists, and actors of his acquaintance, his medical colleagues were a most outstanding
brood. Parry, Fosbroke, and Faulkner were competent versifiers;
Trye and Ring were excellent classical scholars; Baron, Christie,
and, of course, Boisragon[64] were able musicians; and every one
of them (except the latter) published books of one kind or another in his time. Jenner dabbled in all these activities.

The death of Dr. Thomas Denman this year at the age of
eighty-two drew attention to the phenomenally brilliant clan of
which he was the head. As the father-in-law of Matthew Baillie
and Herbert Croft he would have deserved a place in medical
history anyway, but his other connections were almost limitless.
There was Joanna Baillie and Croft's father, the eccentric Sir
Herbert (who wrote *Love and Madness* and helped Johnson with
his dictionary). Greatest of all, however, was the doctor's eldest
son, also Thomas, who not only defied the King in espousing the
cause of Queen Caroline but lived to be Lord Chief Justice of
England. Beside all this the old doctor's position as obstetrician
to the royal family for over thirty years fades almost to a modest
status. Perhaps the death of so old a medical colleague made
Jenner realize how he alone, of the loyal group who had cam-
paigned for the first parliamentary grant, had remained un-
honored by the state. Even his election to the Royal Society all
those years back had not been for his work in medicine but for
his study of the cuckoo.

We do not know whether Jenner knew Robert Southey, who
was appointed Poet Laureate in 1813, but it is likely that he did.
The poet, a Gloucestershire man, came to Cheltenham occasionally and in 1815 wrote his long vaccination poem, *A Tale of*

Paraguay. The opening stanzas are an eloquent tribute to Jenner and his work, but since it was not published until 1825, the doctor never saw it (unless he was shown the manuscript).[65] Alone, perhaps, among the poets, Southey had a firsthand memory of smallpox inoculation and relates a strange experience that may have been peculiar to the west of England at the end of the eighteenth century.

I was inoculated at Bath at two years old and most certainly believe that I have a distinct recollection of it as an insulated fact, and the precise place where it was performed. My mother sometimes fancied that my constitution received a permanent injury from the long preparatory lowering regimen upon which I was kept. Before that time she used to say I had always been plump and fat, but afterwards became the lean, lank greyhound-like creature that I have ever since continued. She came to Bath to be with me during the eruption. Except the spots upon the arm, I had only one postule; afraid that this might not be enough, she gave me a single mouthful of meat at dinner, and *before night, above a hundred made their appearance,* with fever enough to frighten her severely. The disease, however, was very favourable.[66]

I cannot find any example, in Jenner's records, of meat being given to increase the extent of the disease. On the contrary, after inoculation—smallpox or cowpox—the physician usually hoped for the mildest effect possible.

Jenner's life in general drifted quietly along with the range of social interests and conversation generally confined to the local scene. Poor Catherine, nevertheless, could not have been other than concerned with the continuing scandals within the circle of her husband's loyalest allies; the explosion that shook society this summer must have strained her toleration to the limit. Nor was the situation helped by the fact that both great families involved were equally committed vaccination patrons. Lady Ann Abdy was the illegitimate daughter of the Marquess of Wellesley. She had married Sir William Abdy when scarcely more than a child in 1806, but when she met Jenner's friend Lord William Bentinck this summer she fell madly in love and an affair ensued. Both families being seasonal residents of Cheltenham the matter was soon common gossip, though actual divorce did not come about until the following year. The debt Jenner owed to the Wellesleys, including Wellington himself, for the vigorous establishment of vaccination in India was more than balanced by the Bentincks' activity in putting through the first parliamentary grant and young Lord William's efforts in Madras. As usual, the unruffled doctor managed to walk the tight rope of the salons very well, apparently offending no one in the bitter acrimony that split society. In fact, both camps continued to support him.

Surprisingly enough, Lord Borington was created Earl of Morley in the 1815 honors list—a rather puzzling gesture of recognition to the vaccination forces. To be sure, he was a Tory—in name anyway—but he had persistently thrown in his lot with the opposition in the upper house on most major issues. His support of Jenner in the face of the known attitude of the Lord Chief Justice and the Lord Chancellor, and his siding with the Regent against the Government in the matter of the household expenses would surely have made him the last person to be honored. What was even more remarkable—he made no secret of his admiration of Canning who was looked upon as a turncoat by the current establishment.[67] When Canning died, in 1827, Borington openly proclaimed himself a Whig, and with the rest of the Cheltenham group helped to put through the Reform Bill in 1832. He never again presented an anti-inoculation bill in the Lords, but the two attempts he made no doubt affected a large number of people—particularly the fashionable doctors. Borington lived to see the practice dropped—not as a result of legislation, but by professional conviction—in its main stronghold, the Smallpox Hospital, in 1822. The Vaccination Act, which made Jenner's discovery the law of the land, was passed July 23, 1840, just four months after Borington's death.

Jenner makes no comment on this elevation of yet another of his friends, and when Catherine rallied in the spring and spent a fairly comfortable month or so he was disinclined to take much notice of the Court circular anyway. He always feared a relapse and seldom stirred far from his house. Undoubtedly the precedent of having meetings of the Literary and Philosophical Society at St. George's Place did give them both a chance to enjoy some social life at home, but even this was halted by a deterioration in her condition during the summer. The worst befell in August when she was attacked by bronchitis, and with her lungs in such a critical state, this was the beginning of the end. She was already so emaciated from years of coughing that her poor frame sank under this new complication. "She was so slender, so attenuated, and so deprived of all vigour of constitution by protracted illness," says Baron, who attended her with her husband, "that she could not have existed except under the most constant care and vigilance. For many years she had lived almost in an artificial climate; and for a considerable time before her last attack she was confined entirely to her room." By this time she fully expected death and seems to have had no fears. After all, she had been an invalid to a greater or lesser degree for the entire twenty-seven years of her marriage. "I visited her at Cheltenham the night before she expired," says Baron, "and when she was in full expectation of the fatal event. The impression made upon my mind by the scene altogether I can never forget. She had long been preparing for her final account and her departure was marked by those accompaniments which generally attend the death of the righteous." She died peacefully on September 14, 1815. She was fifty-four years old.[68]

Jenner's grief was beyond description. He had worshipped the gentle Catherine who was so different from him in every conceivable way. "Up to the hour of her death," said young Fosbroke, "he always carried about with him a withered rose which had been given to him by his partner in life."[69] Baron came over from Gloucester the following day and found him inconsolable. "He grasped my hand with great emotion and said, 'Baron, I am a wretch.' "[70]

He took Catherine to be buried at Berkeley among the long generations of Jenners, and with her burial a great part of Jenner was buried also. He never really recovered from his grief and seems to have been merely waiting for the time when he could join her in the same grave. His immediate reaction was to withdraw completely from public life and seek solitude in his cottage. Even his medical practice was forgotten and for the next two years only the call of his vaccination commitments or some other purely humanitarian work could draw him from his shell. His eagerness to meet the great ones of the earth in the interest of his crusade completely evaporated. The idea of any kind of social activity was more than he could contemplate, and the stream of influential figures who poured into Cheltenham following the peace were allowed to depart again unseen and unapproached.

Later in the autumn Jenner did drag himself back to Cheltenham, where young Fosbroke was covering the practice, to meet some gentlemen who may have turned his mind ever so briefly from his sorrows. They told him how vaccination had reached one of the few spots on earth that had remained untouched: the wild and recently revolted areas of the erstwhile French West Indian colonies. He wrote to Moore some time later:

In my list of patients last autumn at Cheltenham, were several gentlemen of respectability settled as merchants at San Domingo. One of them, a Mr. Windsor, informed me how much it was the wish of Petion to establish a regular vaccine institution there. I promised to furnish him with vaccine materials but was prevented by what befell me at that period. Mr. Windsor took instructions for calling on the National Establishment, but as you say nothing of the matter, I don't imagine you saw anything of him. All the gentlemen whom I have seen from the island speak of Petion in the most exalted terms as one possessed of great intellectual powers, and who employs them for the best of purposes. Now, what shall we do in this matter? I must leave it to your discretion. Mr. Windsor's address was at Messrs. Peel, Turner and Scott, 109, Cheapside: but I fear he has gone.

By the end of this letter, however,—which was written from Berkeley on December 3—the nagging heartache has returned.

You ask me to come to town. The quiet of this place suits my mind much better at present. But I call into action all the reasons I can muster, and I have always company in my house. These privations are very dreadful and make a man wish he had never existed. But wishes of this sort should be banished and give way to patience and resignation.[71]

Although he had his daughter with him, this Christmas—the first without his beloved Catherine—was almost more than Jenner could bear. The wound seemed to grow deeper rather than to heal. In a letter written to Baron, probably in January, he says,

"I know no-one whom I should like to see here better than your-self, and as often as you can find a little leisure, pray come and exercise your pity. I am, of course, most wretched when alone; as every surrounding object then the more forcibly reminds me of my irreparable loss." And this, as far as vaccination research went, was virtually the end of the road. He did stir abroad when his conscience forced him, but his pen was idle until that last surge of activity preceding his death.

∽ X ∽

The Cheltenham Vaccination
Convention and After
1816-1818

There is no knowing how long Jenner would have remained in melancholy seclusion had not his status as magistrate dragged him from the Berkeley cottage back into the world. On January 18 there was a fight between a gang of poachers and a group of Lord Segrave's[1] gamekeepers. Unhappily one of the latter was killed, and for the second time in his life Jenner was involved in a murder trial. It was doubly tragic in that he was probably not in sympathy with the prosecution. The case of Mrs. Reed had at least related to a sordid and evil murderess, but the young men involved in the poaching affray were men of good character and background who had been goaded beyond endurance.

On November 28, 1815, a young farmer named Thomas Till had been killed by a spring-gun secretly planted by one of Lord Ducie's gamekeepers. This, under the law, was a case of willful murder, even though the gun was fired on his lordship's own land, and the countryside was roused to anger. There was a wide breach between the inhabitants and the landowners of the Vale of Berkeley because of the ruthless enforcement of the game laws in the face of the economic depression that followed the peace. The death of Till, therefore, called for a rigorous example to be made of the people responsible. Instead of any prosecution, however, a verdict—"Found killed by a spring-gun"—was brought in by a coroner's jury composed of the landowner's tenants; that, they hoped, was the end of it. Understandably, this grossly improper verdict caused great indignation among the respectable young farmers in the district. Under the leadership of John Allen, a local athlete, they decided upon retribution. On January 18, 1816, the day set aside for National Thanksgiving for the end of the war, they arranged to raid the preserves of some of the local landowners. The lack of murderous intent was shown by the fact that Allen sent the lady of Hill Court, Miss Fust, whose preserves were to be the target of the first raid, a note warning her to confine her keepers to their cottages. At first it seemed a sporting affair. No firearms were used and the keepers were armed only with sticks. During a hand-to-hand struggle, however, someone amongst the raiders fired a gun and other shots followed. It was then that William Ingram, who had been in the Berkeley service for five years, was killed on the spot, and six of his colleagues were wounded. At this point twenty more keepers arrived on the scene and the raiders dispersed. It was not hard to round them up since they were all well known and of good family. Allen surrendered himself freely when the officers came to his house, upon which Colonel Berkeley twice struck him to the ground with his cudgel.[2]

The pompous Baron tells us: "Dr. Jenner as a magistrate was obliged to exert himself on this occasion and he assisted materially in procuring and arranging that chain of evidence by which the guilt was most clearly brought home to the murderers"—a statement that completely misrepresents the doctor's feelings over the affair.

In April, Jenner went to Gloucester for the trial and stayed with Baron. Inevitably all twelve prisoners were sentenced to death, but all were reprieved except Allen and a man named John Penny who was said to have actually fired the fatal shot. Baron concedes that Jenner "was very much affected by the result of it [the trial]. Most of the culprits were young men and sons of respectable farmers; and though he laboured for the punishment of the guilty, he could not but lament the consequences of the tragedy, which carried such lamentation and woe into so many families in his neighbourhood." The ten prisoners who were reprieved passed through Cheltenham two months later on their way from Gloucester Prison to London where they were to be shipped to a penal colony for the rest of their lives. Despite the fact that the Berkeleys ruled Cheltenham, the *Chronicle* relates, "On their way through the town public commiseration was evinced by offering the unfortunate men pecuniary assistance." It was June 27, when the Gloucestershire countryside is as near paradise as the poets can describe, that ten young men in chains were sent to pay for that foolish lighthearted raid in some remote corner of the antipodes until death released them.[3]

Jenner remained in Gloucester with Baron until the execution was over. He wrote to Gardner:

I am still in Gloucester under the roof of my friend Baron, and have been detained here the whole of this tremendous assize. My intention is to quit this place (rendered dreary by the tragic scene this instant about to be acted on the horrid platform) tomorrow and go to Berkeley; but what renders my return home a little uncertain is a bad catarrh accompanied by sore throat and headache. If Monday, then, was the day you fixed on for coming to Berkeley, pray do not put it off; my motive for writing being nothing more than taking off the fear that you might possibly go to Berkeley and be disappointed, for you might feel hurt at being neglected by an old friend. I should like for you to collect the feelings of the country respecting the execution as I must go deeply into the consideration of the case when we meet. They certainly did not go out with the intention to commit murder. But it is somehow expected that the meanest individual in the state is to be acquainted with our penal laws and all their intricacies. But, in my opinion, this is unreasonable, for no general provision is made for engrafting this knowledge on the mind. An outline might be imparted by our clergy, by reading to their congregation four times a year a sketch of these laws; at the same time they might be blended with moral instruction; so that the laws and the evil consequences of breaking them might be committed to memory at the same time. In short, the Village peasant knows no more at present of the laws which are to act as restraints on his vicious inclinations—that is, when they move into the paths of intricacy—than the village doctor does of the animal economy.[4]

While the tragedy of the Berkeley poachers engrossed Jenner's mind, a tragedy of a totally different kind closed one of the most cheerful Cheltenham homes of his acquaintance. When he returned to the town he would no more be able to stroll up the High Street with William Hicks to Belle Vue House after a sitting of the magistrates. For months it would be dark and shuttered until finally new faces and new voices—strange voices— reawakened it. The Hickses never came back again, and the melancholy cause of the tragedy was a perfect textbook example of the blight of smallpox on those it did not kill.

Ann Hicks was William's infant daughter who had been stricken with smallpox the year Jenner came to Cheltenham. It was rarely that infants ever survived the disease in those days, and undoubtedly her parents had been overcautious in her upbringing. Her cousin, Michael, mentioned that the child's health was a family topic, and averred that "Ann would be very well if her mother did not force her to drink asses' milk." The family anxiety can be well understood, because besides being the only child (following an earlier childless marriage on the part of Sir William) she was twice an heiress. In addition to her father's estate she was due to inherit the fortune of her uncle, Thomas Lobb Chute, whose four children had all died childless. Poor Ann can never be said to have recovered from the sorry start she had in life. At maturity she was less than five feet tall, and, as the family chronicler states it "from first to last, from childhood onwards, she was ugly—that is harshly definite; but she was, in fact, a feminine replica of her father, if without the stutter. And her 'Prospects'—her background—dwarfed her hopelessly."[5] She does not seem to have been either cautioned about or protected from fortune hunters, and as soon as she was old enough she was unwisely thrown into the brilliant Cheltenham season of 1815–16. Balls, banquets, hundreds of handsome new faces and temptations made her forget her physical limitations. The inevitable happened. A dashing but impoverished Irishman, heir to a baronetcy, persuaded her to elope with him—and elope she did, to Gretna Green. He was William Lambert Cromie, and his antecedents did not impress the girl's parents at all. The *Chronicle* reported on February 29, 1816:

A great sensation was excited in the town last week by the sudden disappearance of Miss H. daughter of Sir. W. H. and sole presumptive heiress to more than one large fortune. The young lady took the road to Scotland by a circuitous route, accompanied by Mr. Cromie, to who, according to a letter received from her, dated Carlisle, she has been united by the Gretna parson . . . a pursuit was ineffectually instituted for the purpose of bringing back the fair fugitive.

On March 16, the couple were married in a more formal manner according to the rites of the Anglican communion at Marylebone Church in London. Lady Hicks decided that the best way to lessen the public awareness of the scandal would be to arrange for the young couple to be absent from the local scene, thus a long honeymoon on the Continent was arranged. With all the good intentions in the world, the poor mother determined her daughter should be accompanied by a competent maid. This turned out to be the most foolhardy thing she could have done. In due course a letter came from Ann in Paris: she was all alone in her hotel room, her devoted husband having absconded with the competent maid. So the pathetic stunted girl returned to Witcombe Park to live out her life in lonely seclusion. Had vaccination been ready but one year earlier, the daughter of his friend Hicks would certainly have been one of the first Jenner would have inoculated. Ann lived to be ninety, but the tragedy of well-nigh seventy years of regret was far in the future when Jenner returned to a changed Cheltenham in May, 1816. The shutters were permanently up at Belle Vue House, but for him the house in St. George's Place was by far the more desolate of the two. Perhaps the Cheltenham vaccination convention came just in time to force him back into the world of his crusade, before his sorrow isolated him permanently.

In the summer of 1815 a new epidemic of smallpox had swept the country and by the following spring had reached proportions sufficient to make it the worst visitation of the century. The west of England—particularly Gloucester and Tewkesbury—was badly affected, but Cheltenham, as usual, remained untouched. This phenomenon drew attention to the town—the one place in the country where Jenner had undisputed medical control—and its nearly perfect vaccination protection. An invaluable addition to the local corps of doctors specializing in epidemic disease was Sir Arthur Faulkner.[6] He not only had the same views as Jenner as regards social conditions and poverty, but his expertise in the professional field was of even more importance. His knighthood had been earned, not specifically for work in smallpox, but for battling another scourge—the plague. A military doctor, he had followed in the footsteps of Marshall in the Mediterranean theater and had been mainly responsible for eradicating that disease from the island of Malta in 1813. His knowledge of isolation and diagnostic techniques in his field was second to none in the country and certainly unchallenged in his own locality. The alleys and courts of the poorer parts of Cheltenham in high summer were not a great deal different at that time from the narrow streets of Valetta, which was also of similar size. With Jenner inactive, Sir Arthur would most certainly have been the most expert man to cope if an emergency did arise, even though all the doctors must have been very apprehensive until their mentor returned.

Faulkner took a great house in the High Street[7] near the corner of Cambray and quite close to Coley and Christie. Here undoubtedly the three men watched uneasily as smallpox swept the countryside in all directions but stopped like a high tide on the fringes of their own parish. Inevitably, the Vaccine Institute was bound to acknowledge the phenomenon sooner or later, but it was well over six months before it did so. What might well have precipitated the decision was the less than cordial relationship between the institute and the doctors of nearby Gloucester, who seemed inclined to turn to Cheltenham rather than to London. There had been complaints about the serum sent out by the institute to Gloucester Hospital, and some of the surgeons there asked Jenner himself for some usable matter. "After using thirty point sent from town," they complained, "not a single postule was produced." Ironically it was the systematic and continuing opposition to Jenner in London and his exclusion from any controlling power in the institute that forced him to concentrate his work in Cheltenham until that place stood out unmistakably and unspotted in a disease-ridden country; so much so that the institute was eventually grateful for the example Jenner's town gave to illustrate the vaccination case.

Their first gesture was to appoint Dr. Coley official vaccinator of the infant poor at the Cheltenham Dispensary, which was now the main inoculating center for the town. He was granted an annual stipend for the post, while the dispensary itself was formally congratulated for its success in the anti-smallpox campaign. Needless to say, Griffith was delighted with this official, if belated, recognition of the town's role and made sure that it had the widest publicity. He urged people to go to the dispensary.

Attendance is given from 11 to 12 o'clock each Thursday and Friday morning at 11, Winchcombe Street. We feel it a duty to make his [Coley's] appointment thus publicly known with a view of inducing the respectable inhabitants to inform their neighbouring poor.[8]

There were, however, a few people who were not so respectable, and, as in 1809, some attempt was made to counteract the gesture from London with new evidence of vaccination failure in Cheltenham. During the next two months rumors were spread and some gossip stirred up but the effort was scarcely worthwhile. Nor did the opposition have a single respected and well-known doctor in their ranks to face the redoubtable Dr. Jenner. Even Jameson was a power in the dispensary now, and any challenge to it was a challenge to him. In fact, the vaccination pioneers were on the offensive. This time there would be no mere defense in the newspaper correspondence columns: there would be a convention of the Cheltenham doctors to destroy the libels by way of a thorough investigation and destruction of whatever the enemy could produce. The Medical Committee of the dispensary decided to arrange a systematic onslaught on the lies and half-truths that were actually attempting to hinder the progress of vaccination during the worst epidemic of smallpox since the publication of the *Inquiry*. And the defense operated from strength because some of the most distinguished men in England were involved, including no less than four doctors to the royal family. (Faulkner had recently been appointed Physician Extraordinary to the Duke of Sussex.) There was, however, one important problem to be settled: the mourning doctor Jenner must somehow or other be persuaded to join them.

It was almost summer before the informal discussions ended, and the town was preparing for the extended visit of the Duke of Wellington. The duke owed a great deal to Jenner, and might well be persuaded to help the cause of vaccination that had played no mean part in the victories of his armies. As to the convention itself, there was enough material in and around Cheltenham to make an exhaustive study, through case histories, of the effects of nearly twenty years of the practice in order to prove "that nothing had occurred which ought to weaken the public confidence in the utility of vaccination." A meeting was held at Winchcombe Street on May 21 to plan the operation. Newell, Boisragon, Faulkner, Christie, Minster, Wood, Seager, Lucas, and Coley attended, but what was more important, so enthusiastic was the general mood that even the skeptic, Jameson, appeared on the scene to do his share. The inevitable resolution was passed to call in Jenner, his retirement notwithstanding, and the investigation was arranged for May 24. It says a great deal for Jenner's tenacity that even in the desolation of his sorrow he could force himself to take part in the convention of 1816 in the midst of the hectic preparation for the great duke's visit. Probably through the veil of his misery he dimly recognized the opportunity for a decisive blow against smallpox inoculation. If less expert judges than he examined the evidence the loss might be incalculable. With all these great doctors about him he was still the master in his field. So after months of inactivity he came back to medicine, not as a reluctant general practitioner but as the judge of twenty years of vaccination in Cheltenham.

Things had changed little during his absence; if his own idyllic love was gone forever, life still hummed around that street full of memories. Perhaps the lower orders will ever ape their betters and Regency Cheltenham was as easygoing in her social habits among serving wenches as among the great ladies they served. The very day before the vaccination conference opened a correspondent in the local press complained of the shameless lovemaking that took place of an evening in the churchyard right behind Jenner's house. But I doubt if it worried him very much, as he prepared his documents for the morrow's events, to look out through his back window and see the lurking shadows among the graves. It was the birth of summer, and he more than most understood these things.

Since the conference was in no way associated with the local authority and was entirely the responsibility of the dispensary, it is strange that Dr. Charles Parry is nowhere mentioned. He, above all, had worked to establish the organization and was in closer social relationship with vaccination's discoverer than anyone else in the town. Even stranger is the fact that there was no record in the press of his being unable to attend. One can only assume that the critical ill health of his father in Bath deterred him from a commitment. Caleb Parry was sinking under the very disease—angina—into which his researches had made him one of the world authorities. Faulkner, despite his royal status and international recognition, did not preside, since he was manifestly too recent an arrival, but it is surprising that the senior vaccination men, Newell and Boisragon, were also bypassed. As it was, the chairmanship of the proceedings fell to Christie, one of the youngest men present but who had come to the forefront on medical affairs in the town during his six years' residence—particularly since his appointment to the care of the Prince Regent. The others were those who attended the preliminary meeting—all committed vaccination men except Jameson. (Lucas is a completely new name about whom I have been able to obtain no information.)

The proceedings opened with a speech by Christie who dwelt at some length upon the current epidemic and the importance of vaccination in countering it. His mission was to reassure the public and remove any apprehensions they might have about the efficacy of the system. The record of vaccination was, of course, phenomenal when one looked at the ravages smallpox had made in the years before Jenner's discovery. Then, before they "proceeded to examine the patients," he gave some account of the background, begging leave to call the attention of the public to the following facts:

In the spring of 1769, one hundred and seventy people were carried off by the Small Pox in this town, although the population at that time was very small; but in the present year, though the Small Pox has been more epidemic and malignant than at any period since the first introduction of vaccination, yet only ten deaths could be ascertained as having taken place from that cause, among those persons who had not been inoculated for Cow-Pox, while the great mass of the Inhabitants who have been vaccinated by Dr. Jenner and others, *not one has died* and very few have been affected with any appearance of Small Pox.

In a society where compulsory vaccination was unknown, these facts may well seem conclusive; but every device and twist of the record was attempted by the opposition. Fourteen cases of alleged failure were reported to the committee and exhaustively investigated. As with the past examples, this clutch of "failures" was as baseless as ever. Two had never been vaccinated at all, five had been vaccinated *from eleven to fourteen years ago,* while in the case of five more there was light eruption but "was of such short duration, and scabbed so speedily that it hardly deserved the name of Small Pox." There are details and names given in the full report of the proceedings, but we need only take a few interesting examples here. What is outstanding all the way through, however, is the duration of the protected period reported. The three-year span commonly accepted today as the period of immunity was not the expectation in 1816. People apparently expected immunity for from ten to twelve years, and in most cases obtained it. The conference went to great pains to explain even the most harmless eruptions that took place a decade or more after inoculation.

Two of the patients only, whose arms exhibited the regular reticulated cicatrix or scar, Maria Williams and Miss Reeves, had mild Small Pox, of nearly the usual appearance; but the former, when vaccinated by Dr. Jenner ten years ago, was affected with a considerable abscess or carbuncle on the shoulder, attended with fever and inflammation, which most probably disturbed the regular progress of vaccination. Indeed, in the family of Williams the committee were gratified with a striking example of the powerful influence of vaccination, in preserving the constitution from Small Pox; the whole of the family seem remarkably susceptible of Small Pox infection; and the only child who had not been vaccinated, died of confluent Small Pox.[9]

There is a considerable amount of material on this Williams family—a very large one—which would certainly not have been in existence but for vaccination. Their mother was disfigured by the disease of many years before, but her brood was clean. We might conclude their story with a postscript to the death of the unvaccinated child mentioned above.

One boy, Thomas Williams, had not been vaccinated until the day before his brother died when he was taken from his side and vaccinated by Dr. Coley, but not without a caution from that gentleman and Dr. Christie, as to its possibly being too late to preserve the child;— luckily, however, he went through the vaccine regularly and favourably without having an hour's illness or a single postule, though long exposed to the most virulent Small Pox contagion and belonging to a family peculiarly susceptible to that disease.

When all the patients had been examined, the chairman was at great pains to make it apparent that the record spoke for itself. Though he was not arrogant, the one thing he felt he had to point out was that nothing had changed and nothing new had been revealed. Dr. Jenner had not deviated one iota from the truth he had promulgated from the very beginning.

After all the circumstances which have occurred during the present Epidemic, the Committee consider it their duty to remind the Inhabitants of Cheltenham that these facts are only such as have been *repeatedly published before by Dr. Jenner and the National Vaccine Institute,* who have remarked that in the earlier stages of the practice, when the disease was less carefully watched than at present, spurious vesicles, giving no security, more frequently occurred, either from the matter being taken from an imperfect postule or at an improper period; or from its regular progress being interrupted by the co-existence of some eruptive or other complaint in the system, which, with the premature or frequent wounding of a single postule, have been found the most frequent causes of insecurity.

As to the activity of the dispensary alone, Christie had only to point to its absolutely perfect record. "Since the commencement of the present year upwards of four hundred of the poor have been vaccinated gratis, by Mr. Coley and other surgeons, who have all enjoyed a *total* exemption from Small Pox."

The findings of the conference, however, did not satisfy everyone. Some felt that the evidence had shown a strong case for the prosecution of smallpox inoculators under the terms Lord Ellenborough described in the rejection of the Borington bill in 1814. But what stirred up the most gossip in the salons during the early part of June was the rumor that someone was actually inoculating with smallpox in Cheltenham itself. To be sure, Jenner never suggested this but some of his supporters were far more militant in voicing their suspicions. A correspondent in the *Chronicle* for June 17 in commenting on the conference wrote:

My object, however, in now addressing you is not to confirm the confidence of the advocates of vaccine-inoculation or to remove the scruples of the doubtful, both of which have been done by much more able advocates than I am, but to take notice of a practice which I have, to my great surprise, heard has been carried on by at least one of the practitioners of this town, that of inoculating smallpox.

After some detailed comment on the illegality of spreading the disease in this manner, he points out that "Gilbert Gurney, an apothecary, has recently been sentenced to six months for doing so by Mr. Justice Leblanc."[10]

Rumor seems to have pointed to a completely innocent man— a humble follower of Jenner who did a great deal of free work for the poor. Griffith corrected this a few weeks later. "In consequence of an erroneous opinion that Mr. Chadborne, surgeon, was adverse to the cowpock vaccination," he announced, "we are desired to state, as a proof of the contrary, that he always has and still continues to vaccinate the poor gratis."[11] After this the poor man was left in peace, and no one seems to have seriously suggested that the evil operation was taking place in the town. It was undoubtedly the enthusiastic reaction of the Cheltenham people to Jenner's ringing and unswerving act of faith that stirred them to look for "traitors."

Never before had vaccination been so effectively vindicated. To even hold such a convention during the worst epidemic of the new century—while contagion on a mass scale was such a universal possibility—was courageous in the extreme. The conclusion of the assembled doctors was put modestly enough by Christie at the end of their deliberations:

The Committee, therefore, impressed with the great importance of this subject, beg leave to express their undiminished confidence in the general preservative efficacy of vaccination, the extended practice of which they earnestly recommend as the only certain means of putting a stop to the present Epidemic, which, *but for the influence of vaccination,* must have been extremely destructive.

He might have added "in Cheltenham," because all over the kingdom in the vast unvaccinated areas it *was* destructive—particularly in London. Indeed, the unmistakable proof of vaccination's efficacy after eighteen years of practice in the town surprised even the faithful, and Griffith's exultation in the *Chronicle* a week later was much bolder than Christie's summation.

The dangerous and vulgar prejudice which has sometimes evinced itself in this town against vaccination will, we trust, be eradicated by a perusal of the Address from the Medical Committee of the Cheltenham Dispensary.—The facts it displays are indisputable, from the high source of their authority, and the consequences of its publication will, we expect, silence every clamour against the immortal discovery.[12]

The pathetic little murmurs against Jenner in the town scarcely merited the thunder of Griffith's invective.

In London the National Vaccine Institute was relieved and happy to hear of the triumph of the Cheltenham meeting. There was still bitter hostility in the capital and every encouraging note of vindication was clutched at eagerly. Three weeks after the close of the conference the *Chronicle* announced: "We rejoice to learn that the Medical Council of our Dispensary has received the approbation and thanks of the National Vaccine Establishment in London for its meritorious exertions in promoting the progress of vaccination in this town and neighbourhood."[13]

During the bustle and excitement of the conference the streets of the town were crowded with the cosmopolitan hordes brought together by the first peacetime summer season. In fact the whole year was a busy one for the lodging house and hotel keepers. The Duke[14] and Duchess of Orleans were at Riddell's mansion, and perhaps more interesting, Jane Austen spent most of May here. Griffith gives a colorful description of the High Street this summer. "All the fashion of this mighty empire, from time to time assembled, brings . . . all the youthful loveliness and grace of Britain, and where beauty is—there will be admirers."[15] Jane's sister, Cassandra, took lodging in the High Street much later in the season, when prices were higher than in May. Jane did not approve of the three guineas a week rent at all, but she was impressed that "the Duchess of Orleans drinks at my Pump."[16]

But for Jenner all this was irrelevant; his mission was accomplished and the house in St. George's Place held only the still fresh memory of Catherine's death. He had no desire to rejoin the world yet—if he ever would have. Soon after the doctors and the guinea pigs had dispersed, it was announced that the Duke of Wellington, with his poor little pock-marked duchess, would arrive in exactly a fortnight, on July 7. Perhaps, before returning to Berkeley, Jenner might discuss with His Grace vaccination's part in the victory.

The preparations for the visit of the great soldier outshone even the earlier ones for the Prince of Wales, and, indeed, George III, in 1788. Not the least pleasing aspect of the town from the duke's point of view was its relative freedom from smallpox at a time of a national epidemic. It was unfortunate when Jenner, who alone of the local medical men was known to Wellington, finally decided not to remain for his visit. So while his colleagues were getting ready to meet the great conqueror and bask in the glory of the late conference, Jenner crept back to his cottage in Berkeley. Yet ironically, in some respects the ducal visit was really a medical occasion: despite the unprecedented array of notables who flocked to the town, the four royal doctors—Boisragon, Faulkner, Christie, and Newell—were in the forefront of all the important occasions. Not only this, but between affairs they are repeatedly reported in the press as being in the duke's company. He must surely have wondered where Jenner was— but perhaps he understood.

Nevertheless, in quietly bowing out of the scene when the vaccination conference was over, Jenner certainly did his crusade a great disservice. To be sure, on the surface, the appearance of Wellington in the town was primarily a social engagement, and all the scrambling for invitations and priorities in the unprecedented splendor of the public functions represented the usual clamber of the snobs. But the line between social inanities and hardheaded promotion of his cause was not fully understood by the doctor, and when he hid in Berkeley until it was all over a golden opportunity was missed. The star of Wellington was in its ascendancy and would increase in brightness until he became Prime Minister of England. His family's important role in estab-

lishing vaccination throughout the subcontinent of India, plus
the daily reminder of the curse of smallpox represented in his
wife, would surely have drawn him into the closest association
with the pioneer himself during those warm summer days when
they would have been living within a few yards of each other.
He was in Cheltenham to rest, relax, and talk. As it was, he had
to make do with the lesser lights: Boisragon, Newell, and Christie. Perhaps no man in the history of medicine knew as many of
the world's greatest figures as Jenner without using them to his
advantage. This particular occasion was perhaps his most serious
example of opportunity lost through apathy. He was actually on
the scene—there need be no new break from his retirement to
make, no travelling to London—he had but to remain in his
house and receive the ducal attentions that inevitably would
have come. Indeed, in his contempt for social—as opposed to intellectual—snobbery, Jenner made repeated errors in judgment
to his dire cost. Too often he leaned backwards to avoid clutch-
ing at the skirts of the mighty, even when there was no risk of
losing face in a rational, common-sense gesture. But, conversely,
he was much more lavish of his time on humble, and, quite
often, unworthy people. "The vanity of inferior talent he smiled
at," wrote the younger Fosbroke. He apparently felt that the
poor man had more excuse to be limited and was patient to a
degree he would never concede to the lordly fool. "He condescended to men of low estate, who had access to him, in a way
that seemed prohibitory of more valuable objects, and never
failed to tell their own stories with the usual circuitous diffuse-
ness." But he would leave it for his colleagues to talk about vaccination with the Iron Duke, and what a field day they had.

With all the great people pouring into the town the most unlikely types attained celebrity; this historic occasion turned out
to be the high point of quack Riddell's social career. Not only
was his splendid house, Cambray, chosen for the noble couple's
residence, but a future king of France—Louis Philippe—va-
cated it for the purpose! With the final eradication of Napoleon's
threat to his credit, the duke was undoubtedly the most esteemed
man in Europe, and he arrived in town on July 7 amid scenes
of the wildest rejoicing.

Ever the ladies' man, Riddell persuaded the duchess to allow him to be her escort to church on Sunday morning where she was "the observed of all observers."[17] Pushing even further, he asked the duke to commemorate his visit by planting an oak tree in the grounds of his house, recently renamed Wellington Mansion. This His Grace was pleased to do, but it was the duchess whom Riddell arranged to have put the final touch on the ceremony—the watering of the young tree. He was the superb public relations man. An unashamed quack and charlatan, he reigned supreme in Cheltenham for nearly twenty-five years on persuasive speech, charming manners, and magic potions. But lest he be misunderstood by the respectable medical establishment, the duke somewhat balanced the ledger, relative to his patronage of quack Riddell, by expressing great interest in the dispensary and making a donation of ten pounds. Nor did the quack doctor's aggressive cultivation of the ducal pair pass unnoticed. Griffith published the following lines by an unknown bard on August 8:

> I arrived just in time, my dear cos, at the place
> To behold Colonel R. and also His Grace
> But before I have time my doggerel to scan
> No doubt you'll have heard of this wonderful man
> Who scorning the arts and deriding the schools
> Calls physicians all asses, their patients all fools.[18]

But while most of the Cheltenham doctors were celebrating the visit of the duke, a small item appeared in the *Chronicle* buried amongst the welter of social news. It was not noticed by Baron, but it told Jenner that one more remote part of the earth was ripe for vaccination. It was, indeed, the King of Haiti's reply to the letter of James Moore of the previous year. It was printed in French but Griffith had given an English translation:

Palace of San Souci,
5, February, 1816.

The King to James Moore
Director, National Vaccine Inst.

Mr. Prince Sanders presented to me the work, bearing my direction, on the subject of the smallpox; I accepted it with pleasure and I feel

infinite obligation for your generous attention and the great interest
you take in the preservation of the Haitians. . . . My intention is to
give all possible latitude to the happy results of that immortal discovery which I have not hitherto been able to put into practice, on
account of the difficulty I experienced in my application to Jamaica,
St. Thomas and the United States relative to this object. . . .

                                                          Henry.[19]

Moore had sent the king the information at the behest of Jenner, as we have seen, but the letter was not the only message
from tropical lands this year—nor the most important. Another
pioneer came to Cheltenham looking for the doctor in August.
Stamford Raffles—later Sir Stamford—had just returned from
Java where he had been Lieutenant-Governor during the British
occupation.[20] He introduced vaccination into that vast island as
thoroughly as Christie had disseminated it in Ceylon, and arranged a system of establishments to cover all the villages in
the country, with certain parcels of agricultural land set aside
for their maintenance. Each vaccinator was called a Sawah Jennerian, and each European surgeon had a certain number of
Sawahs under his jurisdiction. The system worked splendidly,
and on his arrival in England Raffles was very eager to meet
Jenner to tell him about it. His wife, Sophia Hull, was a Cheltenham woman and a writer of some accomplishment who had possibly known the Jenners in the earlier days.[21]

It was Coley, as the new official vaccinator, who met the governor when he arrived and explained that Jenner was not in town
but that he would get in touch with him and arrange a meeting.
Typically, the doctor was unable to come just then. He wrote
to Coley:

I certainly would pay my respects to him (Raffles) at Cheltenham were
I not at present so entangled with a variety of engagements. It would
doubtlessly be gladly received if a copy of the governor's letter were
sent to the National Vaccine Establishment, which is too complimentary for me to think of sending myself.

By evidence of what follows, Jenner was not the least bit jealous
of Coley's official position as the town's vaccinator. In fact Jenner commends his colleague almost as though he were his employee.

I cannot conclude without thanking you for your laborious exertions during the late epidemic of smallpox in Cheltenham; but how shocking it is to think that the labours of any medical man should be called forth *at the present period* on such an occasion; and in a town where, for a long series of years, I daily offered my services gratuitously to the public.[22]

Instead, Jenner invited Raffles to visit him in Berkeley—which he did. A covey of vaccination people—Lord Rous, Mr. Rose of the Establishment, and Dr. Saunders arrived in Cheltenham the same week as Raffles—looking for Jenner one would assume; but they did not exert themselves to go on to Berkeley. Undoubtedly the glorious weather and the Wellington celebrations were too much of a temptation. So Jenner and Raffles discussed vaccination and natural history on the banks of the Severn where time stood still, far from the bustle and gaiety of the Cheltenham revels.

Undoubtedly Jenner's wealthiest patients, collectively speaking, were the Berkeleys. He served two generations of them loyally, both in his country days and his Cheltenham days. As we have seen, he was not concerned about their private life, and he catered alike to mistress or wife. After seeing the old earl into his grave in 1810, however, Jenner found the family rather more of a problem. The dowager—whom he had attended both as Mary Cole and the Countess of Berkeley—remained good-natured and warmhearted to the end, but Colonel Berkeley—the new *de facto,* if not *de jure,* head of the family—was a great source of worry. He had more or less deserted Berkeley for the fleshpots of Cheltenham in 1809, and his wild life somewhat shocked local society. Nevertheless, he seems to have depended upon the very proper Jenner a great deal both as doctor and—more important —family friend. The two trials in which he was involved—one to fight for his legitimacy and the other involving the poachers (which did more damage to his reputation than any other event of his life)—both demanded the assistance of Jenner in a manner in which the doctor would have preferred to have had no part. Catherine had never concealed her disapproval of the Berkeleys' free and easy morals, and as long as she lived Colonel Berkeley, it seems, never visited St. George's Place. The very year after her death, however, all this changed. He took Chester House almost opposite to Jenner House on a lease, on November 14, 1816. Jenner was in Berkeley at the time, but when he returned to Cheltenham in December, the wicked colonel was comfortably ensconced with his latest and most beautiful young mistress, the eighteen-year-old Maria Foote, an actress he had discovered at the Theatre Royal.[23]

In Regency Cheltenham people accepted rakes, but not brutes. In contrast with Berkeley, among Jenner's landowning circle, the impact of postwar depression led to kindness and relaxation of the game laws: the Duke of Norfolk, for example, who was also Mayor of Gloucester, reduced all his tenants' rents by twenty to twenty-five percent. As for the game laws: on one occasion a man caught snaring game on Sir Michael Hicks's estate at Witcombe was fined ten shillings, and, in actuality, he did not even pay that. With a cold winter in the offing he elected to take the ninety days in Northleach Bridewell instead. Unlike his father, Colonel Berkeley had all the arrogance of great wealth, and it is conceivable that he still smarted under the refusal of the House of Lords to recognize him as his father's successor. After the Duke of Beaufort he was the richest man in Gloucestershire with an income of some £18,000 from his lands alone. By comparison, Lord Sherborne received £10,000. On the other hand, it is interesting to note that Astley Cooper earned £22,000 per annum from his medical practice, and Baillie £10,000.

A man of violent temper, and later secret regrets, Berkeley was not the ideal for the magistrates' bench, and cases that took place during Jenner's absence did not help the colonel's public image. One example is the case of two little boys who were sent to prison for raiding Ballinger's orchard in St. George's Place. When the doctor returned, we find him listed as Magistrate for Cheltenham alone.[24] All other justices serving the area acted for at least two parishes, but Jenner either decided to curtail his participation because of his many domestic problems, or concentrated his effort on the town because a gentler—not to say more just—hand was needed.

As it happened, Jenner's seclusion in Berkeley had not turned out to provide the rest for which he had hoped. If new problems and shocks could help his numb state of sorrow, then he should have been over his ordeal. But when the autumn set in he was as desolate as ever. The first intrusion on his solitude had been the well-meaning Baron, who was stricken by a sudden attack of illness during a visit to Chantry Cottage in October. "I was seized with violent rigours, headache, and all the signs denoting the approach of a severe and acute disease." Stupidly enough his one idea was to get back to Gloucester and go to bed, but Jenner forbade him to move and took him in charge at once. "Luckily for me," wrote the grateful patient, "I was prevented [from going home] and to his determination on this occasion and his subsequent kind and judicious medical treatment, I probably owe my existence." This particular incident is very interesting since it is the only time, of which I am aware, when a patient of Jenner's actually describes in a professional and knowledgeable manner the treatment he received.

The disease turned out to be inflammation about the pharynx, the fauces, and the tonsils. During the whole of it I had many, many opportunities of witnessing the admirable qualities of this truly great man. His assiduities to myself were unceasing. He punctured my throat three different times; and as an ordinary lancet was rather too short for the purpose, devised an ingenious contrivance for obviating this difficulty.[25]

But scarcely had Baron been treated than a call came from farther afield. "While I was at his house an express came to him from Bath, announcing the alarming illness of his friend Dr. Parry. He went off the next morning and returned the same evening, as he was uneasy about me; I having been delirious in the night."

Caleb Parry was very ill indeed. He had been seized with apoplexy, which left him paralyzed for the rest of his life. When Jenner entered the sick room his friend knew him but could only speak with his eyes. "He looked at me earnestly for some time, then grasped my hand and by piteous moans and sighs expressed how strongly he felt his situation." Poor Parry was six years Jenner's junior and had only just published his greatest work: *The Nature Cause and Varieties of the Arterial Pulse.*

Now, at the age of sixty-one his career was finished—though he
did linger on for another six years. Baron in the meantime was
nursed back to health by Jenner and returned to Gloucester
where another doctor was engaged in the parliamentary election
campaign.

Astley Cooper was helping his brother Bransby against Edward Webb. Though Cooper never aspired to a political career
himself, he seems to have been extremely concerned about this
campaign; certainly another voice to support vaccination in
Parliament was much to be desired. Gloucester was a radical
Whig stronghold—even farther to the left than the Berkeley establishment—and Webb was a popular man. The Cooper brothers on the other hand were uncompromisingly Tory, and were
bitterly resented by the mob as being the creatures of an unpopular government. Astley Cooper came to the district at the
beginning of September and was probably in Cheltenham while
old Dr. Saunders and Mr. Rose were there. There were no party
lines in the vaccination school, and if Colonel Berkeley would
tend more toward Webb politically, Lord Borington (now the
Earl of Morley) would naturally encourage Bransby Cooper.
Others among Jenner's clan who supported the Tory candidate
were the Hicks at Witcombe Park, Dr. Newell, and the De la
Bere's of Southam. To be sure they were hopelessly outnumbered by the Whigs—Lord Sherborne, Lord Ducie, Lord Dunalley,[26] and virtually all the Cheltenham doctors added their weight
to the massive wealth of the Berkeleys; but the contest was none
too easy for the heavier battalions even though Cooper was defeated. There was no Member of Parliament for Cheltenham itself as yet, so the contest roused great local interest.

Astley Cooper sadly returned to London, leaving his brother
to fight another day. As a matter of fact, he did and was duly
elected M.P. for Gloucester in 1818. Just after the election a
London friend of Astley Cooper's, Sir John Hayes, who was
Farington's current physician and something of a gossip, had met
the diplomat from Haiti who was in charge of the negotiations
with James Moore relative to the introduction of vaccination
into that country. Hayes apparently had not been impressed.
Farington wrote:

Hayes called and dressed my leg. He told me he had lately dined in company with Prince Saunders, the Black Agent of Christophe, King of Haiti, at Mr. Carpues's, the Surgeon, and from his conversation thought but moderately of him—He appeared to be a vain man,—he has been much in request among persons of High Life, and has been invited to many fashionable parties. Such is the effect of novelty.[27]

Farington's entry—referring to something that had occurred "lately," is dated August 22—and the letter of the Emperor of Haiti was not printed in the Cheltenham Chronicle until the twenty-ninth, so it would appear that Moore was leisurely entertaining the emissary upon his arrival in the capital. Since Carpues was a Catholic he would be a natural host for the gentleman from a former French colony. As a matter of fact the worthy ambassador let the lavish hospitality go to his head. He rashly commissioned artists and sculptors to return to Haiti with him to undertake vast works in the new capital. It turned out that he had no authority from his government for these things, nor was there any money. Poor Rossi, the sculptor, was one of the people thus hoodwinked at a time when he was sorely pressed financially. The vaccination commission, however, was completely genuine, and the necessary serum was eventually sent to the island. But it is easy to understand why the envoy made a poor impression. Jenner makes no further mention of the Haitian embassy after his meeting with the emissaries the previous autumn in Cheltenham.

The final collapse of Caleb Parry, while perhaps not unexpected, had a profound effect upon his son in Cheltenham, who was something in the nature of a foster son to Jenner. The doctor realized the need for a double therapy—concern for the father and consolation for the son. A letter written at this time rather suggests that Jenner felt he could give some kind of comfort by reminding Charles of the wretchedness that existed for most of them (though it might well be that the new blow inflicted by Caleb's stroke was responsible for bursting the floodgates of his own sorrows). After commiserating the young Parry on his grief, Jenner continues:

No bolts and bars will shut afflictions out. It is the lot of man and as familiar to him as the light. Why should it be so, for a certainty, who can tell? . . . Those dear relations with whom I spent so many social hours, where are they? Gone, to an individual, and I (the worst off of the whole) am left forsaken and forlorn. Providence has certainly provided me with many valued friends. It is with relatives alone we feel that unity which allows us unreservedly to exchange thoughts. What misery, in the progress of human life, is in any way to be compared with this. . . . It is the dreadful *for ever*.[28]

This letter, which, I believe, is printed for the first time herein, is the most poignant and desolate cry we have from Jenner during his years of loneliness and grief. It reveals what he undoubtedly felt at the time: the utter and complete hopelessness of his lot. The sight of his friend paralyzed and helpless only showed that another tiny spark of comfort had been taken away from him in the blackness of his despair. But these especially bad periods passed, and Jenner usually returned to his self-imposed tasks at least outwardly resigned and patient. He got a great deal of consolation from writing letters and was always eager to hear news of the great outside world of medicine. While he never returned to London after 1814, many of the greatest London doctors had close ties with Gloucestershire, and undoubtedly when he was in Cheltenham he would meet them still.

The first complete postwar year led to a winter that threatened to be extremely severe. Most of the soldiers and sailors had been demobilized and were without employment—a condition which led to almost open insurrection in the large towns. Even in non-industrial Cheltenham the cold weather must have brought its problems of poverty and hunger, if not of public health. Both Jenner and Faulkner were identified in the common mind as great humanitarians, and their efforts, combined with the work of the dispensary, probably gave the local medical profession, as a whole, greater esteem than that of any English resort in an age of "society" medicine. The poorest clown in Cheltenham could well be attended by one of the royal doctors.

Significantly enough it was a former patient of Jenner's who was indirectly responsible for such substantial poor relief as the town received aside from the regular channels. On Mrs. Entwistle's death the previous year her daughter Harriot, now Mrs. Coutts, preserved her mother's memory by an annual fund for the relief of five hundred families. She was humiliated whenever she came to Cheltenham, however, by the disreputable behavior of her stepfather, who never failed to embarrass her, even though he lived well upon her bounty. Undaunted by resentment in her husband's family, as well as by her stepfather's churlish behavior, Harriot never ceased to strive for social prestige. Poignantly enough she begged Sir Isaac Heard to hunt for some noble Mellon in her ancestry—no doubt hoping that, as Garter King of Arms, he might stretch a point—but all was in vain. He was a chivalrous old gentleman, but he could not betray his trust. In the end her problem was deservedly solved and in the most salutary manner. After the death of old Tom Coutts she married the Duke of St. Albans in 1832, thus adding to the banker's millions a ducal coronet. The little stagestruck girl—who had walked the Cheltenham paths trying to sell tickets to her benefit—became a duchess and outranked all in the land except the royal family itself. A fairy tale indeed. When she died she bequeathed all her vast wealth to the Coutts children even though they had, by and large, treated her very cruelly.

While Jenner was away, a very distinguished doctor and medical scholar settled in Cheltenham soon after the conclusion of the vaccination convention. Dr. William Gibney, physician-in-ordinary to the Duke of Cumberland,[29] arrived with his family to be physician to the Cheltenham Dispensary. His twin interests were similar to Jenner's—vaccination, as opposed to inoculation, and the mineral springs. He believed in the therapeutic value of natural beauty and saw the invalid in a position "where his mind will be gratified by the beauty of the surrounding scenery and his health invigorated by the bracing and stimulating property of the atmosphere." He set up practice in the house on the corner of North Street and High Street where General Lefevre had lodged and soon became an important figure in local society. His researches on the Cheltenham waters ultimately led to the work on the subject that displaced Jameson's book and which was published three years after the latter's death.

At almost the same moment of the Gibneys' settling in, their neighbor in the High Street, Henry Ruff, went bankrupt. News of his failure appeared in the *Chronicle* on June 26. With his commercial eclipse poor Ruff completely fades out of history; his death passed practically unnoticed, though in his day he had dominated the town's literary life, published Jenner, Jameson, and Dibdin, and founded the first newspaper. His bankruptcy perhaps brought home the realities of the postwar economic problems more than anything else in Jenner's immediate circle. The doctor's own financial situation was sound enough, and most of his colleagues were still either rich or quite well-to-do. But Ruff was an old friend and a close neighbor now ruined and penniless.

Despite the efforts of Harriot Coutts, the months ahead looked very bleak. Some of the country girls—undoubtedly attracted by the festivities surrounding the duke's visit—joined the ladies of pleasure by making a living in the traditional manner. On October 24 Griffith's wrote:

By the inflexible conduct of our magistrates the number of unfortunate females who formerly paraded our streets are greatly diminished. Within the last six months the constables, Allen and Cozzens, have apprehended upwards of forty, most of whom were committed to prison or sent to their respective parishes. Sunday night, the above officers proceeded round the town and its precincts and apprehended the following noted characters for keeping disorderly houses: John Wood, Mary Wood, Elizabeth Davis, William Hooper, John Dovey and Sarah Dovey.

Some—or indeed all—of these must have appeared before the magistrate Jenner in the ensuing days and perhaps prompted him to the action that followed. Fortunately, there was now a fair-sized winter community in the town, and the rector, Mr. Jervis, in conjunction with Father Birdsall—with an eye to the Irish peers—called a meeting to organize a relief campaign and deter the local maidens from a return to prostitution. It is interesting to note that despite the fact that the press gives an account of the town clergymen's initiative, the whole business was actually in the hands of the doctors. Colonel Berkeley, Colonel Riddell, Probyn the local M.P., and Sir William Hicks are not even mentioned. Agg and Morhall were Jenner's friends, of course, and the two parsons would be necessary in any kind of charity project in those days. The *Chronicle* reports:

At a meeting of the residents and visitors of Cheltenham held at the
Public Rooms on Tuesday, Dec. 10th, the Rev. Charles Jervis in the
Chair, it was resolved unanimously that a society be formed . . . to
be called *The Society For The Relief of The Deserving Poor* . . . and
that a committee be formed to consist of the following gentlemen:

Dr. Boisragon	Dr. Fowler	Mr. Morhall
Rev. J. A. Birdsall	Dr. Jenner	Dr. Newell
Dr. Christie	Dr. Jameson	Dr. Seager
Dr. Coley	Dr. Lucas	Dr. Wood
Sir Arthur B. Faulkner	Dr. Minster	James Agg, Esq.[30]

A poignant note is introduced here when we read that someone
on the committee suggested that the campaign be started off with
a collection by a group of ladies in the parish church. It was the
kind of gesture that would have appealed to Catherine Jenner,
but as it was, the wives of Newell and Faulkner led the collectors,
and the takings amounted to £400—a sum unsurpassed on any
previous occasion in the town's history. "It was curious that the
collection was made by a number of ladies," observed Goding,
"and perhaps this may account for it."[31] The enormous collection—the present equivalent of £4,800 (approximately $10,000)—
was not spent upon any kind of moral uplift, however; it was solely
devoted to food and fuel.

As the dean of the local medical profession, Jenner was undoubtedly the spirit behind this project. It kept the town relatively well-fed and warm in a terrible winter that saw riots even
in nearby Gloucester. In his first year without Catherine, he had
led the Vaccination Convention and now he led his colleagues in
this winter relief movement despite his heartbreak, or perhaps,
since she was always in his thoughts, because of it. At the end of the
Colonnade, Dr. Newell and Mr. Jervis operated a soup kitchen
where for a penny the hungry might enjoy a steaming bowl of
soup and all the bread they could eat.[32]

Save for his part in the relief campaign there is no record of
Jenner's own Christmas this year, nor do we know of any letters addressed from either Berkeley or Cheltenham before the
middle of February. In January, however, one of his earliest disciples from overseas arrived in Cheltenham after an exile of many
years.

"I have thought that this short account of the state of vaccination in Russia would be acceptable to you," Alexander Crichton had written from St. Petersburg in 1812, in one of the most welcome letters Jenner had ever received. It had dealt with millions of inoculations—not thousands—and no doubt the two men would have dearly welcomed a long session of comparing experiences. Five years later—years of war, bereavement, and social unrest—Crichton appeared on Jenner's doorstep in the suite of the Grand Duke Nicholas of Russia who arrived in Cheltenham on January 17, 1817.[33] It was the most unusual time of the year for royalty to appear and the fact that they occupied most of the Plough Hotel rather than a private villa, which would have to be prepared beforehand, suggests that there was some special reason for the visit. Those members of society who patronized the resort in midwinter did not come for the waters, but for the social activities of their own county circle. It seems highly improbable that the Grand Duke would undertake the long, uncomfortable coach journey through the winter weather to the west of England when all the grandeur of royal entertainment was available to him in London. It would seem, like Governor Raffles before him, he was seeking out the celebrated cowpox doctor. On the other hand, there is no mention in any of the family records that Jenner and Crichton (or indeed, the duke) ever met. It is conceivable that the pomp and panoply of the ducal entourage might have been too much for the doctor to face in his present state of mind; but he had come out of his shell for the Vaccination Conference the previous year, and a meeting with Crichton was surely just as important to his cause. The tremendous esteem with which he was held in Russia through war and peace would make such a journey on the Grand Duke's part quite plausible —particularly if specially urged by Crichton, whose stock at the Imperial Court was scarcely less than Jenner's. Crichton had been with the Emperor for thirteen years and was the main pillar of what must have been the most comprehensive vaccination campaign up to that time. (When he finally returned to England many years later he was knighted for his service to medicine.)

The need to implement the decisions of the relief committee might have kept Jenner busy until Crichton's arrival in the town, which was as free of civil strife during the terrible winter of 1816–17 as it was of smallpox. The arrangements worked very successfully, and the able among the unemployed were given maintenance work on the roads until the warmer months made their normal outdoor occupations possible. Since from the actual meeting on December 10, we have no record at all of Jenner's activities until well into February, it seems likely that he did, indeed, meet Crichton in the cosy warmth of the Plough Hotel, or —shrinking from the ducal formalities—the two men might have chatted in the more intimate atmosphere of St. George's Place. As exemplified in his solitary meeting with Raffles, Jenner did not shrink from welcoming his friends from overseas provided it was in private and away from a crowded social function.

In due course Crichton returned to London, and it is known that Jenner was at his cottage in Berkeley by the middle of February. Despite his desire to be alone in his sorrow he had been forced abroad in the past year through the mandate of law and his sense of duty, but in 1817 he hoped he might be left alone to recover in his own good time. Young Catherine stayed with him when she was not visiting the Kingscotes, but Robert was away at Oxford, so that Jenner spent many hours completely alone. Nevertheless, if the old social life was finished, Jenner— when he was to some extent over his grief—continued his interest in vaccination research. He still kept up both houses in St. George's Place, and Dr. Coley kept him informed of the progress of the anti-inoculation campaign. Young Fosbroke, now twenty years old, assumed the role of junior partner in the Cheltenham practice, while the Berkeley practice remained in the hands of Henry.

Jenner's avoidance of social gatherings continued, and when the new Masonic Temple was opened in Portland Street, he declined to attend. The occasion was almost entirely centered around three of his closest friends: Colonel Berkeley was the guest of honor, Boisragon was installed as Master, and Coley as Senior Warden. Yet perversely, Jenner was miserable away from the old life. "I suppose it will be my fate to summer amongst my oaks and elms (if I summer at all)," he wrote to Moore in the spring.[34] In the meantime, Coley did not let the grass grow under his feet after his national recognition, and it was he rather than Jenner who wrote an account of Governor Raffles's vaccination campaign in Java for the *Medico-Chirurgical Journal* for February 1817.

Inevitably, after the Vaccination Conference, Jenner's continued inactivity once more played into the hands of his enemies. The practice of smallpox inoculation increased and a great deal of the new cowpox vaccine was impure. The result was that smallpox began to spread and with it the attacks on Jenner himself. He wrote to Coley what he should have written to the outside world. From the conference until his "Letter to Dillwyn" at the end of 1818 (which came out in Philadelphia), he published nothing. Yet he seemed to enjoy reminiscing and reminding Coley of the old triumphs in St. George's Place. He was, alas, lecturing to the converted. He wrote:

I have searched in vain for a record respecting the person you name to me who has had smallpox after being vaccinated by me ten years ago. From the date you fix, it probably took place at the time I permitted persons of all descriptions, not only those of the town, but from the districts around, to come to me weekly. The smallpox was as their heels, and this drove them to my house in immense numbers. I was literally mobbed, driven to a corner, and made a prisoner, necessitated to submit to their will. "The man shall do me next." "No, he shan't; he shall do me," was the language I was often obliged to hear and submit to. For many successive inoculating days, the numbers that assembled were, on average, about three hundred. The taking of notes or the observance of anything like order and regularity was out of the question. However, I persevered with patient submission and completely gained the grand point I aimed at: the smallpox was subdued in every direction. Though this was the fortunate result, yet it would be absurd to suppose that out of this vast body all could go through the disease with that correctness which protects them from smallpox infection; in numerous instances, indeed, they did not afford me an opportunity of judging their security by ever returning to show me their arms; and this teasing occurrence not infrequently happened among the common people of Cheltenham, when I vaccinated on a reduced scale. But now, sir, more immediately to the consideration of your communication. Let us admit that the individual in question went through the vaccine in all its stages with the most perfect regularity, and that, at the expiration of ten years she became infected with the smallpox, and had that disease with as much regularity as if she never had been under the influence of vaccination. What then? Is the smallpox itself a perfect and constant guarantee against future infection? Where is the medical man possessed of experience in his profession, and of an enquiring mind, who will not answer this question in the negative? Cheltenham is certainly not exempt from this deviation in a general law of the animal economy, as it exhibits abundant testimony of the contrary; one instance, indeed, is so very remarkable, that it is worthy of being recorded. I allude to that of the lady of Mr. Gwinnett who had had the smallpox five times.[35]

In many respects Jenner was like a pied piper to Cheltenham, and now, more than a century later, he has inherited the same ingratitude. It was his presence that had attracted the great number of distinguished doctors to the town in the postwar years— a movement that continued well after his death—and such medical talents would, in turn, attract a number of wealthy invalids. In other respects, however, the peace radically changed the social scene. As in 1802 people could again go to the Continent, and some very familiar faces were seen no more. Byron never returned, and Mrs. Jordan died at St. Cloud on July 6, 1816. When the Hardwick's daughter Elizabeth married Sir Charles Stuart, British Ambassador to France, the Lord and Lady moved to Paris and took Mary Berry with them. There a large part of the old Cheltenham circle made its home, and Celia Lock with her daughters entertained Mary Berry and members of the Leinster and Ogilvy families for a period of three years' residence on the Continent. Those who still came to Cheltenham undoubtedly brought back all the current news, but it was Angerstein who was the permanent link between these two worlds. He maintained contact with Jenner right up to the period of his death. I do not know whether he ever visited Berkeley, but he was certainly in Cheltenham every summer.

The physical character of the town was also changing with the end of the wars. Building became more sumptuous, and many great families settled as permanent rather than seasonal residents. The Dunalley, Clonbrook, and De Saumerez clans

joined the Suffolks in houses that long bore these family names,
and a vast retinue of artists, intellectuals, and craftsmen joined
the migration of doctors to serve them or seek their patronage.
The painter John James Chalon[36] set up at 35, High Street in
the summer of 1817, apparently feeling, like the younger Engleheart, that it represented a viable change from the overcompeti-
tive London scene. The name that dominates this surge of expansion following the war, however, is Lansdowne, and undoubtedly the man responsible for the interest of this great
family, the erstwhile pillar of smallpox inoculation, was Dr. Jenner. The grace and majesty of the building that went on during
the war was dwarfed by the scope of the Lansdowne development. Great boulevards and terraces, some veritable palaces,
stretched over hundreds of acres. It is interesting that this most
sumptuous area of Cheltenham should be named after the Lansdowne family since, among the nobility who were seasonal residents of the town, the Suffolks, Sherbornes, and Berkeleys in-
vested far more money in property. The value of the Lansdownes
was undoubtedly their prestige and the wealthy crowds they drew
in their train, though there is no record of their presence at all
before the advent of Jenner. As a young man of twenty-five, Sir
Henry Petty, the third Marquess of Lansdowne had been fascinated by the miracle of vaccination, but it was the influence of
Ladies Crewe and Devonshire that changed him into one of the
most dedicated supporters of the movement in general and Jenner in particular. Steadily after the turn of the century, the
Lansdowne clan became entrenched in the social life of the town,
and from their seat at Bowood in the adjoining county of Wiltshire they moved easily back and forth, usually bringing a train
of followers with them. The poet Moore, the greatest of the Lansdowne protégés, was only one of the distinguished company they
brought to Cheltenham, and incidentally, into friendship with
Jenner. And now, with the doctor in a state of defeatist apathy
and would-be retirement, the energetic young peer—he was still
only thirty-seven—was as concerned as ever in the cause. He was
not at all pleased with the irresolute attitude of the National
Vaccine Institution, and as the doctor glumly remarked to Baron:
"The present constitution of the National Vaccine Institution is

bad. The Marquess of Lansdowne and myself had arranged an excellent plan; but the change of the Ministry knocked it on the head, and George Rose and Sir Lucas Pepys concocted the present imperfect scheme."[37] Nothing was done and the institution bumbled along in its inefficient way. Rose was an able enough man but knew nothing about medicine, while Pepys, at the age of seventy-four, certainly allowed jealousy of Jenner to cloud his ailing judgment. Interestingly enough, Pepys, who lived to be eighty-eight, actually came to Cheltenham himself years after Jenner's death, and his wife died there in 1852.

But with the end of the year we move from the world of medical debate to the crueler realm of professional prestige and one great tragedy. The power of the Denman dynasty seemed destined to go on forever, and since the principle actors in the case consisted of one of Jenner's closest friends, Matthew Baillie, and a very old acquaintance and ally, Sir Richard Croft, I feel the story has a place here. In addition, other friends like Astley Cooper and Sir Henry Halford were obliquely concerned. Fortunately old Dr. Denman was already in his grave. Almost alone of Jenner's colleagues, Richard Croft's success went somewhat to his head, and he became arrogant and inflexible even to his royal patients. Possibly his recent inheritance of the baronetcy on the death of his brother also inflated his ego, but he made it clear that he considered himself the sole arbiter in the affairs of the royal family and, understandably, made most of the great doctors his enemies. Almost inevitably, as the leading accoucheur in the kingdom, following the death of his father-in-law, he was appointed to deliver the child of the Princess Charlotte, heir presumptive, and the only child of the regent. At the age of fifty-five Croft was rich, confident, and not without challengers. With Matthew Baillie long established at court, one had the rare example of two brothers-in-law, both physicians-in-ordinary to the Crown, at the same royal bedside, a family pressure force that did not set too well with many of those near to the throne. In this case such doubts were justified. With his haughty, almost brutal, procedures both the princess and her infant died, and Croft blew out his brains.[38]

Given the caliber of the distinguished doctors involved, the tragedy of Princess Charlotte shook the medical establishment and had a dire effect on Matthew Baillie in particular. Even though he was not in charge he had been in attendance and thus was forced to watch the princess's mad fight for life. He confessed that, medical man though he was, the experience had profoundly shocked him. Within weeks of the princess's death a Mr. William Cook published a pamphlet, *An Address to British Females on the Moral Management of Pregnancy and Labour—Suggested by the Death of Her Royal Highness Princess Charlotte Augusta of Wales. With a Vindication of Her Royal Highness's Physicians, Sir Michael Croft, Dr. Baillie and Doctor Sims*. If the intention of this work was to exonerate the three doctors in the public mind, it also, subtly, implied that they were equally responsible.

Baillie himself was a sick man. Ironically, he was now bedeviled by a liver complaint such as had brought so many people to his care during his Cheltenham seasons. Now his presence at the Wells was in the interest of his own health also. He was physically exhausted; one of the hardest working doctors in England, the strain of the royal ordeal had been almost too much. After a period of reflection he decided that he must for the future avoid the long shaking coach journeys to the west country by acquiring a permanent home there. The following year he purchased Duntisbourn House, some twelve miles out of Cheltenham, on the road to Cirencester. It had belonged to Lord Radnor, Sir Henry Mildmay's kinsman, and Baillie had undoubtedly enjoyed its hospitality many times during the early vaccination days. Here he would not only be near Jenner but conveniently placed to visit his friends Hicks at Witcombe Park and Russell at Charlton Kings. Only Baillie and Jenner were left of the original vaccination pioneers of the Hunter days—Parry was paralyzed, Trye was dead, and Clinch in his remote Newfoundland exile. For the remainder of his life Baillie was no longer a seasonal patron of the Cheltenham Wells; he was now at home here, leaving his London practice to seasonal visitations. When he was in the capital, he continued to work at an unhealthy pace, however, which was in some part responsible for his relatively early death. In any event, there is no doubt his migration added a great deal to Jenner's last days. The two had been friends for thirty-eight years when Baillie moved to Duntisbourn House.

By and large, vaccination and its supporters had reached a crisis point by the winter of 1817–18. The smallpox epidemic that had been steadily spreading for the past year both in England and the Continent was sufficiently severe to shake the confidence of many of Jenner's own circle. Despite the wide dissemination of cowpox vaccine the disease was manifestly gaining, and an increasing number of erstwhile believers doubted the good doctor's insistence that it was not vaccination that had failed but the expertise of the vaccinators. To make matters worse, the fathers of the movement were no longer as strong as they had been. Baillie was not the only invalid: Lysons was a very sick man and Farquhar at the age of eighty was rapidly failing.[39] Now in his seventieth year Jenner himself was very tired after nearly a quarter of a century of struggle.

To be sure the parliamentary situation might have been improved somewhat when Astley Cooper's brother took the Gloucester seat from Webb on his second attempt in June of this year,[40] but by this time Jenner was apathetic to political activity and support in the Lower House. Most of his friends in Parliament were peers of the Whig persuasion, and in this particular poll for Gloucester his friend and patient Colonel Berkeley was a third candidate. Either of these two friends would have been of equal value to Jenner in the house despite their bitter antagonism in politics, but there was to be no more legislation related to vaccination in his lifetime. In all probability, when the defeated Berkeley returned to St. George's Place he found his neighbor more preoccupied with the declining health of his old allies than with the advent of new ones in the House of Commons.

Nor were these older comrades the only casualties. It had been a terrible shock when, of all people, that great champion and friend J. E. Griffith died at the age of thirty-four in the spring of 1818. It was the last thing anyone had expected—particularly Jenner. "What could destroy poor Griffith?" he wrote to Worthington on May 2. "It could be fulness in the head. When his successor is established and all the new arrangements are completed, then for a complimentary reply to a certain paper."[41] What was meant by his comment on "a certain paper" is not known but the successor he was concerned about ensured the immediate future. Griffith's younger brother took over with some initial assistance from his mother, and there was no change in policy on vaccination. Nevertheless, Jenner felt some apprehension. J. E. had been more than an editor; he had been an eager, fighting crusader. Add to this the fact that the two men had been personal friends who had even been connected in financial transactions and the gap left becomes all the wider. Nevertheless, the fact that the paper remained in the family was some consolation at a time when Jenner's morale was very low. There were indeed other blows to follow and with Lettsom gone and the virulence of the enemy increasing, the situation was not helped when Sir Thomas Bernard died in the spring. Nor was the local scene untouched, with all the new doctors coming in, and even Charles Parry left Cheltenham to settle in Bath with his ailing parent. He was offered the position of Physician to the Royal Hospital in that city, and, under the circumstances, was wise to take it.

Nor was the disintegration of a good practice the only erosion in his world; familiar *things,* also, were going. The *Chronicle* was not the same, somehow, with his old friend no longer running it, and Jenner did not bother to read it unless there was something special to interest him. "The Cheltenham Chronicle certainly appears here weekly," he told Worthington, "but I seldom see much more of it than its cover. On searching I have found your second and third number, but shall defer my critique until I find the first." In periods of sorrow and apathy newspapers are all too often left on the mat, as it were. But as far as journalistic support was concerned he need not have worried. Young Griffith was a tower of strength and eventually outstripped his late brother as a journalist and scholar. Under him the *Chronicle* was to become a legend for honest reporting, and he also published one of Jenner's last pamphlets. Perhaps an anonymous tribute quoted by young Fosbroke sums up the esteem people eventually had for the new editor:

> After my death, I wish no other herald
> But such an honest chronicler as Griffith.[42]

In the meantime the smallpox continued to spread and at length the tiny community of Berkeley was hit. "We have at last imported the disease into this place," wrote Jenner to Worthington. His nephew Henry, a good enough physician but not overly endowed with common sense, was a great trial to him. On his increasing commitments in Cheltenham and later, in his retirement, he had not been very assiduous in monitoring the younger man's handling of the Berkeley practice. For some years now things had not been running too successfully.

Henry Jenner who, though he has seen nearly half a century fly over his head, has not yet begun to *think,* perched himself in the midst of a poor family pent up in a small cottage. It was the abode of wretchedness, had the addition of pestilence been wanting. He was infected, of course; and his recovery is very doubtful. I am told to-day that he is very full of an eruption, the appearance of which stands about midway between smallpox and chicken-pox.[43]

Hennry Jenner, despite his lack of caution, did not succumb to smallpox, and continued to run his uncle's old practice in a rough and ready style. Jenner was tolerably content in his quiet life as long as his daughter Catherine was with him, but she was called away to her mother's former home early in 1818 to care for one of the Kingscote children, who had been badly burnt in a domestic accident. Her absence left a great gap in her father's life. "You speak to me, my dear doctor, about indulging hope," he wrote to Worthington.

I have almost done with this business and it is very odd that one should continue to grasp at it so long when it is as slippery as a pig's tail. . . . About corporal strength and animal spirits. The corporal is in tolerably good condition and fit for service; but of the latter, if I give any account of it at all, it must be such a miserable one, that I will spare the feelings of a friend and say nothing. . . . Catherine is still on the hills at the ill-fated house of Kingscote, where she officiates as first nurse. I begin to think that the burnt girl will recover.[44]

And recover she did, but the perpetual struggle against the forces of darkness soon buried this small domestic incident. As the years drew out after 1816, his last great vindication was forgotten, and he had to endure the sight of continuing smallpox inoculation and a steady return of mass smallpox deaths. Cruelly enough this situation led to further bitter attacks on Jenner because the disease was manifestly on the increase despite vaccination. In addition, complaints began to come in from all over the world about the *quality* of cowpox vaccine. Without the most rigorous care the serum injected could become unsterile or stale; in this state, when mixed with the bloodstream it could cause harm rather than protection. In vain did the loyal faithful repeat their unswerving contention that vaccination properly conducted was the sure preventive of smallpox. "Dr. Coley alone has vaccinated more than a thousand persons without a case of subsequent failure," observed John Fosbroke.

Even though Jenner still spent too much time in self-imposed solitude, he now began to travel about a little more and was required in the persuance of his desultory vaccination work to maintain steady consultation with young Fosbroke in Cheltenham.[45] Nothing in the way of serious writing had come from his pen since the death of his wife and even his correspondence seems to have petered out. The continual stream of letters from the doctors and celebrities all over the world, which had been so important a part of his life even in the leanest years, simply dried up. For the entire year of 1818, with one exception (save for relatives), his correspondence was restricted to Baron and Worthington. While this may be explained by his increasing personal contacts—there is no record of any letter *ever* having been written to John Fosbroke, for instance—set against his avid and lengthy letter-writing in the past, it is also a measure of his sagging enthusiasm.

The exception we mention was brought about by his own gradual, if belated, awareness of a weakening on the part of many natural allies in their faith in vaccination. And the erosion had started in the hitherto unsullied area overseas—North America, to be precise. Returning to England in the middle of the worst epidemic of smallpox since the introduction of vaccination, a Mr. William Dillwyn, who was staying at Highnam Lodge, Walthamstow, Essex, expressed some doubts as to the effectiveness of the cowpox inoculation to stop it. It was a bad time for Jenner to be vulnerable on the American front, but fortunately he was goaded rather than discouraged by the situation and returned to the fray with something of his old vigor. Not only did he write the doubter a twenty-page letter, but he ransacked the files for supporting evidence on an international scale, which consisted of a copy of the letter from the President of the National Vaccine Establishment to Lord Sidmouth dated July 15, 1814, with a report on the state of vaccination in Sweden on February 10 of that year. In addition he enclosed the two pamphlets Ruff had brought out in Cheltenham in 1806—the Supplement to the *Madrid Gazette* dated October 15, 1806, with Lord Lansdowne's translation, and a copy of *Varieties and Modifications*. The whole impressive dossier was sent off from Berkeley on August 19, 1818. In his letter, Jenner emphasized the international success of his system and pointed out the impressive record in Ireland, where it had been allowed a free hand. With no suggestion of apology or explanation he concluded with the italicized statement, *"My confidence in the efficacy of the vaccine, to guard the constitution from the smallpox is not the least diminished."*[46]

This forceful reaction to Mr. Dillwyn's doubts apparently served its purpose, for when that gentleman returned to America, he passed the letter, with the papers, to the Philadelphia Vaccine Society who published it before the year was out. Dillwyn stirred Jenner from a serious phase of lethargy that could have become complete defeatism. As it was, with this renewed clarion cry from one side of the world to the other, the patient doctor embarked on his crusade once more with a zeal and determination that only ended with his death.

In Cheltenham John Fosbroke was doing his best to keep up the practice and also indulge in vaccination research. Indeed of all Jenner's protégés, after the appearance of Christie's book, he was the only one who made a serious study of vaccination—as opposed to merely administering it. He appears to have had very little money, and his father continued to assist him as best he could for the remainder of his qualifying period. There obviously would not be very lavish remuneration for the young man, still only a trainee, who was trying to deputize for the great Dr. Jenner. Nevertheless, he was respected by the other doctors and his ideas were taken seriously. He was deeply interested in his mentor's theory of a kind of "secondary smallpox"—almost a separate and even milder eruption than cowpox—that occasionally appeared after vaccination and, as a result, made the patient completely immune from smallpox itself. But as was so often the case, this very phenomenon was distorted from a boon to curse by the anti-vaccinationists as soon as they heard about it.

In Philadelphia at the time that Jenner's letter to Dillwyn was published was the irascible pamphleteer, William Cobbett.[47] He had left England the year before under the threat of a number of lawsuits from various public figures. Indeed most of his life had been spent moving from one side of the Atlantic to the other depending upon the degree of pressure he felt as a result of his latest escapade. He had been fined £5,000 at the turn of the century for libel on the distinguished Doctor Benjamin Rush[48]— an experience that may well have colored his opinion of doctors. More important was his violent hatred of vaccination, and the power he exerted over mob opinion. He was a friend of Riddell's "patient," Sir Francis Burdett, who may have informed him of the secondary smallpox theory. As far as Cobbett was concerned, it was an admission from Jenner that it was possible that vaccination did not always immunize from the more serious disease. Crookshank, the anti-vaccination apologist, quotes Cobbett in this context. "Vaccination in 1818 stood in great need of some excuse for failure; hence the ingenious doctrinal fiction of modified smallpox." In a work of his, *Advice to a Young Man,* Cobbett wrote, "Quackery has always a shuffle left. Now that the cowpox has been proved to be no guarantee against smallpox, it makes it milder when it comes. A pretty shuffle indeed, this!" He returned to England a few months later, bringing with him the bones of Thomas Paine, for whom in later years he had assumed a fanatical reverence. But this formidable man was nothing if not consistent, and much as he apparently hated Jenner and the vaccination movement, he hated its headquarters even more. "This place," he wrote, referring to Cheltenham,

appears to be the residence of an assemblage of tax-eaters. These vermin shift about between London, Cheltenham, Bath, Bognor, Brighton, Tunbridge, Ramsgate, Margate, Worthing and other spots in England, while some of them get over to France and Italy. . . . Soon after quitting this resort of the lame and lazy, the gourmandizing and guzzling, the billious and the nervous, we proceed on. . . .[49]

On the other hand he possibly did not realize that during his absence the dispute between the Princess of Wales and the Prince Regent had assumed very formidable proportions and that the Whig peers of Cheltenham included some of her loyalest supporters. Cobbett, too, was a devoted follower of her fortunes and looked upon her as something of a martyr. When the investigation into her life in Italy was launched two years later, he is said to have placed his very able pen at her disposal. It is ironic that Jenner, too, saw eye to eye with the vitriolic hater of vaccination in this particular matter.

But Jenner, as he girded his loins for the last phase of his life's work, could expect no mercy from the enemy. Just as in the early stages of the campaign otherwise intelligent men like Moseley and Birch had professed to believe that cowpox injection would reduce one to a bovine appearance, so the most unrelated phenomena were used to attack at this time when the cause appeared to be weakening. Even Jenner's relatively uninteresting and prosaic routine in administering the town's affairs offered promising possibilities for exploiting the vices of the "cowpoxers." One thing in particular that Cobbett and his like linked with vaccination was, extraordinarily enough, gaslighting. The noxious fumes, which were supposed to pollute men's lungs, were compared to the poisonous matter that Jenner injected into man's bloodstream. As a born-and-bred country man and nature-lover it is probable that the doctor disapproved of this form of illumination, but the facts again conspired to confirm his enemies' views of the latest "delinquency." This new and vastly superior street lighting was introduced into Cheltenham on September 23. "In 1818," wrote the local historian, "some of the influential inhabitants went to Parliament for a Gas Act."[50] But, in fact, the Town Commissioners, including Jenner, were not at all happy about it, and even after the lights were in use they continued to argue hotly. Again Jenner found himself willy-nilly on the wrong side, because the populace was entranced by the system. "On the 19th we were gratified by seeing the whole of the High Street illuminated by this beautiful light, which assumed its usual brilliancy toward midnight, when the atmospheric air had escaped from the main pipes."[51] He seemed fated to have the worst of both worlds. As a commissioner he appeared to oppose the popular will; to the hostile medical hierarchy he was supporting the pollution of the air with poisonous gas fumes. With it all, however, the lights were a good thing and made the town a safer place after dark. At least the anxious Mr. Morhall's task of controlling vandalism was made easier.

Having been brought back into active service, as it were, in the autumn of 1818, Jenner began to plan new strategies for the coming year. Perhaps his awareness of his age made the remaining time seem more precious, and there was still so much to do. Fortunately, with all the disruptions and changes in his society, the solid, dependable John Fosbroke was always awaiting him whenever he went to Cheltenham. Between them they had a great deal of work to accomplish in the days that were left. In going over the records of this time the young man appears to be closer to the role of son than the happy-go-lucky, fox-hunting Robert Jenner, who seems to have spent far more time at Berkeley Castle than with his father.

Fosbroke lived in lodgings in Winchcombe Street about half a mile from Jenner's house. Since from this time on the doctor's literary work depended more and more on the assistance of the younger man, we may assume that most of the writing would have been done at St. George's Place, where Jenner had his fine library and where he is listed as resident in the directories of 1816 and 1820. During his long periods of seclusion at Berkeley, however, he had few visitors. "I am in perfect solitude, and have been so this six weeks," he wrote to Worthington.[52] "Mr. Fitzharding (his son Robert) is grousing in the Highlands and Catherine is in Yorkshire." Nevertheless, Jenner kept himself busy and never spent the hours idly brooding.

In the course of the year he was able to see Phipps move into a brand new cottage—planned, sited, and laid out by the doctor himself. Baron tells the story:

When travelling with him towards Rockhampton, the residence of his nephew, Dr. Davies, he observed, "It was among these shady and tangled lanes that I first got my taste for natural history." A short time afterwards we passed Phipps, his first vaccinated patient. "Oh, there is poor Phipps,"[53] he exclaimed; "I wish you could see him. He has been very unwell lately, and I am afraid he has got tubercles in the lungs. He was recently inoculated for smallpox, I believe for the twentieth time and without effect." . . . at a subsequent visit (October, 1818), I found lying on his table a plan of a cottage. "Oh," said he, "that is for poor Phipps; you remember him: he has a miserable place to live in: I am about to give him another. He has been very ill but is now materially better." This cottage was built, and its little garden laid out and stocked with roses from his own shrubbery under his personal superintendance.[54]

It was but a tiny place—one room up and one down—but it gave poor Phipps a clean, dry shelter in which to live out his remaining days, which were not, alas, to be very long.

But, in the nature of things, occasionally one of Jenner's opponents also passed away. Lord Ellenborough's life came to an inglorious end on December 11. It was perhaps poetic justice that this arrogant vaccination renegade who had ridden roughshod over so many good people in the courts should have been reduced to the most humiliating and helpless state before his death. "He is now very weak both in body and mind," wrote Farington on November 15, "and is lifted into his carriage . . . about four days ago he had a paralytic stroke. . . . The decline of his mental faculties was known to Sir Samuel Romilly."[55] Jenner made no comment at the time of his old enemy's death; after the failure of Lord Borington's 1814 bill, he had spoken bitterly and with more passion than he usually showed: "Why should Lord Ellenborough or any other earthly lord, when the Lord of all has commanded us as it were to get rid of this pestilence, sanction its continuance?" Pride, indeed, goeth before a fall. As a final humiliation, this hitherto all-powerful Lord Chief Justice of England was reported by Lysons to be "in such a state of weakness and mental debility as not, it was thought, to be competent to make an alteration in *His Will*. The consequence will be very serious to his second Son who is married and has a family."

A year younger then Jenner, Ellenborough left a handsome brood of nine children, all of whom had been protected by the doctor's unappreciated remedy, and who outlived him by many years, as did a daughter born out of wedlock. He was not, however, deeply mourned. The enthusiasm with which he had been

received in the Cheltenham salons after the acquittal of Hastings
had long been forgotten. Farington did not feel that his lordship
would leave much of an estate.[56] "He is not supposed to be rich,
he having lived liberally." In fact, he left £240,000.

If the ominous signs of discouragement among vaccination's
English supporters disturbed Jenner's apathy, the departure of so
formidable and powerful an enemy as Ellenborough cannot have
done other than comfort him. In fact the chapter of woes that
the year 1818 represented concluded on an optimistic note. Certainly the letter to Dillwyn marked the end of the post-Cath-
erine slumber, and the aging pioneer returned to his pens and
paper. It was as though the reality of his declining strength had
suddenly made itself apparent. Most of the original zealots were
dead—before it was too late Jenner himself would have to get
back into the battle.

❧ XI ❧

The Last Sally
1819-1823

The renewed tenacity of Jenner, aided by the youth and energy
of John Fosbroke, made the prospects for 1819 far rosier than
they had been for some time, and in the new year he gained a
new neighbor and perhaps ally from the most unexpected quarter, albeit an ally by default. While attending to his many financial and "medical" projects in the capital, the quack Riddell had
acquired interests in various products that today would be called
patent medicines. In the course of the winter, Riddell appears
to have met some opposition from the Royal College of Physicians. He decided that it would be easier to defy them away from
their home ground, and therefore returned to Cheltenham where,
like Jenner but on a lesser scale, he had a respectable following.
He arrived soon after Christmas in a very militant mood, his long
resentment of the medical profession bolstered by the secret
awareness of his irregular status and the humiliation that would
have been his lot had he been a poor man. Happily in his case his
policy could be comfortably based on the confidence bred of a
great wealth. He had no official status that could be taken away,
nor any ideals that could be frustrated. In short, no one could
hurt him except through his vanity, and, indeed, despite his
shameless charlatanism, he had never been submitted to the bitter attacks that were Jenner's lot. But even a wealthy man's
pitcher can go to the well once too often, and so in the new year
of 1819 he found himself, surprisingly enough, on common
ground with Jenner in being criticized by the Royal College.

A rich man in his own right, after operating as a quack for

nearly twenty years in the highest ranks of society, he must have made many thousands of pounds. In the years following Wellington's visit he had spent a great deal of time in London and had acquired a product called James' Powders,[1] which he maintained could cure any kind of fever no matter what the cause. His wealth and influence were too great to have his activities halted, but they were frowned upon by an increasing number of important people, and he came back to Cheltenham in a very angry mood. Perhaps, compared with the haughty doctors of the metropolis, he considered his medical "colleagues" in the town relatively bearable. He came right into the heart of his old territory and took lodgings at 6, St. George's Place, next door to Jenner.[2] It is not certain whether he still owned any property in the street, but he is listed in a contemporary directory as a tenant at Dr. Fowler's house, which had now been divided between several occupants. Apparently his feelings toward Jenner, Fowler, Newell, and company were now friendly, or he would scarcely have chosen to live among them. On January 14 he announced defiantly in the *Chronicle:* "Be it known to the Royal College of Physicians . . . I can subdue any fever known in this country in a few hours." The announcement seems to have been ignored by the college, but some time later, Riddell challenged them again. He had been letting Wellington Mansion for lucrative sums during the past two years but had also built himself a delightful cottage in Cambray. It is hard to understand, therefore, why he took lodgings next door to Jenner fourteen years after he had sold his house there to the doctor, unless he now wished to be identified with the local hierarchy. To be sure, he fancied himself a writer, and he was currently doing "research" on his remedy for typhus. Thus in the evening of his days, Jenner found himself neighbor to his old landlord, each defying the Royal College from St. George's Place. It was a sign of the new mood. With Ellenborough dead and Riddell apparently neutralized the vaccination cause was stirring almost imperceptibly from its lowest fortunes.

Unlike Jenner, Riddell got the best of his confrontations with the Royal College. Whatever the great ones of the earth thought of him privately, they treated him with the greatest respect in public, from the Duke of Wellington downwards. When he had completed his research on typhus he immediately went up to London. It was announced:

At the Mansion House Colonel Riddell of the East Indian Company's service, waited on the Lord Mayor to inform him that he had a sovereign remedy for the typhus fever which seemed prevalent in the metropolis. The Lord Mayor said that he was happy to hear it, and begged the Colonel would not delay so important a communication. Riddell replied, "If I had your authority for its introduction, my Lord Mayor, I am confident that the contagion would soon depart." The Lord Mayor said that he did not himself know much about fever but why did not the Colonel draw the attention of the Medical Faculty to his specific. "The medical faculty! If I cured a whole hospital of patients, the physicians would take no notice."[3]

Which remark aptly weighed up his scorn of the profession. Soon after, Riddell inherited the family estates from his mother and lost all interest in medicine. Years later, when Jenner was in his grave, Riddell's wife returned to Cheltenham and claimed the whole terrace in St. George's Place from Robert Jenner, maintaining that her husband never had any authority to sell, but the claim failed.[4]

With the publication of the letter to Dillwyn—news of which could not have reached England until the new year—Jenner started the last phase of his vaccination pamphleteering that was to continue right up to the time of his death. Despite the fact that the main load of his medical practice in both Berkeley and Cheltenham was borne by his younger partners, he was himself loaded with additional responsibilities by what appeared to be the well-spaced passing of his most active lieutenants. Spring brought the death of one of the most powerful of them all— Sir Walter Farquhar, who passed away on March 21. A wise old man of eighty-two, it was he who urged Jenner to settle in London all those years ago right after the publication of the *Inquiry* and thereby had inspired the doctor's spirited defense of his decision to stay in Cheltenham. A lot of water had passed over the dam since then: Who is to say which of them was right? Perhaps, had he persevered in the London struggle Jenner would have fared better. At the same time, the capital could have been another Berkeley where his ideas might have died on the vine from ridicule and malice.

The capital was still unpredictable, and, indeed, not always logical. Certainly, it must have puzzled Jenner at this late point in his life that despite the two parliamentary grants——tacit admissions of his contribution to medicine—he had not been called upon to vaccinate a single member of the enormous royal family. He, the ultimate authority and discoverer of the system, had always been passed over in favor of a lesser expert. However, in 1819 the great senior figures among the royal physicians, and, in particular, the vaccination pioneers among them—Lettsom and Farquhar, both older men than Jenner—were dead. Should a further opportunity within that highest domestic circle arise, Jenner would be the only safe possibility. The country had been in a very anxious state since the death of Princess Charlotte, lest an heir to the throne should not be forthcoming. None of the royal princes appeared likely to beget children as they advanced in years. Then after some miscarriages the Duchess of Kent was brought to bed and delivered of a daughter on May 24. Perhaps now, as a long overdue honor, the pioneer himself would vaccinate the future Queen of England. But it was not to be Jenner—nor was it Baillie or Ring; the man chosen was the youngest favorite of them all: the twenty-eight-year-old Pettigrew.[5] This then was the end; there were no more royal children, and the Duke of Kent only survived the birth of the Princess Victoria by a few months. But Jenner's friends continued to scale the heights, and in some cases, at least, helped draw attention to the forgotten man in England.

In what might be called an unconscious "embassy" from the Vale of Gloucester to the Roman Campagna, the painter Lawrence wrote in mid-February, 1819, that "he was preparing to go to Rome to paint a picture of the Pope, and one of Cardinal Gonsalvi,"[6] thus drawing into the select company of his sitters the two great Catholic churchmen who had supported Jenner through these difficult recent years. Nor did Lawrence receive any remuneration, and perhaps, during the long sittings this generous man talked of his friend, the doctor, and of how the cowpox battle was still raging in England. Lawrence, more than most great artists, enjoyed painting his friends. Among the vaccination people—in addition to Jenner—Lysons, Farington, Angerstein, and poor John Worgan's first employer, Richard Hart Davis, had sat for him. The portrait of this latter gentleman, incidentally, was judged by the critic, Sir John Beaumont, as the painter's greatest work.

But if these tenuous threads stretching to Philadelphia and Italy in some measure helped to keep up Jenner's morale, he still had a difficult and determined opposition at home. The difference now was that he was eager to fight again. He worked with John Fosbroke on the subject of secondary smallpox, and the young man wrote a paper based on their joint findings, which appeared in the *London Medical Repository* for June, 1819.[7] It was only twenty-two pages, and the author conceded the considerable part that had been contributed by Jenner. It is important as being the beginning of their joint literary activity. In the meantime, Fosbroke senior in his Herefordshire parish was organizing materials for a biography of Jenner based on their friendship of nearly twenty-five years. The wheels were definitely turning again, though the road was still difficult and the way as frought with sorrows as ever.

This same month of June brought another bereavement that bore away yet another very old friend. Samuel Lysons died on the thirtieth after many years of indifferent health. He had been a remarkably energetic man and had never accepted his liver condition as a reason for an easy life. Travel was most irksome to him, yet he moved constantly between Cheltenham, Gloucester, and London. Only in January he had become Antiquary to the Royal Academy, a most responsible position. "Lysons called," wrote Farington on January 16, "having arrived early in the morning in one of the night coaches from Gloucester. He showed me a letter written to him by Howard, the Royal Academy Secretary, informing him officially of his being unanimously elected Antiquary to the Royal Academy. . . ." (As a matter of fact, Farington had been responsible for his appointment.) Six months later he was stricken with a heart attack in Gloucester, and an effort was made to take him to his brother's house at Rodmarton. At Cirencester, however, he collapsed again and had great diffi-

culty in breathing, whereupon he was put to bed at the **Ram Inn**
where the doctor declared that he was in extremis. According to
Farington he did improve somewhat:

But on Monday, twenty-ninth of June he seemed to be somewhat better so as to afford faint hopes, and he, himself, thought he should recover so far as to live some time longer. Between three and four o'clock
in the morning of Tuesday, June 30th, he expressed a desire to rise
and be seated in an armchair, and he walked to it better than could
have been expected. The person attending went to his brother's room
to inform him of Mr. Lysons being up. On returning he was found
reclining against the back of the chair and he was dead.[8]

Lettsom, Griffiths, Farquhar, Bernard, and now Lysons—all
gone within two years. Jenner's world continued to disappear before his eyes, but he persevered in his new initiative. Coley helped
things along at the dispensary when he deserted surgery entirely
to concentrate on his vaccination duties. He rather belatedly obtained his M.D. this year, as Jenner had done twenty-seven years
earlier, deciding that he could only concentrate on the one field.
Perhaps by way of encouraging this imitative step, Jenner himself gave ten guineas to the dispensary this year instead of his
usual subscription of two. The establishment was, indeed, thriving, and in September it was announced that no less than 4,280
patients had been cared for during its six years of operation since
1813.[9] The Secretary, Mr. Morhall, had these figures ready to be
released on September 16, but unhappily he did not live to see
their publication. "At half-past twelve on the 15th September
while he was attempting to mount his horse in the Gloucester
Road" he was thrown violently and sustained fatal injuries.[10] The
animal was described as a "skittish brute" and had thrown him
only a month before, but on that occasion he had escaped with
merely a broken rib. This time, however, his skull was fractured,
and he lost a profuse amount of blood before medical help
reached him. The accident had occurred a short distance from
his house, where he was carried on a chair while Drs. Seager and
Lucas were sent for. They could do little for him. The degree
of respect in which he was held is revealed by the fact that two
doctors to the Crown, Faulkner and Boisragon were then called
in; but all was in vain and the poor man died without regaining

consciousness. Jenner himself was in Berkeley at the time, and
when he returned to Cheltenham his friend had been dead
nearly three weeks. The death of Morhall was in some respects
a more intimate grief to Jenner than that of many of the great
doctors who had supported him. Morhall was the soul of depend-
ability and, in effect, always on the doorstep. Also, in addition
to being Secretary to the Dispensary, he was Secretary to the
Literary and Philosophical Society that the doctor had founded
so hopefully six years before. Nor was that the extent of Morhall's
usefulness. To Jenner he represented, in more mundane fields,
support on the Board of Commissioners, the willing ally in those
plans of a comprehensive sewage system for the town, and the
man who helped to make St. George's Place a comfortable and
livable home for Catherine and the family through the years.
Altogether, an eager, warm, and, most important of all, familiar
figure. For Jenner there would soon be no one left.

So, as summer gave place to autumn, the doctor plodded on his
way, determined to keep up the good fight. He still had no intention of extending his renewed cowpox campaign into the
realm of his social life. Those days, he felt, were past.

In his years of bereavement while young Fosbroke knew him,
Jenner's normal life style, even in Cheltenham, was very different
from the old regime. In Berkeley he had practically no visitors
as his lonely letters reveal; in Cheltenham—aside from Fosbroke—relatively few.

Temperate in his habits, he retired early to his couch, and the breakfast hour found him busied with his coffee at the parlour fire. A scrap
of paper transferred from the toilet and inscribed with the first im-
promptu ideas that his genius may have caught on the wings of the
morning, embraced some new speculation into the laws of nature,
the growth of subterranean seeds, for formation of hyatids into
tumours, analogies between coralline bodies and men; or some reflexion hurried down like a Cretan note, or the fruit of an epigram-
matic vein, incited by some singularity of human character. It may
have happened that the morning shall have brought some curious
stranger from a distant country and the time passes in a domestic pre-
lection upon the rules of vaccine security; or some rural son of
Esculapius may have arrived to discuss a particular case, and in nine

instances out of ten noontide will have found the intelligent idler calmly revelling in the beloved regions of favourite speculation.[11]

Things were not so grand any more—no ducal drawing rooms, no soirees. But the reference to the "stranger from a distant country" suggests that people from abroad still sought Jenner out when they were in the town. These visitors would not be aware of his withdrawal from society, and he might, indeed, have welcomed them since they were from that overseas world to which he owed so much, and were no part of the old life he was trying to forget. All through the wars he had been above politics and owned to no national enemies. He had shared Charles James Fox's appreciation of Napoleon, though not for the same reason. His was the reaction of gratitude, and it is significant that in his audience with the foreign monarchs in 1814 he had made no attempt to meet the restored Bourbons of France. After all, Napoleon had treated him with far greater esteem than his own government. It is of special interest, therefore, to notice, on the list of arrivals for September 2, a stranger from a very distant country indeed, the Island of St. Helena: Dr. O'Meara,[12] who had been dismissed from the Navy the previous year for alleged conspiracy with Bonaparte to effect an escape from the island. He was undoubtedly devoted to the deposed Emperor, and, as his personal physician, had attained closer intimacy than any of the other captors. He also loyally supported the Princess of Wales, an affiliation that would have somewhat compensated in the Cheltenham salons for his association with Napoleon. If he had come to meet Jenner, however, he would have had a month's wait, since the latter did not arrive until October 4.

When he did return to St. George's Place Jenner found himself in the midst of an increasing group of vaccination forces, such as had not been seen since the death of Catherine. Laymen, for the most part, they had been arriving all through the autumn and continued right up to Christmas. Perhaps it was a part of Jenner's last serious effort to push the anti-inoculation campaign while he still had the strength, though it is more likely to have been accidental, since it seems to have started with the inauguration of the Cheltenham Races. Fortunately, the key figures in this event consisted of his neighbors in St. George's Place, the Duke of Gloucester and Colonel Berkeley, together with his relative by marriage, Lord Rous. The latter, who was probably the most respectable and long-standing vaccination ally left, arrived with sundry other Peytons on September 2. His lordship's horse Zenith, a two-year-old, came in second in the first running of the Cheltenham Gold Cup and his Lupus won the Ladies' Plate. Some days later Sir William Inglis (to whom Jenner had poured out his heart by proxy over the De Carro-East India Company business) arrived. Old Lord Fauconberg's daughter Charlotte returned after many years, bringing with her several younger members of the family, and Thomas Farquhar, the new baronet, with his family all arrived in October. The delightful and unrepentant Lady Lucy Foley and her Admiral appeared just before Christmas (he was now a Cheltenham magistrate), and last but not least came the very sorely missed Thomas Lettsom's widow and her children.

With Matthew Baillie now a permanent resident at Duntisbourn House and all the royal doctors on the spot to aid him, Jenner had a formidable medical phalanx of support besides the noble vaccination amateurs. Undoubtedly it was this gathering of the clans, such as had not been seen since the days preceding the Prince of Wales's visit, that prompted Jenner to bring out a new edition of his first Cheltenham vaccination tract, *Varieties and Modifications*. Poor Ruff, the original publisher, was no longer in business, so the job was given to William Roberts, the Gloucester printer who had handled the work for Bransby Cooper's election campaign the year before. It is strange that Griffiths was not employed, but there must have been a good reason because, far from being put out, he did his usual part in stirring up the visitor's enthusiasm. On November 11 he printed a trenchant reminder of the inroads smallpox had made in London during the past month and pointed out what a shocking situation they themselves might be facing "had that beneficial discovery not been generally adopted."

Jenner possibly spent Christmas in Cheltenham this year since he makes no reference to the great pike-headed whale that was washed up on the coast near Berkeley on November 18. It was a unique event in the natural history of the district, and only the phenomenal rise of the tide in the Bristol Channel at that time of the year could have moved the giant beast ashore. The vague accounts of the time describe the creature's length as being up to fifty feet, whereas the whale Jenner had sent to Hunter in 1776 had been a mere sixteen feet. One can only assume that he had not yet returned to Berkeley at the time, since an event of this nature would have drawn him to the spot no matter what his preoccupation. Perhaps he remained in Cheltenham because so many of his old friends were there. Certainly Griffith would have meant him to see the news item he printed in the *Chronicle* on December 23. It was a fitting Christmas greeting after the year of renewed vaccination campaigning. "For the last eight years not a single case of smallpox has occurred in the dominions of the King of Denmark. The whole of the inhabitants have been vaccinated. Herein is one good effect which has resulted from the arbitrary power of the King of Denmark." It provided an encouraging note on which to face the New Year even at the age of seventy.

The new year of 1820 was dominated by old George III's death on January 29. Despite all the vicissitudes of his sixty-year reign, he had been popular among the mass of the people, and many communities all over the country held meetings to mourn his passing. Late in February, Jenner, William Hicks, and Bransby Cooper—who had recently moved to Matson House a few miles out of Cheltenham—announced a meeting to be held at the Shire Hall in Gloucester to "explain their deep feelings of respect" and also to express their faith in the new monarch. This meeting is interesting for the fact that we first see the name of Robert Jenner appearing in the notice of a public function. He had just come down from Exeter College, Oxford, where he had achieved no particular celebrity, yet there he was, listed beside his father among the great ones of the county, in the *Gloucester Journal* of February 28. He appears to have been a somewhat innocuous young man who was happy to leave the family's vaccination fight in the hands of his cousins George and Henry. For him the pleasures of the hunting field took first priority, though he eventually took a commission in the army and lived out his life in relative obscurity. Sadly enough, he is mentioned very little in his father's correspondence, and as he grew older continued to prefer the company of county society. It is possible that when he came down from Oxford he had not yet made up his mind as to his part in the family crusade, and perhaps Jenner arranged to have him on the platform at Shire Hall as a kind of introduction to public life. There was no further gesture of this nature during the doctor's remaining years, however. Robert was something of a lost cause as far as his father's plans were concerned.

One person who entered the new reign with confidence and hope almost amounting to arrogance was young John Fosbroke. The marked concern and trust shown to him by Jenner undoubtedly went to his head, and although he was still two years away from qualifying at Edinburgh, he took himself very seriously as a result of the joint research in which he had been engaged by the master. Despite Jenner's increasing dissociation from general practice there is no evidence to indicate that his unique power of diagnosis had lessened during his later years. Nonetheless, by 1820 his assistant felt capable of challenging some of the older man's judgments. "Being once on a visit to the Rev. Rowland Hill," Fosbroke wrote, "a woman at Wotton-under-Edge in whom he was charitably interested, was so affected, and given up by Dr. Jenner and a surgeon for Pthisis [that] having formed a contrary opinion I recommended a change of place; she went to Weymouth and returned well."[13] But Jenner seems to have been very good-natured about the pretensions of his pupil and was shrewd enough to see the real potential under an overfamiliarity that was merely a manifestation of youth. Significantly enough most of the other established doctors in the town also accepted the young man on an equal footing—a phenomenon that was forcefully illustrated at the time of Jenner's death a few years later when most of the work relative to a memorial and other tasks were left in John Fosbroke's hands. Judging by his own description, he considered himself "in practice at Cheltenham" from the year 1816—or from the age of nineteen.

For the rest, the research combination of age and youth worked very well. There were three areas of study: the continual assembly of evidence of the effectiveness of vaccination, the dangers of smallpox inoculation, and the investigation into artificial eruptions. This latter project consisted in the reexamining of work carried out through the years from as far back as 1794 in the days of Dr. Fewster,[14] long before Fosbroke was born. It was actually a development on the theme of Jenner's first published work, *Emetic Tartar,* and considered the therapeutic value of this substance, in ointment form, as a counter irritation agent. From more recent sources the work of George Jenner and of young Fosbroke himself was investigated. With the pressures of more immediate needs, however, the work did not appear in print for another two years.

Fortunately Jenner's tutelage of his assistant had made a collaboration easier than it might have been. Unlike Baron, Fosbroke's interests were almost identical with his mentor's, and he was not by any means the dull worshipper we find in Baron. If master and pupil argued over many things, they were always within a wall of esteem that surrounded the older man in Fosbroke's subconscious. In an age when for a quarter of a century practically every great man in the country spent at least part of the year in the town, the younger man wrote without equivocation in 1826: "Of those who have added a superior presence to Cheltenham, our late friend, Dr. Jenner stands highest."[15] And if imitation is the surest form of esteem there was no ambiguity in the situation whatsoever. In his adult years—from 1816 to 1823—when the great premises in St. George's Place were empty for the long periods of Jenner's lonely meditation in Berkeley, Fosbroke became more and more indispensable in carrying on the doctor's plans. Inevitably, his interests were oriented toward vaccination, liver complaints, and the mineral waters so that, intellectually speaking, Jenner had made the youth into a fair replica of himself. One interesting task Fosbroke undertook was to test the effect of the waters on the various maladies that passed through this hands, including complaints that would not normally be related to Spa treatment. Again, like Jenner, he found that there was a marked difference in the way various forms of mental sickness were affected. Nor was he sufficiently the blind supporter of the town's reputation to ignore those conditions that the waters would not help. In recommending muriate of lime, he observes, "There are cases of so obstinate constipation of the bowels, the torpid liver, that it might be well to try it. In these, frequently the Cheltenham waters do *not* suffice."[16] Moreover, he depended entirely on his own observations "drawn from the actual application of the waters, *by the author,* to various diseases" (Fosbroke's italics), rather than merely absorbing Jenner's ideas even though the end results were in many cases identical. This precocious young man remains our principal Boswell for the period—at least in Cheltenham—and there was no one at all reporting from Berkeley save for what emanated from Baron on the occasional social call. Fosbroke himself was disinclined to visit Jenner in Berkeley for health reasons. He did attempt one sojourn to the village during the summer of 1820 but apparently did not repeat it. All of which would make their joint researches a rather one-sided effort geographically speaking, with the older man having to do all the travelling whenever he was not actually resident in Cheltenham. Perhaps, in some respects he was a healthier man than either of his young protégés. "When residing with Dr. Jenner in the interval between my studies in London and Edinburgh," wrote Fosbroke,

I suffered much from dyspepsia in the low and damp wooded vale about Berkeley. Going from thence to Bath to make a stay with my learned and ingenious friend, the present Dr. Parry, I lost the dyspepsia; and departing thence to Edinburgh, a bolder atmosphere, recovered entirely. Dr. Parry himself had recovered by a removal from Bath to Cheltenham.[17]

There is no question but what he was convinced of the healthy character of the latter place.

Cheltenham is not, as it has been ignorantly supposed, a dock for un-shipped livers merely; but the active member of the senate, the man of science, of fancy, the commercial man, the speculatist, the lover and the poet form a great proportion of those who compose the morning visitors of its numerous physicians and quaff the spring which the earth here so bountifully affords. After all, however, neither these nor the salubrious rides nor walks, nor its bold Cotswell air have exclusively obtained for Cheltenham pre-eminence over other British watering-places, and stripped Bath of its gaudy day as a place of the like description; but it is the potent charm of its moral as well as of its natural advantages which have helped to prevail.

This of course is all good publicity—chamber of commerce stuff —but Fosbroke does admit, realistically, that there is a place for the voluptuary at the Spa. "In those diseases which spring from illicit Venus, the waters avail much."[18]

At least one "illicit" patient of Jenner was doing very nicely at his St. George's Place menage with the beautiful Miss Foote. Colonel Berkeley continued as her patron and protector for eight years, and she in her turn repaid him with two handsome daughters, with Jenner, one would assume, presiding at the confinements. As a result of her association with the noble family of Berkeley her stage career prospered out of all proportion to her actual acting ability; she was, frankly, more beautiful than talented, and she is said to have amassed some twenty thousand pounds while still in her twenties. Though unkind things were said about her lover at the time of their separation in 1823, in this particular case he seems to have been honest enough according to contemporary standards.

As for Jenner, his melancholy moods seem to have been reserved for Berkeley where he was near Catherine's grave and the solitude that gave him too much time to think. When he was back with his old friends in Cheltenham, he cautiously allowed himself at least a modicum of social intercourse. Here there was company and conversation if he wanted it. He was the arbiter. Undoubtedly the increasing musical activity exemplified in Boisragon's Philharmonic Society and several other groups helped to fill an important element of his life. Baron writes of these days: "I have seen him in his latter years after his renown had filled the world and after the many cures attendant upon vaccination had often weighed heavily upon him, shake them entirely off, he would then take up a humorous strain, and sing one of his own ballads, with all the mirth and gaiety of his youthful days." Unhappily, however, these occasional reversions were the exception rather than the rule. At his age it was almost impossible to really adjust to any new bereavement since they now occurred too frequently. He was never allowed more than a month or two of unrelieved peace, let alone happiness.

Matthew Baillie, who had attended the King on his deathbed, was undoubtedly the most active practicing physician of the old Cheltenham group. Still making his ten thousand a year, he numbered not only the Duke of Gloucester but several other members of the royal family among his patients. The death of Warren Hastings in 1818 in no way lessened His Royal Highness's interest in the town, and with the establishment of the Cheltenham Races the following year, he extended his annual period of residence until early winter. Inevitably Baillie still served a considerable practice in London, but so many of his distinguished patients frequented Cheltenham that his home at Duntisbourn made him readily accessible even when he was ostensibly relaxing. For Jenner, of course, having his old friend nearby was a great boon in these later years. Baron describes seeing Jenner at Baillie's house in the summer of 1820 and remarks that he "never saw him more happy." For the first time—after five years—he seemed to be in some way reconciled to the loss of his beloved Catherine. "He had much recovered from the impression left by the death of Mrs. Jenner and all the recollections of his youth, his intercourse with Mr. Hunter, together with many of the remarkable incidents which were connected with his own life formed animated themes for conversation."[19] From his remarks it would seem as though this was Baron's first visit to the house.

It was cheering to see the great London physician mounted on his little white horse, riding up and down the precipitous banks in the vicinity of his house, or trotting through the green lanes and opening the gates, just after the manner of any Cotswold squire. Nothing could exceed the relish of Baillie for the ease and liberty and leisure of a country life, when he first escaped from the toil and stress of his professional duties in London.

And there were other diversions during this pleasant summer—perhaps the happiest since Catherine's death. In connection with his work with Fosbroke, Jenner's main preoccupation remained the study of artificial eruptions, though he occasionally harked back to earlier work from happier days. Nor was it necessarily work immediately related to smallpox. Just as he had reprinted *Varieties and Modifications* the previous year, he now decided

to reprint another work of 1807—though to be sure it was one
of the least of his efforts, and it is difficult to understand why
he chose it. "Classes of Intellect," which Prince Hoare had published in *The Artist* all those years ago, was issued in pamphlet
form by Griffiths late in the summer. It is possible that it was
printed for distribution to West Country friends as Le Fanu suggests, but it is also likely to have been a charitable gesture extended to Griffiths to help keep his presses running while he
was going through a temporary period of financial embarrassment. On August 15 he wrote to W. Vizard, a prosperous miller
of Dursley, begging him to renew his advertising in the *Chronicle,* an account which had apparently lapsed.[20] Jenner's pamphlet,
a poor little effort of seven pages, differed only from the London
issue in that it bore the new publisher's name, S. V. Griffiths,
Printer, Chronicle Office, Cheltenham. (The advertising account
of Mr. Vizard, incidentally, was resumed the following year.)

All through the summer Queen Caroline's trial had been
heatedly discussed in the salons, and a number of former supporters had discreetly changed sides when her guilt seemed likely
to be proved. Jenner's coterie, however, remained strictly loyal.
Her solicitors-general were Mr. Sergeant Denman, Baillie's
brother-in-law, and Mr. Brougham[21] (later the great Lord
Brougham), a close friend of Sir Arthur Faulkner's. Lord Lansdowne chivalrously supported her to the end as did Hutchinson's
brother—Lord Donoughmore—and Lord Grosvenor. Among the
royal dukes it is significant that while Clarence and York felt
obliged to support their brother, Sussex and Cumberland refused
to vote and the one royalty who lived in Cheltenham, the Duke
of Gloucester, openly supported the Queen—such was the force
of the local current. The whole business of forcing a royal divorce
was eventually dropped when the Prime Minister, Lord Liverpool (a Gloucestershire man) dropped the proceedings in the interest of keeping the peace. Public opinion was increasingly on
the side of the Queen whose outrageous permissiveness was forgotten by a people who were deeply shocked by her humiliation
and suffering.

But Jenner was away from it all when the end of the trial
came. In August he returned to Berkeley and his memories. He

had accomplished a great deal, however, and the groundwork
had been laid for what was to be his last book. Strangely enough
there were a few people who tried to dissuade him from pursuing
this particular field of research, even though it had been based
on a lifetime of observation, and it was the fierce tenacity of
John Fosbroke that finally gave the work to the world. "The
publication of the Essay on Artificial Eruptions," wrote the
young man, "was opposed by eminent friends and urged by
others. In this affair, I believe I gave the casting vote myself,
which decided its appearance."[22]

But the complete solitude that was Jenner's lot at Chantry
Cottage in his lonely periods of retreat was downright dangerous
as he grew more frail and, on one occasion at least, could have
proved fatal. On August 6 on his return to Berkeley he collapsed
in his garden and lay there alone and unconscious for some time
before he was able to crawl into his house. He was eventually
found with his clothes covered in earth and his poor hat lying
on the ground outside. Baron reported:

An express had been sent for me, but I did not reach Berkeley till 2
a.m. He was then asleep and I did not, of course, disturb him. Next
day I had the satisfaction of finding that although the attack had been
threatening, it had not left any permanent trace of its nature. There
was no paralysis, no confusion, no indication of serious mischief having been done to the brain. He was, however, depressed and thought-
ful, as became one who had been saved from great peril. Death and
its consequences formed an interesting part of our conversation, and
his mind on that subject was tranquil and firm. He recurred to the
loss of his dear wife, remembered her patience and resignation.

Nevertheless this narrow escape did not deter him from his
path. The work he had mapped out continued even through his
lowest periods of depression. Nor did he arrange to have anyone
in attendance in case of a further collapse. Perhaps he even
looked forward to death in order to be reunited with Catherine.
In the meantime the fight against smallpox had to continue unabated; and there was at least one friend who was determined
that the fight should be recorded for posterity. Now, when he
was so near the end of his days Jenner had received pathetically
little gratitude for the patient, tireless work he had devoted to

the conquest of disease. Often tactless to the wrong people, he was nevertheless, after so many years of struggle, the soul of tolerance to those so often given preference and honors that should have been his. Even though great sorrows such as the loss of his eldest son and of his devoted Catherine might have strengthened him to withstand continual rebuffs, his last seven years were essentially ones of fairly unrelieved sadness. Consequently the unexpected flash of gratitude[23] or appreciation gave him tremendous pleasure as he grew older.

The first biography of Jenner—in book form as opposed to periodical literature—came from his old friend Thomas Dudley Fosbroke, perhaps one of the most prolific antiquarian writers of his time. This elder Fosbroke was still short of money, but he never gave up hoping for a lucrative best seller. He was a far greater scholar than Dibdin but never managed to produce a *Bibliomania,* or anything approaching its profits. Nevertheless, in his comfortable parish in the Wye Valley at Walford, Herefordshire, he managed to make a living, and bring up his brood of ten children as well as do the thing he enjoyed more than anything else—write.

After vaccination had swept the world and his friend had received the verbal thanks of the allied sovereigns, it occurred to Fosbroke that his long association with Jenner, and the intimate knowledge it represented, would be material for a book. He appears to have pondered the matter for years before the work actually appeared in 1821, and as early as the summer of 1818 he decided to broach the subject to John Nichols,[24] the publisher and editor of the *Gentleman's Magazine.* At the time, he was planning a volume on the history of Berkeley Castle with selected passages from Smythe's *Lives of the Berkeleys.* He knew that Nichols was particularly interested in this manuscript because Fosbroke's last Gloucestershire work had sold extremely well for an expensive folio publication. He therefore decided to incorporate a life of Jenner in the same deal, because it was by no means certain that an essentially antiquarian publisher would also be interested in the life of a modern doctor. His letter is a masterpiece of bluntness:

Walford, Oct. 16, 1818.

. . . In reply to yours I have to observe that about 240 of my *Glouces-tershire* was subscribed for; about twenty sold afterwards (on my account) and that the 50 Large Paper were eagerly subscribed for: by the Principal Nobility and Gentry . . . the next step is to adjoin the History of Berkeley Castle with extracts from Smythe's lives of all that is important in them, in reference to family, general matter, etc., *and a Life of Jenner.* I reckon this a hundred copies saleable.[25]

Nichols was no enthusiast for Jenner, but he was extremely deep into business commitments with the antiquarian and he put the best face possible on the deal. There were other works involved, past and projected: "I shall beg your acceptance of Leo Roy," he wrote back, "in return for the History of Berkeley Castle, and Extracts from Smythe:[26] for the life of your celebrated Dr. Jenner, for which if you can make room in the proposed quantity (56 sheets) by omitting less interesting matter, so much the better."

The work went forward through the winter and spring, but after six months Fosbroke was obliged to ask his publisher for some financial assistance. He was apparently still helping his son John, in Cheltenham, at this time.

Walford, May 9th, 1819.

Dear Sir,

Owing to my having one son going to the hospitals and another to Cambridge, I am induced to solicit an act of kindness i.e. permitting me to draw for the money for the *Gloucester* at two months. . . . With your approbation, I will draw for £13, leaving the odd shillings and future proofs to cover the advertisement, which I wish to be repeated next month.[27]

With all the involvements of other literary transactions with Nichols, it was another year before the Jenner book was ready. Fosbroke the elder is mainly valuable for the details we have about the doctor's very early adult years and also the description of the meetings with the various foreign royalties in 1814, obviously obtained from Jenner himself. The advantage that this author has over all the other biographers of Jenner is that he could verify all his facts with his subject personally. Fosbroke was in correspondence with a young man named Marklove, whom he greatly admired as an artist, and sent him—apparently for his comments—a "profile" of Jenner that was to appear in the book. Marklove, sensibly enough, took the illustration round to the doctor for *his* comments. Poor Jenner was not impressed at all and wrote a postscript to the young man's reply to Fosbroke:

Mr. Marklove has just called to show me a profile which it seems you have some inclination to prefix to your intended work. Pray do not introduce so bad a thing. We can get you a better thing. Will you have some Epigrams to introduce instead of the Ass? I do not feel bold enough to publish the paper on eruptions.

E. Jenner.[28]

The last sentence here, incidentally, suggests that the letter was written before young John Fosbroke had persuaded him to publish his last work—the work on artificial eruptions entitled *Letter to Parry.* Fosbroke took heed of the doctor's advice, and the idea of the profile was dropped. Unfortunately, however, no other portrait was put in its place. Moreover, we might be forgiven for suspecting that a great deal more of the work was dropped also, for in the final result such a tiny fraction of the book was devoted to Jenner that the title scarcely represents the actual contents. It came out early in 1821 with the following impressive title: *The Berkeley Manuscripts: Abstracts and Extracts of Smythe's Lives of the Berkeleys, illustrative of ancient manners and the constitutions, including all the pedigrees in that ancient manuscript. To which are annexed a copious history of the Castle and parish of Berkeley, consisting of matter never before published, and biographical anecdotes of Dr. Jenner, his interviews with the Emperor of Russia, etc.*

Nevertheless, disappointing though the long-promised work may have seemed at the time, it was, indeed, the first book on Jenner to appear with his name on the title page. Also it is definitely a first-hand record, and, together with the work by John Fosbroke that appeared five years later, is the most dependable record we have of the doctor's life. We hear no more of the rejected profile. Possibly Fosbroke hoped that Marklove—whom, he remarked, "draws and paints as well as S. Lysons"—

would offer an alternative portrait. But with all its limitations Fosbroke's work was a labor of love, and it was he, of all Jenner's friends and relations among the clergy, who delivered the doctor's memorial sermon little more than two years later.

In the meantime Jenner, too, was busy writing. At the age of seventy-one he had become a literary man rather than a practicing doctor. He had not taken part in routine medical practice since the Cheltenham Conference, and, encouraged by the zeal of John Fosbroke, he determined to devote the remaining time he had to completing the vindication of his discovery; it was a kind of renewal of youth and strength. The two eternal commitments dominated him as the winter of 1820–21 set in: acceptance of vaccination as the sole destroyer of smallpox and the eradication of variola inoculation; and all that was needed to achieve both these ends was an insistence upon the correct operative procedure. Ever since 1804, when Ruff had printed his "Madrid" pamphlet, Jenner had harped upon the need for the *exact following of the procedure* laid down by him, and ever since 1804 every Tom, Dick, and Harry had operated as he pleased with any serum he could get hold of. Because of his dedication and confidence Jenner had never been moved by the libels and abuse that implied his system was a failure. Over and over again he cited Cheltenham or Ireland as examples of smallpox-free areas where vaccination was correctly performed. And now, as Christmas came and went, he and Fosbroke planned the last foray.

It is interesting that in the evening of his days Jenner worked more and more with the two young doctors whom he had taken under his wing in Cheltenham. Fosbroke and Charles Parry were the sons of his two oldest friends—Parry might easily have been his son, Fosbroke his grandson, and it is possible that he identified with them owing to the loss of his own boy. As we shall see, the last work of Jenner's life was linked to Parry in its title; the work that went out in 1821 was linked to John Fosbroke.

Early in the new year Jenner received a letter from a lady in Devizes, Wiltshire, which particularly irked him since she questioned him at length on aspects of vaccination that he felt were undebatable. She even asked him if he himself was still convinced of its efficacy, assuming, no doubt, that even he must have been shaken by the duration of the 1816–1820 epidemic. It would appear, from the dates involved, that this correspondence initiated the project of 1821.

With Fosbroke he decided to write a *Circular Letter* that would be sent to all the leading vaccination people and centers in the country. His case was that vaccination could only be effective if carried out correctly, and he asked for a reply to the following questions:

1. Whether the vaccine vesicles under contingent circumstances of herpetic or other eruptive states of the skin, go through their course with the same regularity as when the skin is free of diseases of this description?
2. Whether such individuals are more likely to resist the legitimate action of the vaccine lymph?
3. Whether you have met with cases of smallpox, or the varioloid disease, after vaccination?[29]

In addition, he pointed out various other important facts that had appeared in his earlier comments on the problem.

The third of these questions was particularly important to Jenner since time and time again some relatively innocuous eruption after vaccination had been described as smallpox. The existence of a very mild form of the disease, so scoffed at by Cobbett and his friends, was a possibility that the doctor always found interesting. Vaccination, even when imperfectly given, might well soften the severity of the attack; as Fosbroke stated: "Cases have occurred, though without fatal results and, chiefly, mild as to character." It was his curiosity about this phenomenon that impelled Jenner to call a meeting of the Cheltenham doctors to investigate the situation. Fosbroke, our informant, does not mention the date, but it must have been in the period before Christmas 1820, since the findings of this conference would have been considered in drawing up the January questionnaire. Fosbroke further states that "An association was also formed to persevere in rejecting the inoculation of smallpox, and pursuing vaccination to the extermination of it."[30] The thought of Jenner sufficiently recovered from his bereavement to be considering his old dream of a Cheltenham Anti-Inoculation Institute is very interesting, but the evidence does not bear it out. There was never any such establishment and no other contemporary authority mentions it. On the other hand, with the marked renewal of enthusiasm on the part of Jenner at this time, he might well have *discussed* it with the other doctors as an eventual possibility. On a more concrete level, he did initiate this circular letter campaign with a letter in the Cheltenham paper. Like the launching of the *Inquiry* in 1798, this last active foray in the cause of vaccination was also from his fortress in St. George's Place.[31]

The circulation of the letter started in mid-January and seems to have had a slightly different title from time to time. Perhaps the most impressive was the one sent to and issued by the Edinburgh *Medical and Surgical Journal:* "Vaccination: Dr. Jenner's Circular to the Medical Profession, pointing out the causes of those affections which have occasionally followed Vaccinia and Variola. Communicated under the author's authority by John Fosbroke, Esq." The movement itself, however, was inaugurated a little earlier. When Jenner wrote his long detailed answer to the lady from Devizes he sent a copy to Griffiths to be printed in the Cheltenham *Chronicle,* ensuring that the campaign was launched *after* the public had been given the opportunity to read the background. The very next day the first of the circular letters was printed in the *Gloucester Journal.* The two documents appearing almost simultaneously formed a perfect question-and-answer pattern for the people in Gloucestershire, and the "Circular Letter" itself went all over England. The Devizes letter has only now been discovered and is worth printing as an example of Jenner's spirited defense of, and belief in, vaccination when he was an old man of seventy-one. Griffiths's introduction is brief and to the point:

VACCINATION.—The following letter on this interesting subject has been addressed by the celebrated Dr. Jenner to a lady resident near Devizes:—

My dear Madam,—You ask me if I have any reason to doubt the efficacy of Vaccination, as a certain preventive of the infection of small pox. Various, you tell me, are the opinions on this subject; I beg for opposing your declaration; be assured there is but one opinion among Medical men, who have conducted the practice with that attention which it requires, according to the rules I have precisely laid down. This island might have been entirely freed from the pestilence many years ago, if its wisdom in this respect had kept pace with many of the Continental kingdoms, where small-pox has been entirely unknown for many years; and for ages previously to the introduction of the new practices, it had frequently raged with uncontrollable fury. I do not know how its merits can be set in a more intelligible, or convincing point of view, than by giving you the substance of a quotation from a very recent publication on the subject, by Mr. Cross, an eminent surgeon of Norwich, where through the folly and absurdity of the people, the small pox lately committed great havoc. He tells us that 10,000 of this population who had been vaccinated, lived in the midst of a contaminated atmosphere, and the exceptions to complete protection, after perfect vaccination, were so few as to be not worth detailing; on the other hand, out of three thousand who had neglected to be vaccinated, 530 individuals died, and some, who had been inoculated with regular small pox, caught the disease a second time!

What you have heard respecting my opinion of re-vaccinating in seven years, has no foundation in truth. Perfect vaccination is permanent in its influence. It is quite terrible to see the obstinacy of the people, but the basis of it rests with the superior orders; coercion however has never a good effect, but quite the contrary. It is shocking to contrast the conduct of people at home with that of those abroad. Let the country be ever so extensive, ever so populous, where vaccination has been solely and universally propagated, small pox has been wholly got rid of, and never brought back again, even after periods of years have elapsed in most instances. I am sorry to find poor people around you are so infatuated, but does not the fault lie with them? I remain, dear Madam,

Very faithfully yours,
Edward Jenner.

Berkeley, Jan. 11, 1821.[32]

After the launching of the letters Jenner experienced a renewed feeling of depression that solitude so often brought about. Waiting to see what the reaction would be was a great strain on an aging man who had been so frequently disappointed in the past. On a gray January day after he had returned to Berkeley he wrote to Baron, adding after the almost routine plea for a visit:

If you do not come, let me have a line soon—I cannot get my nerves in good order. Certain sounds such as I am frequently exposed to, still irritate them like an electric shock. The blunt sounds such as those issuing from the bells in the tower, two pieces of wood striking each other—indeed *obtuse* sounds of any kind—do not harm me; but the sharp clicking of teacups and saucers, teaspoons, knives and forks on earthen plates, so distract me that I cannot go into society which has not been disciplined and learnt how to administer to my state of distress.[33]

Undoubtedly, his condition was a reaction from the enthusiasm with which he had been imbued when planning the operation with Fosbroke, but once he was alone again his increasing physical frailness discouraged him. He was a doctor and knew he might not live to see these last efforts bear fruit. A month later his melancholy state was little changed. "I have written but seldom lately, my dear doctor," he states to Worthington, "for I have met with very little worth writing about." And so somehow the weeks dragged on into spring.

But that season, always a period of renewed hope, brought some surcease from his defeatism. The campaign gathered force as it went along, and in the middle of this surge of activity every problem seemed, for the moment, to disappear. When the letters started circulating all over the kingdom and being printed far and wide, the King became aware of Dr. Jenner once more (it had been fourteen years since the theater party at Cheltenham). Very belatedly—his life was almost finished—Edward Jenner was appointed Physician Extraordinary to the King on March 16, 1821. It was, however, at least in time for him to have this splendid designation on the title page of his last book. Almost inevitably, his friends, most of them already the recipients of many awards, received much higher honors. Sir Everard Home, already a baronet, became President of the Royal College of Surgeons, and Astley Cooper was made a baronet. Nevertheless, some official recognition had finally come even as the country became aware of the crusader's new offensive.

On March 21 the letter was reprinted for the national audience in the *New Monthly Magazine*[34] to coincide with the London appearance of the "Circular Letter" in the *Medico-Chirurgical*

Review. This widespread and vigorous presentation of the vaccination case had a profound effect on general as well as learned
opinion. In addition to the belated appreciation that came from
the Court of St. James, Jenner had the satisfaction of seeing the
circular published in Berlin and Philadelphia before a year had
passed. Undoubtedly he and Fosbroke were an effective partnership—even though the young man had occasionally to be kept in
check. Perhaps the rash enthusiasm his friend exhibited was a
good balance to the recurring melancholy moods that plagued
Jenner even when things were going well. But it was apparent
now that the trouble was also tangible physical sickness rather
than the pangs of memory alone. In mid-1821, Jenner had a mere
year and a half to live.

He spent the summer in Berkeley rather more content than he
had been for some time, and his physical condition had improved
as a result of advice from Worthington with whom he kept in
correspondence. He was particularly concerned about the resurgence of inoculation with smallpox in Wotton-under-Edge in
defiance, it would seem, of the "Circular Letter." He wrote to
his friend on July 16:

Twenty in that small town already slain by the poisoned arrow of
variola! Is not this too shocking. Can you forbear saying a word or
two to these murderous people? . . . Look back and invoke the same
genious of inspiration that nestled in your heart when you penned
the pathetic appeal to the humanity of Cheltenham. You need not be
in a hurry. I fear the mystery is not finished. These death deeds will
go on as long as some of the faculty in Wotton can get a fee for their
perpetration.[35]

In the same letter he changes to a lighter topic—Worthington's
dog. "We will endeavour to keep your white terrier till you
return. The animal is promising, but, at present, in a rather
shapeless state, which, I understand, is to be modelled into the
beautiful by the hand of Time." Within a fortnight, however, the
old mood had returned. He was lonely, bored, and pessimistic.
"While you have been enjoying luxuries of all descriptions
(among the rest the luxury of woe) I have been a fixture in this
joyless spot, and here I am likely to remain till moved one way
or another." But move he did. It was probably time for further

consultation with Fosbroke anyway, since the basic work on the eruption essay was just about ready. He and Baillie appeared at Baron's house in Gloucester on August 30 probably on the way from Duntisbourn to Cheltenham. The good-natured Baron was delighted to see them and insisted that they stay the night. "Jenner in the interval had sustained a serious illness," he said in his usual confused chronological pattern.

He was in pretty good spirits and his ardour for knowledge unabated. I remember he brought in his pocket some fossils and one of the vertebrae of the back of a horse, to show the nature of the change which takes place in that disease called spring halt. I fondly hoped that from the vigour which they both then exhibited that their lives might have been spared for many years; but before two were over it was my misfortune to see them both laid in their graves.

At Cheltenham in the meantime, Fosbroke was letting things go to his head. He was obviously not consulting his master as he should and seems to have come in for a scolding when Jenner met him. Something had gone wrong with the preparation of the manuscript. In an undated letter Jenner wrote to his nephew in the autumn he says: "I very much want to see you on account of *the book*—the copies (500) are all printed off by a hasty mistake of Fosbroke"; which rather looks as though the manuscript was sent to the printer before it was ready—or before Jenner had a chance to approve it. Then he adds, "But 'tis well the work is not published, for much of it must be new modelled. I am very unhappy about the book and fear that the whole must be cancelled, for a slice of one's purse is as nothing compared to a shaving taken from one's reputation." Internal evidence reveals the probable cause of the trouble. "The title page is inscribed for *Mr. Fosbroke,* and there are a number of manuscript corrections through the text, *which were not all used*" (my italics).[36] The young man had become very bold indeed if he felt that he could ignore the corrections of his master. The incident, however, seems to have had no permanent effect on their friendship. Fosbroke was still looked upon as Jenner's collaborator in the work. "During the progress of these last labours," wrote Baron, "he was assisted by Mr. now Dr. John Fosbroke for whose suc-

cess and well-being he always expressed an anxious concern."
Anxious seems rather a strange word to use here, incidentally;
Fosbroke was well able to take care of himself. A proof copy of
the work was printed in the autumn of this year, by John Nichols,
but it was never actually released for publication; the final, corrected edition was not published until the following year—a
delay that must certainly be laid at Fosbroke's door. In the
meantime Jenner left Cheltenham for Berkeley, visiting his
nephew, at Ebley, on the way. It was here that he sat for his
portrait for Hobday,[37] who was the last of the old masters to
attempt the doctor's likeness. It shows him honestly as an older
man and as having put on a considerable amount of weight. For
what it is worth, Hobday was the only painter to whom Jenner
wrote a poem, unless we include the whimsical lines addressed
to that most modest practitioner, Stephen Jenner.

The King was due in Cheltenham within a few days, and it
may seem strange that Jenner did not wish to see him—particularly after receiving His Majesty's formal recognition six months
before—but the situation vis-à-vis the royal family was a very delicate one in the town at the moment. Queen Caroline, who had
only died on August 7, had been barred from her coronation
mainly through the efforts of Lord Eldon and was considered a
martyr by most of the nation. When Dr. Denman,[38] who had so
tenaciously fought for the Queen's right to be crowned, came to
Cheltenham, presumably to visit his brother-in-law Baillie, there
had been ugly demonstrations against the King and all who
supported him. About the only people who sided against the
Queen were Sir Isaac Heard, automatically because of his office,
and the local parson, Mr. Jervis, who unwisely refused to allow
the bells to be rung in celebration of the distinguished lawyer's
arrival.

The populace, however, met Dr. Denman at Charlton Kings and taking his horses from the carriage dragged him through the town to
his lodgings at No. 5 Crescent, from the balcony of which house he
addressed the people for three quarters of an hour. The mob then
proceeded to the church, and, arming themselves with weapons from
the site of the subsequent Public Offices, burst open the belfry door
and regaled their visitor with a merry peal. On the same evening the

street lights were put out, and afterwards the mob attacked Mr. Jervis's house, broke the windows and did other damage. . . . it was no wonder if public opinion ran high in the town.

Nor was it any wonder that when His Majesty did arrive on September 14 he elected not to stay overnight.[39] He was on his way home from Ireland and looked ill. No doubt a rest would have been very welcome, but he decided to press on, noticing— or perhaps not—the paucity of rank in the group that greeted him. Not a single member of the peerage or any other of the distinguished residents were there except Sir Isaac Heard. The chairman of the reception committee was Rev. Mr. Jervis assisted by a Mr. Marshall, the Master of Ceremonies, and Mr. P. Kelly, "one of the proprietors of the Rooms."[40] The nobility of Jenner's Cheltenham fortress was distinguished by its absence. The Berkeleys, the Ducies, the Suffolks, the Lansdownes, and the rest were nowhere to be seen. Even the Lord of the Manor, Sherborne, dared to stay away. Had Jenner been an opportunist he may well have taken a place in the depleted line that welcomed the King, but being the man he was and bearing in mind the special circumstances of the situation, he too stayed away. After all, he had accepted the unhappy Queen's watch.

In any case the Cheltenham days were over. He was too tired for any further civic duties, and even though he kept his houses and property in the town, he withdrew from the Cheltenham Board of Commissioners in 1821. It was the end of the chapter.

The year 1822 opened with the bleakness inherent in obituary notices and the sickroom bulletins. The departure from Cheltenham became academic when the society that Jenner had helped to create there itself passed away. The young men had taken over completely with just one or two of the older ones patiently waiting out their remaining days. Matthew Baillie was a very sick man, and the sour, disillusioned old Dr. Jameson was bedridden. But the vaccination fight went on; the younger men—Newell, Gibney, Coley, McCabe, Christie, Faulkner, and a score of newcomers—were Jenner's legacy to posterity, and eventually Baron came back to Cheltenham and joined them. There was no case of the captain leaving behind a sinking ship. The sadness was in the change—new faces where the familiar ones had been—not in the collapse of a crusade. But even if Jenner had come to consult with John Fosbroke during the little time he had left, it would be to a place of more memories than friends.

Farington, at the age of seventy-four, died tragically on the last day of the year while leaving Didsbury Church in Cheshire after the evening service. He slipped descending the stairs from his pew in the gallery, and, striking his head on the stone floor, was killed instantly.[41] But much as he must have felt the passing of as old a friend as the diarist, Jenner received an even greater shock some two weeks later. In the middle of January Caleb Parry died. He had been bedridden for the last seven years, and his passing had been expected by most of his friends; but still he was a link with schooldays and youth. "Poor Parry," Jenner wrote to a friend. "I have just returned from Bath, where I went to attend his remains to the silent tomb. The manifestation of regard and affection exhibited by all ranks from Sion Hill to the Abbey, bore unequivocal testimony to his worth and talents." Parry was sixty-seven but Sir Christopher Pegge who died in harness at Oxford the same year was only fifty-seven. On the other hand the two old stalwarts who followed them to the grave this melancholy year—Tom Coutts and Sir Isaac Heard—were eighty-seven and ninety-two, respectively. Soon Jenner would be all alone as far as his own generation was concerned. But he buried his loneliness in work. Not only was his *Letter to Parry* finally finished, but he did a great deal of revision on his *Migration of Birds,* which was eventually published after his death. According to Fosbroke Jenner had a further book in mind on vaccination. On the day "that I advised the publication of his latest discoveries in vaccination which I had arranged for him, he said 'Alas, they will be received like the oracles of Cassandra; the second rising of the sun will not be like the first.' "[42] Nothing ever came of Fosbroke's suggestion, however, and the *Letter to Parry* proved the final work.

All the Cheltenham friends of Jenner's generation were now dead except Creaser and Baillie. The appointment of Physician to the Crown was the last honor that he could ever hope for in his own country where so many of his lesser colleagues had attained wealth and title. He was sick and tired and felt very old.

He had but to bring out his book and his work would be done. At least he had lived long enough to see smallpox inoculation abolished at the Smallpox Hospital in London in 1822—twenty-three years after Dr. Aspinwall closed his Smallpox Hospital in Brookline, Massachusetts.

During his last year, low fever, poor health, and a recurring sense of loneliness confined him to his Berkeley cottage where at least his relatives could occasionally see him. I would rather think that Fosbroke made the necessary journeys back and forth from Cheltenham during this time to make final arrangements for the publication of the book, since there is no record in the local press of Jenner's being in the town after leaving the Board of Commissioners. The work was finally published by Baldwin Cradock of Peternoster Row; the date on the title page is 1822. Despite the years of work that went into it, it only ran to sixty-seven pages, but they were potent and challenging in their implications. (Had he lived longer he may have branched out in totally new directions. I cite in particular Jenner's observation: "I suspect that dysentery in the first instance is an affection of the brain.") The new publication did not cause a great deal of comment in England, but it was, typically, published immediately in America and the Netherlands.

With this final vaccination call sounded, Jenner's work was completed, and his last real interest in life was removed at the end of the summer.

His domestic happiness after the death of Mrs. Jenner was necessarily much impaired. Another bereavement, though of a different kind, which occurred not long before his death rendered his state still more desolate. His only daughter, Catherine, was on the seventh of August, 1822, married to John Yeend Bedford, Esq., of South Bank, Edgebaston, near Birmingham. The day that this event took place, he sent me the following note:—"Pray don't desert this forlorn cottage, but come sometime and chase away my melancholy hours."[43]

He engaged in a great deal of correspondence to temper his loneliness, much of it with his younger relations to whom he always showed a brave front, but his sadness is apparent in letters to others. "I am in solitude here," he wrote to the Misses Worthington on September 15. "Caroline at Bath and Robert lives at the Castle." Even his writing—letters or otherwise—was not always a consolation. Two weeks before his death he wrote to his niece Emily Kingscote on January 10, 1822.

In earlier days, indeed, at any period of my long life, I do not think there was ever a period when I worked harder. It is no bodily exertion, of course, that I allude to; but it is that which is far more oppressive, the toils of the mind. I am harassed and oppressed beyond anything you can have a conception of. In the midst of these embarrassments I have not a soul about me who can afford me assistance, except, indeed, my two good-humoured nieces who copy letters for me and would willingly do more if they could.[44]

It was bitter cold on the morning of January 23, and Jenner walked over to Ham, a tiny settlement near Berkeley, to arrange for fuel to be sent to some poor people of the parish. Afterwards he visited the studio of his nephew Stephen whom he considered his pupil. The young man was singing at his work as the doctor arrived. It was a popular Scottish air. "Jenner heard the notes as he entered the room, and detected an inaccuracy in the tune. 'Oh,' said he, 'you are singing but not in the right way let me tell you: this is the manner in which you ought to do it;' and he than sang a stanza or two."[45] Since it was cold he then went downstairs and brought up a bucket of coal, good-naturedly remarking that his nephew had a servant.

The following day Baron was called from Gloucester and arrived there at about two in the afternoon. Edward Jenner was dying. Baron relates:

I found him in bed lying in a complete state of apoplexy. The right side was paralysed, the pupils of the eyes contracted to a point and unaffected by a strong light; the breathing stertorous with a general insensibility to almost every external expression. Every effort was employed to arouse him from this condition: but the fatal character of the malady became more and more apparent and he expired about three o'clock in the morning.

It was January 25, 1823.

Sir Gilbert Blane attempted to interest the government in a state funeral at Westminster Abbey, and poor Jenner's remains waited—as *he* had always waited—nine days for such a fitting recognition; but it was not to be. The government pointed out that something might be arranged if the family bore the entire cost. This, of course, was a much easier reply than a point-blank refusal. The transportation, the arrangements for a state funeral in London, and interment in the Abbey involved the kind of expenditure that no private family is ever called upon to incur. So Edward Jenner was interred in the vault of Berkeley Church on February 3, beside his beloved Catherine. Perhaps it was better that way, after all.

Aside from his relatives and Colonel Berkeley few people attended the funeral. Creaser, Fosbroke, and Parry, the loyal contingent of "Cheltenham doctors," were, of course, present along with Baron and Thomas Pruen; but the great world went on with scarcely a ripple on the surface that gray February day. As in his life—so in his death—it was the people of Cheltenham, its doctors in particular, who were concerned and insisted that a fitting memorial be raised to him. Undoubtedly as their carriages rumbled through the gas-lit streets during those bleak winter nights, when the day's practice was over, these doctors of Cheltenham fondly thought the same activity was taking place all over the kingdom. As the key figure, Newell was in charge of the operation from his house in St. George's Place—with the tall, deserted facades of Jenner's own dark and empty houses just two doors away. It was convenient enough for those who turned out in the bitter weather: Boisragon, Wood, and Seager were within walking distance, and young John Fosbroke, who certainly had no carriage then, may well have been picked up on his way from Winchcombe Street by Gibney whose High Street house he had to pass. All the others had their carriages to bear them in relative comfort to the rendezvous where plans were made for a meeting on a countrywide scale to raise funds. It was all very optimistic, and Baron confidently suggested that Baillie get in touch with some of the leading doctors in London. "It was specially thought," he said, "that all the leading members of his own profession would have eagerly seized such an opportunity of burying in oblivion every hostile feeling . . . in order that a conspicuous monument might be erected by them to the memory of Jen-

ner." Only nineteen days after the funeral the first formal
meeting was held at the King's Head, in Gloucester. It was considered appropriate that the memorial be sited in the great
cathedral of the doctor's native county. As far as general interest
went, however, it might have been more appropriately placed in
the Cheltenham High Street; it turned out to be almost a purely
local venture. Dr. Newell accepted the Chairmanship and Fosbroke was Hon. Secretary—which meant that he did most of the
work. All the Cheltenham doctors but Jameson subscribed. (The
latter, however, was a very sick man and died himself within the
year.) "The design was", continued Baron,

> that this object should altogether be accomplished by the contribu-
> tions of professional gentlemen in different parts of the Kingdom; and
> under the expectation of a large number of contributions, a small
> sum was fixed upon as the amount to be subscribed. Our calcula-
> tions proved erroneous. We did not find that extensive cooperation
> either among the learned bodies of the profession, or among in-
> dividuals, which we anticipated.

Nor was the rest of Gloucestershire particularly interested. On
February 17, just a few days before the meeting, Sir William
Guise of Elmore—the county M.P.—had urged the government
to vote a contribution toward the cause. It would have been a
splendid announcement for the opening gathering had he succeeded, but aside from polite words the administration offered
nothing. From the House of Lords, however, the Cheltenham
peers Ducie, Berkeley, Sherborne, Lansdowne, and others contributed as generously as the local doctors.

By April 3 the situation looked very poor indeed. On this
date a further meeting was held, and in an ensuing issue of the
Chronicle a report appeared including the contributions to date.
Only two doctors from the City of Gloucester, counting Baron,
had contributed by that time. On the other hand, Jenner would
have been moved could he have seen the list from his fortress of
Cheltenham. They were all there—his friends as well as the newcomers who scarcely knew him: Baillie, Creaser, Murley, Boisragon, Newell, Wood, Gibney, Christie, Coley, Seager, Minster,
etc. Among the younger men was Charles Averill who that year

published his much translated *Operative Surgery*, which was re-printed in Philadelphia by Dr. Bell.

With all the good intentions the money raised in Cheltenham would not, alone, raise a statue to Jenner by any reputable sculptor, and on April 29, Fosbroke wrote anxiously to Nichols at the *Gentleman's Magazine* begging him to print a letter in his next issue.

A very numerous and respectable meeting of medical men and of private individuals of the County of Gloucester (Dr. Newell of Cheltenham in the Chair) was held on the third of April, at the City of Gloucester for the purpose of promoting the erection of a Provincial Monument, by subscription, to the late Dr. Jenner.[46]

After explaining that the apathy so far manifested by the profession might be from a "misapprehension," he pleaded for general support and concluded with the proud statement, "Among those who have already marshalled themselves in the list of subscribers stands the name of Dr. Baillie." Nichols, however, never printed the letter, and it looked as though the memorial would either never materialize or be on a very humble scale. The situation was helped somewhat when the Royal College of Physicians of Edinburgh sent £50, and the same city's Royal College of Surgeons another ten pounds.

We probably see the hand of Newell, Boisragon, and Coley in the idea of a special Masonic service at Gloucester Cathedral some eight months after Jenner's death.[47] These three were prominent masons, and Thomas Fosbroke, whose own son was Hon. Secretary of the memorial fund, undertook to preach a sermon in memory of his old friend. Both the donations received at the service and the revenue from the printed edition of the sermon would go to swell the fund. It was a joint Gloucestershire and Herefordshire enterprise, since the elder Fosbroke had long lived in the latter county, even though he was the father of a Cheltenham doctor. The service was held on August 19. Fosbroke preached his long sermon (it came to twenty pages of type) before the Provincial Grand Lodges of Gloucester and Hereford. It was attended, we are told, by "a very numerous and respectable assemblage of the craft."

But with all these efforts the money was very slow to appear. There would certainly be no chance of a Westmacott, Chantrey, or even Rossi chipping out poor Jenner's image in Gloucester Cathedral. By the end of 1823 the lists of subscribers to the fund that appeared at rare intervals in the Cheltenham and Gloucester papers ceased altogether. One notice did appear in the *Gloucester Journal* soon after the doctor's death that announced the family had placed all the correspondence and papers in the hands of Dr. John Baron who was thereby designated as the writer of Jenner's official biography. In fact, Baron seems to have been the first choice of the family for the organizing of the memorial fund, but he almost immediately withdrew in favor of Newell and young Fosbroke. Perhaps it was just as well, all things considered, since the completion of the biography took him some fifteen years.

Fortunately there was a young sculptor, still in his twenties, who had exhibited at the Royal Academy in 1822, Robert William Sievier,[48] and he agreed to produce a statue at a cost they could afford. And so it was that the doctors of Cheltenham, with the Royal Colleges of Edinburgh, made it possible for Jenner's image to stand in all its dignity in the nave of Gloucester Cathedral. Almost opposite is the sculpture of Charles Brandon Trye by Lord Egremont's protégé, Rossi. Jenner joined his friend in the Gothic splendor of Gloucester on September 25, 1825, where they now stand in perpetual companionship.

APPENDIX

Address to the Inhabitants of Cheltenham, on the Subject of Vaccination

May 24, 1816—Thomas Christie, Chairman

Christie's address was issued as a broadsheet, but I can trace no copy now extant. I did discover, however, what is manifestly the entire text in the *Cheltenham Chronicle* for May 30, 1816. Christie must have arranged for Griffiths to reprint the newspaper report for separate circulation. The description in Hyett and Bazeley's *Bibliographer's Manual of Gloucestershire Literature* (Gloucester, 1896) is as follows:

Address to the Inhabitants of Cheltenham on the subject of Vaccination (signed) Thomas Christie, Chairman, May 24, Griffiths Pr. Cheltenham Chronicle Office s.sh.fol. W.P. The Address is from the Medical Committee of the Cheltenham Dispensary to the effect that nothing has occurred which ought to weaken the public confidence in the utility of vaccination. (vol. 2, p. 54)

The initials W. P., which indicate the ownership of the copy examined by the authors, stand for William Phelps, Esquire, Chestal House, Dursley, Glos.

The version given below is exactly as it appeared in the Home News section of the paper.

Cheltenham Chronicle May 30, 1816
Home News

BIRTHS.—On Sunday last, the Lady of Captain Ricketts, R.N. of a son.—At Woodchester, in this county, Mrs. Hawker, wife of Major General Hawker, of a son.

MARRIED.—Thomas Morris, esq. of Thornbury, in this county, to Ann, youngest daughter of G. Buckle, esq. of Chepstow.

The dangerous and vulgar prejudice which has sometimes

429

evinced itself in this town against Vaccination, will, we trust, be eradicated by a perusal of the Address, from the Medical Committee of the Cheltenham Dispensary, inserted in a subsequent column. The facts it displays are indisputable, from the high source of their authority, and the consequence of its publication will, we expect, silence every clamour against the immortal discovery.

Address to the Inhabitants of Cheltenham, on the Subject of Vaccination

The Medical Committee of the Cheltenham Dispensary having held a Meeting on the 21st of May, to investigate some supposed cases of failure in Vaccination, present: Dr. JAMESON, Dr. BOISRAGON, Dr. NEWELL, Sir A. B. FAULKNER, Dr. CHRISTIE, Mr. MINSTER, Mr. WOOD, Mr. SEAGER, Mr. FOWLER, Mr. LUCAS, and Mr. COLEY, and the meeting having been adjourned to the 24th, when they had the assistance of Dr. JENNER, proceeded to examine the Patients, and to enquire into all the facts connected with this subject; and after mature consideration are unanimously of the opinion, that nothing has occurred in the present Epidemic which ought to weaken the public confidence in the general utility of Vaccination, as the safest preservative against Small Pox; and, with a view to remove any false apprehensions on this subject, beg leave to call the attention of the public to the following facts:—

In the Spring of 1769, one hundred and seventy people were carried off by Small Pox, in this town, although the population was at that time comparatively very small; but in the present year though the Small Pox has been more epidemic and malignant than at any period since the first introduction of Vaccination, yet only ten deaths can be ascertained as having taken place from that cause, amongst those persons who had not been inoculated for Cow Pox, while of the great mass of the Inhabitants who have been vaccinated by Dr. Jenner and others, not one has died, and very few have been affected with any appearance of Small Pox.

Of fourteen cases reported as failures to the Committee, it ap-

peared on enquiry, that two, Charles Newman, and Martha Greville, had never been inoculated at all; and that five other Patients who have had the regular Small Pox, in a severe though
not fatal form, had certainly been inoculated for Cow Pox, at
the distant period of eleven, twelve, and fourteen years, when
Vaccination was less understood than at present; but in all five,
it appeared from the marks in their arms, that the disease had
been irregular in its progress, and in three of the name of
Hawkins, this had been notified to the Friends of the Patients
by Mr. Jukes, of Stourport, the inoculator, who urged them,
without success, to submit to a second operation, as stated by the
Patients, and confirmed by Mr. Jukes, who had been written to
on the subject. In proof of the irregularity of this first inoculation, it ought also to be mentioned, that the Mother, Mrs.
Hawkins, who was likewise subjected to it by Mr. Jukes, at the
same time with her children, was, on the first of them being
taken ill with Small Pox, again vaccinated by Mr. Coley, passed
through the Cow Pox regularly, and has, in consequence resisted
the contagion of Small Pox, although constantly exposed to it in
nursing her three children.

In five other Patients examined by the Committee, there was
a slight eruption which might probably have been produced by
the contagion of Small Pox, in the way that nurses who have
passed through that disease, are often affected; but it was of such
short duration, and scabbed so speedily, that it hardly deserved
the name of Small Pox.

Two of the Patients only, whose arms exhibited the regular
reticulated cicatrix or scar, Maria Williams and Miss Reeves,
had mild Small Pox, of nearly the usual appearance; but the
former, when vaccinated by Dr. Jenner, ten years ago, was
affected with a considerable abscess or carbuncle on the shoulder,
attended with fever and inflammation, which most probably disturbed the regular progress of Vaccination. Indeed, in the family
of Williams, the Committee were gratified with a striking
example of the powerful influence of Vaccination, in preserving
the constitution from Small Pox; the whole of this family seem
remarkably susceptible of Small Pox infection; and the only
child who had not been vaccinated, died of confluent Small Pox,

a short time ago, while the mother, who is much marked with that disease, which she had severely when young, was, from nursing the infant, affected with smart fever, which confined her to bed 2 days, and was succeeded by a second eruption of Small Pox Pustules. The children of the family who had been previously vaccinated, were either altogether preserved, or had it only in the mild form above mentioned. One boy, Thomas Williams, had not been vaccinated till the day before his brother died, when he was taken from his side and vaccinated by Mr. Coley, but not without a caution from that gentleman and Dr. Christie, as to its being possibly too late to preserve the child;—luckily, however, he went through the Vaccine regularly and favorably, without having had an hour's illness or a single pustule, though long exposed to the most virulent Small Pox contagion, and belonging to a family peculiarly susceptible of that disease.

After this candid exposition of all the circumstances which have occurred during the present Epidemic, the Committee consider it their duty to remind the Inhabitants of Cheltenham that these facts are only such as have been repeatedly published before by Dr. Jenner, and the National Vaccine Institution, who have remarked, that in the earlier stages of the practice, when the disease was less carefully watched than at present, spurious vesicles, giving no security, more frequently occurred, either from the matter being taken from an imperfect pustule, or at an improper period; or from its regular progress being interrupted by the co-existence of some eruptive or other complaint in the system, which, with the premature or frequent wounding of a single pustule, have been found the most frequent causes of insecurity.

It has also been admitted, that in some rare instances the disposition to Small Pox is so great, that even the perfect vesicle will not give an absolute security, but that Small Pox or an anomalous eruption, proceeding from that contagion, will occasionally occur in vaccinated Patients, in the same way as the disease has been known to occur, in a great variety of well-attested cases, a second time after inoculated or even natural Small Pox.

The Committee, therefore, impressed with the great importance of this subject, beg leave to express their undiminished confidence in the general preservative efficacy of Vaccination, the extended practice of which they earnestly recommend as the only certain means of putting a stop to the present Epidemic, which but for the influence of Vaccination, must have been extremely destructive.

Since the commencement of the present year, upwards of four hundred of the poor have been vaccinated gratis, by Mr. Coley, and other Surgeons, who have all enjoyed a total exemption from Small Pox; and as Inoculation for Cow Pox continues to be practiced at the Dispensary, and at the house of Mr. Coley, who is appointed Vaccinator for this District by the National Institution, it is earnestly entreated that such Inhabitants of Cheltenham as have not yet been Vaccinated, may lose no time in applying for that purpose, in order that they may be secured against the ravages of Small Pox, which is perhaps the most destructive and most loathsome malady to which mankind is subject.

Published by Order of the Committee.

THOMAS CHRISTIE, M.D.

May 24, 1816   Chairman.

NOTES

Abbreviations

AA   *Mrs. Jordan and Her Family. The hitherto unpublished correspondence of Mrs. Jordan and the Duke of Clarence,* ed. A. Aspinall, (London, 1951).

B&C   *Bath & Cheltenham Gazette,* 1812–1823.

BGS   *Transactions of the Bristol & Gloucestershire Archeological Society,* 1877 to date.

BL   John Baron, *Life of Edward Jenner, Physician Extraordinary to His Majesty George IV, etc.,* 2 vols. (London, 1827–1838).

BP   *The Berry Papers. Being the correspondence hitherto unpublished of Mary and Agnes Berry (1763–1852)* (London, 1914).

CC   *Cheltenham Chronicle,* 1809–1826.

CPL   Cheltenham Public Library, Gloucestershire Collection.

DG   *Georgiana Extracts from the Correspondence of Georgiana, Duchess of Devonshire,* ed. Earl of Bessborough (London, 1955).

DNB   *Dictionary of National Biography* (London, 1921).

EL   *Letters of Mary Nisbet of Dirleton, Countess of Elgin* (London, 1926).

FD   *Joseph Farington Diary,* 8 vols. (London, 1923–1928).

FJ   John Fosbroke, *Contributions towards the Medical History of the Waters and Medical Topography of Cheltenham* (Cheltenham, 1826). The work forms the last and major section of Rev. Thomas Dudley Fosbroke's *Account of Cheltenham.* John was Thomas's son and Jenner's assistant in the Cheltenham practice from 1816 to 1823.

FTh   *Thomas Dudley Fosbroke Biographical Anecdotes of Edward Jenner . . . . his interviews with the Emperor of Russia etc.* (Published with same author's *Berkeley Manuscripts—abstracts and extracts* of Smythe's *Lives of the Berkeleys*) (London, 1821).

GC   *Gloucestershire Collections.* comp. Roland Austin, "Books, Pamphlets, and Documents in the Gloucester Public Library relating to the County, Cities, Towns, and Villages of Gloucestershire."

GH   Gwen Hart, *History of Cheltenham* (Leicester, 1965).

GJ   *Gloucester Journal,* 1752–1825.

GN&Q   *Gloucestershire Notes and Queries* (London, 1881–1911).

GRO   Gloucester Records Office.

HR   Henry Ruff, *History of Cheltenham* (Cheltenham, 1803).

JA   John Anstey, *Poetical Works of the late Christopher Anstey, Esq., with some Account of the Life and Writings of the Author by his Son, John Anstey, Esq.* (London, 1808).

JCL   *Memoirs, etc. . . . . of John Coakley Lettsom with a selection of his correspondence,* ed. Thomas Joseph Pettigrew, 3 vols. (London, 1817).

JG   John Goding, *Norman's History of Cheltenham* (Cheltenham, 1863).

LN   Duchess of Sermonetta, *The Locks of Norbury* (London, 1940).

MD   *Diary and Letters of Madame D'Arblay. Edited by her Niece,* 7 vols. (London, 1842).

MK   Michael Kelly, *Reminiscences,* ed. Theodore Hook, 2 vols. (London, 1826).

PhJ   Mrs. Zoë Jenner Phoenix: Jenner family records.

PS   Powell Snell, *Poetical Effusions from Fairy Camp,* 2 vols. (Tewkesbury, 1803).

PWL   *The Prince of Wales' Letters,* ed. A. Aspinall, 8 vols. (London, 1938).

RB   Robert Bloomfield, *The Works* (London, 1864).

RS   *Life and Correspondence of Robert Southey,* ed. Caroline Southey (London, 1849).

SM   Simon Moreau, *A Tour to Cheltenham Spa* (Bath, 1793).

SR   Samuel Rudder, *A New History of Gloucestershire* (Cirencester, 1779).

TC   Hartley Coleridge, *Life of Thomas Coutts,* 2 vols. (London, n.d. [1852?]).

TCh   Thomas Christie, *An Account of the Ravages Committed in Ceylon by Smallpox, etc.* (Cheltenham, 1811).

W&H   Edith Humphris and Capt. E. C. Willoughby, *At Cheltenham Spa or, Georgians in a Georgian Town* (London, 1928).

WL   William Le Fanu, *A Bio-bibliography of Edward Jenner, 1749–1823* (London, 1951).

Chapter I

1. Sir George Cranfield Berkeley (1753–1818): Burke's Peerage (1893, p. 129) credits him with a knighthood but the DNB does not. Joined Royal Navy at thirteen. Sailed under Capt. Cook in survey of Newfoundland coast and mouth of the St. Lawrence River, 1769. M.P. for Gloucestershire 1783–1810.

2. GN&Q, vol. 3, pp. 538–39. M.A. Magdalen College, Cambridge, 1753.

3. Thomas Bruce (1729–1814): 1st Earl of Aylesbury.

4. SR, pp. 700–701.

5. Ibid., p. 667.

6. BL, vol. 2, pp. 304–5.

7. GJ, Oct. 5, 1756.

8. Sir Astley Paston Cooper (1768–1841): One of the leading surgeons of his day. Created baronet 1821.

9. GJ, March 21, 1758.

10. GC, 12050. Joseph Bence (fl. 1768–1808): Publisher of a sermon by Thomas Newton, Bishop of Bristol, and an editor of the works of Milton.

11. SR, p. 309. Samuel Rudder (1726–1801) was a near contemporary of Jenner and ran a printing house in Cirencester for fifty years, including the period of Jenner's residence there.

12. PhJ.

13. GJ, March 21, 1758.

14. Joshua Parry (1719–1776): A well-known West of England pamphleteer. Minister of Presbyterian Church, Cirencester, from 1742 to his death.

15. B&C, vol. 11, p. 126, "Cirencester Grammar School" by the Reverend E.A. Fuller, M.A.

16. Ibid.
17. Rev. Daniel Lysons (1762–1834), *Sketch of the Life and Character of Charles Brandon Trye* (London, 1812), pp. 6–8.
18. BL, vol. 1, p. 21.
19. Ibid., p. 27.
20. CC, May 30, 1816.
21. Mrs. William Hicks Beach, *A Cotswold Family, Hicks and Hicks Beach* (London, 1909), p. 286.
22. John Hunter (1728–1793): Surgeon Extraordinary to George III 1796.
23. Sir Joseph Banks (1743–1820): President of the Royal Society from 1778 to his death.
24. Sir Everard Home (1756–1832): F.R.S. 1785. Surgeon to St. George's Hospital 1793–1827. Baronet 1813. As executor of John Hunter's estate was condemned for destroying all the great surgeon's papers.
25. Matthew Baillie (1761–1823): Physician to St. George's Hospital 1787–1799. Physician Extraordinary to George III. Declined a baronetcy in 1810.
26. William Hunter (1718–1783): Elder brother of John Hunter. M.D. Glasgow 1750. Physician Extraordinary to Queen Charlotte 1764. F.R.S. 1767. First Professor of Anatomy, Royal Academy 1768. His *Anatomical Description of the Human Gravid Uterus* (1774 in Latin) was edited by Baillie 1794.
27. Ann Home (1742–1821): Her works were published 1811. Greatly admired by Burns.
28. Mainly slanted to anatomy. Hunter's was a stern regimen. "He rose at six to dissect." DNB.
29. BL, vol. 1, p. 59. Hunter's letter was on May 24, 1775.
30. BGS, vol. 36, p. 314; A.N. Welch, *Old Arle Court.*
31. BL, Vol. 1, p. 68.
32. GN&Q, vol. 3, p. 540.
33. Sarah Siddons (1755–1831): While born in Hereford, is supposed to have lived for many years at Lydbrook in Forest of Dean, Gloucestershire. The Coffee House Yard Theatre, where she was discovered in Cheltenham, was a converted malt house.
34. SR, p. 337.
35. Thomas Campbell, *Life of Mrs. Siddons* (London, 1834), vol. 1, p. 77.
36. Sir Henry Bate-Dudley (1745–1824): Assumed name Dudley late in life. Distinguished journalist. Founded *Morning Chronicle* in 1780. Had previously edited *Morning Post.* Writer, amateur boxer, and finally Prependary of Ely. Died in Cheltenham.
37. Samuel Lysons (1763–1819): F.S.A. 1786. F.R.S. 1797. Barrister Inner Temple 1798. Treasurer of Royal Society 1810.
38. Charles Moore (1762–1810): Barrister Inner Temple. Confidant and friend of Siddons family. Brother of James Carrick Moore.
39. Sir Thomas Lawrence (1769–1830): Born in Bristol. President of Royal Academy 1820. Leading portrait painter of the day. Painted many of the vaccination pioneers.
40. BL, vol. 1, p. 86.
41. This creature was the subject of Hunter's "largest and most memorable zoological paper." WL, p. 7.
42. Robert Bransby Cooper was M.P. for Gloucester 1818–1830. Medical Officer at Cheltenham 1832.

43. Sir Francis Milman (1746–1821): Came under the patronage of Duke of Gloucester as a young man, having graduated from Exeter College Oxford at age of seventeen. Elected to a Fellowship 1765. Radcliffe Travelling Fellow 1771. Physician to Middlesex Hospital 1777–1779. Physician Extraordinary, King's Household 1785, and to the King 1806. President Royal College of Physicians 1811–1813. Created Baronet 1800. Married 1779, Frances Hart of Stapleton, Gloucestershire, a girl many years his junior. According to DNB, his medical ability scarcely matched his high honors.

44. FJ, pp. 289–90.

45. Sir George Baker (1722–1809): A gracious and highly cultured man. Excellent classical scholar. Settled in London 1761. Wrote *An Enquiry into the Merits of a Method of Inoculating the Smallpox*, 1766. F.R.S. 1776. Created Baronet and Physician in Ordinary to King and Queen 1776. Staunch supporter of vaccination.

46. Madame D'Arblay, nee Frances Burney (1752–1840): Novelist and Second Keeper of the Queen's Robes 1786–1790. MD, vol. 4, p. 142.

47. Dorothy Jordan (1762–1816) was of Irish parentage. Debut at Drury Lane 1785. Excelled in Shakespeare's comedy roles.

48. William Duke of Clarence (1765–1837): Second son of George III. Ascended throne as William IV, 1830.

49. WL, pp. 1–21.

50. PhJ.

51. WL, pp. 2, 16–17, 79.

52. FTh, p. 226.

53. GC, 12302 (peerage trial).

54. There were no university medical schools in England. All doctors served apprenticeships.

55. Powell Snell (fl. 1803): Cheltenham dandy. Barrister Inner Temple. Came of a distinguished legal family. Ran for Parliament against George Selwyn.

56. FTh, p. 230.

57. PS, p. 24.

58. Joseph Farington (1747–1821): Landscape painter. Royal Academy 1785. Secretary to the Royal Academy. His *Diary* is the most copious private record of the late Georgian era. Was particularly intimate with Cheltenham society and Jenner's circle.

59. GJ, April 18, 1796. 7071. *Trial of Mary Reed for Petit Treason* in *poisoning her husband William Reed, gent,* of *Berkeley* .... *at the Assizes holden at Gloucester, March 28th 1796, before Sir Soulden Lawrence, K.C. Gloucester,* printed by Robert Raikes. RR.41.810962 (15).

60. WL, pp. 15–16.

61. FTh, p. 229.

Chapter II

1. John Parker, 2nd Baron Borington (1772–1840): Succeeded father 1778. F.R.S. 1795. D.C.L. Oxford, 1779. Created Earl of Morley, 1815.

2. John Ingenhousz (1730–1799): Born in Netherlands. After three years in England, 1765–1768, returned to the Continent and patronage of royal houses of Austria and Russia. Granted annual life pension of nearly £600 from Russian Emperor. Returned to England 1778.

3. John Fosbroke (1797–1845): M.D. Edinburgh 1821. Jenner's literary assistant and junior partner in Cheltenham practice 1816–1823. Son of Thomas Dudley Fosbroke.

4. FJ, pp. 295–96.

5. Ibid., p. 296.

6. GJ, Sept. 2, 1802.

7. Mary Berry (1763–1852) and sister Agnes, a year her junior, were the protégées of Horace Walpole. He took up residence in 1791 at Little Strawberry Hill, which he left them on his death in 1797. The sisters, with their father, were entrusted with editing Walpole's works, 1798.

8. The Locks of Norbury, Surrey, prominent patrons of the arts. William Lock (1732–1810) was a wealthy banker. William Lock the younger, his son, is said to have promoted the marriage of Fanny Burney to Gen. D'Arblay.

9. William Bagshaw Stevens (1756–1800): A poet and translator of some ability. He was indolent and happy-go-lucky despite patronage in high places. Both Coutts and Sir Francis Burdett sponsored him for his brilliant mind and conversation, but he failed in everything he touched. During his headmastership of Repton School (1779–1800) he almost ran the school into the ground. He died of apoplexy allegedly brought on by a fit of laughing.

10. George Monk Berkeley (1763–1793): Lawyer Inner Temple, LL.B. Dublin 1789. Better known as a minor poet.

11. Dr. John Moore (1729–1802): M.D. Glasgow 1770. A wealthy and fashionable physician. Also a prolific man of letters. Edited the complete edition of his friend Smollett, 1797.

12. James Carrick Moore (1763–1834): M.C.S. 1797. After Jenner, possibly the leading authority on smallpox. Wrote *History of Smallpox,* 1815.

13. Edward Law, 1st Baron Ellenborough (1750–1818): Fellow, Peterhouse, Cambridge 1771. K.C. 1787. Attorney General 1793. Knighted 1801. Lord Chief Justice and created peer 1802. One of Jenner's first supporters.

14. Joseph Pitt (1759–1842): A self-made man. Bailiff of Cirencester 1790. Partner of Jeremy Wood in Cheltenham and Gloucester Bank. Planned and built a large part of Cheltenham.

15. John Burns Rous of Dennington (1750–1827): His sister, Lady Frances Rous, was wife of Catherine Jenner's cousin by marriage. Lady Peyton was Catherine's sister-in-law.

16. Thomas Newell (1763–1836): Surgeon Extraordinary to George IV. Practiced in Cheltenham for forty-one years.

17. Prince Hoare (1755–1834): Painter turned playwright. Hon. Foreign Secretary to Royal Academy, 1799.

18. GN&Q, vol. 3, p. 637.

19. BL, vol. 2, pp. 418–19.

20. Charles O'Hara (1740–1802): Fought in American War of Independence. Captured at Yorktown.

21. FD, vol. 1, p. 166.

22. William Frederick, Duke of Gloucester (1776–1834): Grandson of George II.

23. SM, p. 46.

24. Christopher Anstey (1724–1805): Educated Eton & Kings' Cambridge. Brilliant satirical poet. Lived his last twenty-five years at Bath.

25. JA, p. 36.
26. Philip James Loutherburgh (1740–1812): Born Fulda, Germany. Member of French Academie Royale, 1767. Came to England 1771. R.A. 1781.
27. FD, vol. 1, p. 165.
28. FJ, p. 285.
29. BL, vol. 2, p. 294.
30. Thomas Minster the younger (1770?–1854): Son of Thomas Minster, surgeon of Stow-on-the-Wold.
31. GH, p. 276.
32. MD, vol. 4, p. 132.
33. Shenton's Cheltenham Directory (Cheltenham, 1800).
34. SM, p. 46.
35. FTh, p. 229.
36. Ibid., p. 230.
37. Lord Fauconberg, 2nd Earl (1743–1802): Bought the newly erected (by Skillicorn) Fauconberg House, 1780, as his summer residence. It was also known as Bayshill Lodge.
38. Mrs. William Hicks Beach, A Cotswold Family (London, 1909), pp. 350–51.
39. Ibid., p. 352.
40. JG, p. 538.
41. Newgate Calendar (London, 1824–1826), vol. 2, p. 177.
42. Sir Soulden Lawrence (1751–1814): Fellow of St. John's, Cambridge 1774. Barrister Inner Temple, 1784. Judge, Court of King's Bench, 1794.
43. GC, 7071, p. 16.
44. Ibid.
45. Ralph Bigland, Historical, Monumental & Genealogical Collections relating to the County of Gloucester (London, 1791), vol. 1, p. 162. The Nelmeses lived at Breadstone, a hamlet of Berkeley parish. In Bigland's time there were at least four family tombs in the church with armorial bearings.
46. Autograph letter at Royal College of Surgeons. There is an illustration of it in Le Fanu (p. 28).
47. Henry Cline (1750–1827): Surgeon-Lecturer in Anatomy St. Thomas' Hospital, 1781–1811. Something of a radical in politics. President of Royal College of Surgeons 1823. His most famous pupil was Astley Cooper.
48. Jenner received letters that might have been replies to his from Cline on August 11, and from the margravine December 1. Le Fanu, p. 128.
49. FJ, p. 152.
50. Ibid., p. 221.
51. FD, vol. 1, p. 165.
52. Michael Kelly (1764?–1826): Tenor and composer. An intimate of Mozart and Gluck. Had distinguished career on the Continent from age of fifteen.
53. James Leigh Hunt (1784–1859), Autobiography (New York, 1850), vol. 1, p. 93.
54. MK, vol. 1, p. 93.
55. BL, vol. 1, pp. 115–17.
56. FD, vol. 1, p. 165.
57. MK, vol. 1, p. 94.

58. Ibid., p. 95.
59. Ibid., p. 97.
60. FJ, p. 284.
61. Ibid., p. 285.
62. FD, vol. 1, p. 166.
63. MK, vol. 1, p. 76.
64. Harriot Mellon (1777–1837): Little is known of her antecedents. Her mother was of Irish peasant stock and worked as a shopgirl in Cork. Nothing is known of her husband, Mellon, who "disappeared" soon after the marriage. Harriot was "a generous and beautiful girl as well as an excellent actress" her contemporaries averred.
65. FJ, p. 294.
66. Jesse Foot, the elder (1744–1826): Practiced in West Indies and Russia before settling in London. Wrote a hostile biography of John Hunter.
67. MK, p. 98.
68. The loss of this entire year was revealed at the Berkeley Peerage trial in 1811. It has never been mentioned by any writer on Jenner or vaccination.
69. GC, 122298. Berkeley Peerage Trial. Minutes of evidence for March 8, 1811.
70. BL, vol. 2, p. 295.
71. FD, vol. 1, p. 272.
72. SR, p. 280. The incumbent was Rev. Thomas Augustus Hupsman.
73. GC. Gardner's *Miscellanies* (Bristol, 1798), vol. 3, p. 136.
74. William Somerville (1675–1742): Poet. Came of an old Gloucestershire family. His *Chase* had wide popularity among rural sportsmen.
75. GC, 12298. Berkeley Peerage Trial.
76. WL, pp. 22–45.
77. John Southey, 15th Baron Somerville (1765–1819): Celebrated agriculturist. Invented an improved plough. Active in local affairs with Jenner and encouraged consumption of cheap fish in Cheltenham. George III made him Minister of Agriculture in 1798.
78. Benjamin Moseley (1742–1819): M.D. St. Andrews 1784. Practiced for many years in West Indies and became authority on tropical diseases. L.R.C.P. 1797. Physician to Chelsea Hospital 1788. Physician Extraordinary to Prince of Wales.
79. FD, vol. 1, p. 186.
80. Daniel Lysons, *Charles Brandon Trye* (Gloucester, 1812), pp. 14–15.
81. Daniel Lysons (1727–1800): M.A. Oxford 1751. Fellow of All Souls 1755. M.D. 1769.
82. Lysons, *Trye*, pp. 16–19.
83. Sir Matthew John Tierney, 1st Baronet (1776–1845): Perhaps the most honored of the vaccination pioneers. M.D. Glasgow 1802. Physician to both George IV and William IV. Created Baronet 1818.
84. James Gregory (1753–1824): A leading medical scholar of his day. M.D. Edinburgh.
85. PhJ.
86. Francis Seymour-Conway, 2nd Marquis of Hertford (1743–1822). BL, vol. 1, p. 602.
87. SR, p. 700.

Chapter III

1. PhJ.
2. Ibid.
3. BL, vol. 1, p. 296.
4. WL, p. 24.
5. DNB (London, 1921), vol. 28, p. 433. Charles Creighton, noted opponent of vaccination, wrote in his article on Ingenhousz, "Ingenhousz formed an opinion adverse to Jenner but confined his opposition to a private letter."
6. Cother went into partnership with his son who carried on the practice at this house after his father's death.
7. Vaccination was not seriously taken up in Ireland until a Cheltenham peer, Lord Hardwick, became Lord Lieutenant in 1801.
8. BL, vol. 1, p. 495.
9. LN, pp. 146–47.
10. BP, p. 198.
11. Georgiana, Countess Spencer (1737–1814): widow of John, the first earl, who died in 1783. Her daughter the Duchess of Devonshire was named after her.
12. Lucan's son married the divorced daughter of Lord Fauconberg of Cheltenham.
13. FD, vol. 1, p. 234.
14. BP, p. 193.
15. DG, pp. 232–33.
16. Anne Seymour Damer (1749–1828): Sculptor. Studied under Carracchi and Cruikshank. Executed statue of George III for Edinburgh Registry Office.
17. William Lock's son married Celia, daughter of the Duchess of Leinster by that lady's second husband. The girl was thus related to Charles James Fox's family through his mother's sister, Lady Holland. Lord Holland was one of the leading vaccination peers.
18. BL, vol. 2, p. 244.
19. William Woodville (1752–1805): M.D. Edinburgh 1775. L.R.C.P. 1784. Was also a distinguished botanist.
20. BL, vol. 2, p. 244.
21. Ibid., p. 304.
22. Sir Walter Farquhar (1738–1819): M.D. Aberdeen 1796. Created Baronet 1796. Physician in Ordinary to Prince of Wales 1796. A wealthy doctor with a fashionable practice.
23. BL, vol. 2, p. 155.
24. FJ, pp. 300–303.
25. FJ, p. 302.
26. George Pearson (1751–1828): Pioneered study of Lavoisier in England by translating *Nomenclature Chinaique* in 1794. Physician to St. George's Hospital, 1787. F.R.S. 1791.
27. Thomas Beddoes (1760–1808): M.D. Oxford. Reader in Chemistry, Oxford 1788–1792. Founded Pneumatic Institute, Bristol, 1798. Married Maria Edgeworth's sister.
28. John Ring (1752–1821): One of the earliest vaccination converts. Active in London from 1799 on.

29. Hugh Scott, 6th Baron Polwarth (1758–1841): Egremont's brother-in-law. John Abernethy (1764–1851): Asst. Surgeon, St. Bartholomew's Hospital 1787. F.R.S. 1796. Surgeon St. Bartholomew's 1815–1827. Continued John Hunter's system of surgery.
30. BL, vol. 1, p. 333.
31. FJ, pp. 303–6.
32. Ibid., p. 304.
33. BGS, vol. 37, pt. 1, p. 157.
34. Ibid., p. 158.
35. Not to be confused with Trye's home at Leckhampton, Gloucestershire.
36. WL, pp. 19–20.
37. Anthony Fothergill (1732?–1813): M.D. Edinburgh 1763. Pioneer in study of Cheltenham Waters. Practiced in Bath 1785–1803; in Philadelphia 1803–1811.
38. BL, vol. 1, pp. 334–37.
39. WL, p. 52.
40. At this time Hanover was still a possession of the British Crown.
41. WL, p. 141. Le Fanu points out that a correction was made by the author after publication.
42. Thomas Bruce, 7th Earl of Elgin (1766–1841): In addition to his fame as vaccination pioneer, he is remembered for bringing the Elgin marble to England.
43. Sir John McMahon (1754?–1817) was later promoted to Colonel.
44. Mary Robinson (1758–1800): Born at Bristol. Became Prince of Wales's mistress at the age of twenty. After her stage career she distinguished herself in the world of letters. One of the most beautiful women of her time, she was painted by the greatest artists including Gainsborough, Reynolds, Hoppner, and Romney.
45. FD, vol. 1, p. 286.
46. Sir Richard Croft (1762–1816) was brother of eccentric writer Herbert Croft, author of *Love & Madness* (1780) and who was condemned for his exploitation of the poet Chatterton.
47. John Julius Angerstein (1735–1823): One of the shrewdest financiers of his day and founder of Lloyds as we know it. His art collection formed the nucleus of the National Gallery.
48. WL, p. 49.
49. Ibid., p. 50.
50. Sir George O'Brian Wyndham, Earl of Egremont (1751–1837).
51. BL, vol. 2, pp. 367–70.
52. BL, vol. 1, pp. 320–22.
53. William Hayley (1745–1820): Studied law at Middle Temple but devoted his life to literature. Wrote lives of Cowper and Romney, both of whom were personal friends. His poetry is largely forgotten.
54. In his *Dictionary of Authors* (Philadelphia, 1859), Allibone lists a *Cowpox and Smallpox* by William Fermor (London, 1800). Though Allibone is usually accurate, I can find no record of this work elsewhere.
55. WL, pp. 54–55.
56. BL, vol. 1, pp. 324–25.
57. JG, p. 135.
58. PS, vol. 2, p. 120.

59. Ibid., p. 121.
60. BL, vol. 1, pp. 287–90.
61. WL, pp. 40–41.
62. BL, vol. 1, p. 396.
63. PS, p. 121.
64. Ibid., p. 118.
65. FJ, pp. 276–77.

Chapter IV

1. BL, vol. 1, pp. 434–35.
2. John Jeffreys, 1st Marquis Campden (1759–1840): Recorder of Bath and Chancellor of Cambridge University.
3. BL, vol. 1, p. 487.
4. *Shenton's Cheltenham Directory* (Cheltenham, 1800).
5. GRO. A bill submitted to Dr. Fowler by one Ballinger, greengrocer of St. George's Place.
6. SM, p. 33.
7. PhJ.
8. *Morning Chronicle* (London), March 17, 1777. Also *London Gazetteer,* October 2, 1776.
9. Charles James Fox (1749–1806): The Uncle of 3rd Lord Holland who became one of Jenner's most powerful patrons and sat with him on the magistrates bench in Cheltenham.
10. BL, vol. 2, p. 305.
11. LN, p. 216.
12. Thomas Haynes Bayly (1797–1839): Popular playwright and songwriter. Wrote "Long Long Ago."
13. Anne Chaworth, boyhood sweetheart of Byron.
14. Johann Friederick Blumenbach (1752–1840): Great German anatomist. Professor of Medicine, University of Gottingen 1778. Member of French Academy of Science.
15. Louis Sacco: Italian physician, author of *Trattato de Vaccionazione,* 1809.
16. Alexander Marcet: Born in Geneva. Graduated from Edinburgh and practiced in London.
17. BL, vol. 1, pp. 452–55.
18. WL, p. 61.
19. Bayshill Lodge was the name by which the local inhabitants knew Fauconberg House.
20. GC, 12370. Autograph letter.
21. Elizabeth, Lady Craven (1758–1820): Later Margravine of Anspach; died in Naples.
22. FD, vol. 1, p. 151.
23. *Memoirs of Margravine of Anspach—Written by herself* (London, 1826), vol. 1, pp. 65–66.
24. Thomas Trotter (1760–1832): Physician to the Fleet. M.D. Edinburgh, 1788.
25. *Dictionary of American Biography* (New York, 1928), vol. 1, p. 395.
26. Cooper had been appointed surgeon to Guy's two years previously, succeeding his Uncle, William Cooper, in the post.

27. BL, vol. 1, p. 473.
28. Ibid., p. 595.
29. Ibid., p. 532.
30. Ibid., p. 471.
31. Ibid., pp. 454–55.
32. Ibid., pp. 457–58.
33. Sir Henry Mildmay (1764–1803): 3rd Baronet. M.P. for Westbury 1796–1807. Lived at Duntisbourn House outside Cheltenham.
34. The entire body of evidence at the parliamentary debate is taken from Baron, vol. 1, pp. 480–510.
35. John Courtenay (1738–1816): Antislavery pioneer, sat in Parliament thirty-two years 1780–1812. One of Jenner's earliest supporters.
36. Thomas Bradley (1738–1816): M.D. Edinburgh 1791. Physician to Westminster Hospital 1794–1811. Revised *Fox's Medical Dictionary*.
37. BL, vol. 1, pp. 480–510.
38. Thomas Dale (1729–1816): M.D. 1775. L.R.C.P. 1786. Helped to found Royal Literary Fund.
39. Thomas Keate (1745–1821): Surgeon to St. George's Hospital 1792–1813. Master of the College of Surgeons 1801, 1809, 1813.
40. William Saunders (1743–1817): M.D. Edinburgh 1765. Physician to Guy's Hospital 1770–1802. F.R.C.P. 1790. Physician to Prince Regent 1807. First President of Medical and Chirurgical Society.
41. John Coakley Lettsom (1744–1815): Born in West Indies. One of the leading international figures in eighteenth-century medicine. Studied at Edinburgh and Leyden. F.R.S. 1771.
42. Thomas Denman the elder (1733–1815): St. George's Hospital 1753. M.D. Aberdeen 1764. Physician Accoucheur Middlesex Hospital 1769–1783. Licentiate in Midwifery College of Physicians 1783.
43. Robert John Thornton (1768–1837): M.B. Cambridge 1793. Worked at Guy's Hospital. Son of the eighteenth-century wit Bonnell Thornton.
44. J. T. Nicholls and John Taylor, *Bristol, Past and Present*, vol. 2, p. 241. The authors, both serious scholars, do not mention their source.
45. Franck went on to Bristol to visit Beddoes. It was apparently an unheralded visit, since the learned Viennese wrote of their meeting: "The first words that he addressed to me were 'Which Dr. Frank are you since there are so many of you.'" G. Cunningham, *The English Nation* (London, n.d.), vol. 5, p. 440.
46. TCh, p. 25.
47. Ibid., p. 19.
48. Ibid., p. 25.
49. Ibid.
50. BL, vol. 1, p. 461.
51. Ibid., pp. 462–63.
52. Ibid., p. 465.
53. Ibid., pp. 401–3.
54. John Ring, "Edward Jenner," *Public Characters* (London, 1802–1803), pp. 37–40.
55. HR, p. 10.
56. BL, vol. 1, pp. 567–68.
57. Ibid., pp. 569–70.

58. Ibid., p. 570.
59. Ibid., p. 575.
60. George, 1st Earl Macartney (1727–1806): Governor Cape of Good Hope 1796–1798. Ambassador to China 1792–1794. Lifelong friend of the Hollands. Married daughter of Lord Bute.
61. John Philip Morier (1776–1853): Born in Smyrna, son of a Levantine merchant. Attached to Constantinople Embassy 1799. Accompanied Lord Elgin to Egypt and published firsthand account of Egyptian campaign.
62. FD, vol. 2, p. 97.
63. EL, p. 199.
64. Ibid., p. 240.
65. *Shenton's Cheltenham Directory* gives an excellent description of St. George's Place when Jenner lived there. (The orchard mentioned belonged to a Mr. Ballinger who was in the fruit and vegetable business.) "The coach road is down St. George's Place and over an arch brick bridge, thro' a pleasant orchard, on the left hand leads to the well and Grove Cottage; on the right hand to Bayshill Lodge the seat of Lord Fauconburg."
66. GRO, *Sherborne Papers*, October 26, 1803.
67. FJ, p. 301.
68. BL, vol. 1, p. 597.
69. GJ, January 19, 1803.
70. *Medical and Physical Journal* (London, 1803), pp. 540–42.
71. James Boaden, *Memoirs of Mr. Siddons* (London, 1827), pp. 331–41.
72. Thomas Campbell, *Life of Mrs. Siddons* (London, 1834), vol. 11, p. 110.
73. RB, p. 313.
74. HR, p. 82.
75. John Hoppner (1758–1810): In addition to being a painter he was a competent musician and poet. The only serious rival of Lawrence in portrait painting of his time. He did portraits of Mrs. Jordan (as a young woman in 1764), the Duke of Clarence, Abercrombie, and Bloomfield, the poet.
76. BL, vol. 1, pp. 586–87.
77. FD, vol. 2, p. 146.
78. John Claude Nattes (1765?–1822): He also drew the sketch of Upper St. George's Place in the Cheltenham Museum.
79. BP, p. 278.
80. FD, vol. 2, p. 146.
81. GJ, Aug. 10, 1803.
82. Charles Burney (1726–1814): A native of the north of England, he spent most of his adult life in Bath. Perhaps the leading musicologist of the eighteenth century. Father of Madame D'Arblay (Fanny Burney).
83. Francesco Bianchi (1752–1810): A romantic figure, he settled in England in 1794 and married a young singer named Miss Jackson. After a brilliant career he committed suicide.
84. Elizabeth Billington, nee Wachel (1768–1818): A child genius who made her debut as a pianist at age six. Wrote two pianoforte sonatas before she was eleven and became opera singer at sixteen.
85. FD, vol. 2, p. 147.
86. Ibid., pp. 157–58.

87. John Hely Hutchinson, 6th Earl of Donoughmore (1757–1832); EL, p. 293.
88. FD, vol. 2, p. 125.
89. PhJ.
90. WL, p. 70.
91. BL, vol. 1, p. 602.
92. EL, p. 293.
93. The other signatories were Oliver Wendell, Simon Howard, John Lathrop, Elyphalet Pearson, John Davis, and Ebenezer Storey.
94. *Gentleman's Magazine*, vol. 75, 1805. Part 2, pp. 673–74.
95. George Cunningham, *The British Nation* (London, n.d.; the last entry is Hannah More who died in 1833), vol. 5, p. 395.
96. JA, p. 4.
97. *Ad Edwardium Jenner*, M.D. Bath, 1803, p. 2.
98. Thomas Frognal Dibdin, *Reminiscences of a Literary Life* (London, 1836), pp. 201–2.
99. GN&Q, vol. 3, p. 445.
100. BL, vol. 2, p. 399.
101. Anthony Addington (1713–1790): M.D. Oxford 1744.
102. GN&Q, vol. 3, p. 448.

Chapter V

1. BL, vol. 2, p. 33.
2. Samuel Bell Labatt introduced vaccination into Ireland. Author of *An Address to the Medical Practitioners of Ireland on the Subject of Vaccination* (Dublin, 1805).
3. GN&Q, vol. 3, p. 338.
4. Thomas Joseph Pettigrew (1791–1865): Medical scholar. Lettsom's biographer.
5. FD, vol. 2, p. 194.
6. Rev. Rowland Hill (1744–1833): Famous and wealthy preacher. Brother of the religious contraversialist, Sir Richard Hill.
7. Rev. Edwin Sidney, *Life of Rev. Rowland Hill* (London, 1834), p. 227.
8. BL, vol. 1, pp. 334–37.
9. PS, p. 76.
10. EL, p. 313.
11. FD, vol. 2, p. 125.
12. WL, p. 146. Le Fanu refers to Goldston as "Dr." in his index. There seems to be no information on record before his vaccination involvement. Jenner addressed some lines in verse to him.
13. BL, vol. 2, pp. 338–39.
14. Anstey's work was published in Bath, but Ring published the translation in London for the national market.
15. BL, vol. 1, p. 340.
16. Henry Hunt, *Memoirs* (London, 1820), vol. 2, p. 139.
17. CPL, Sarah Fox, Diary and Correspondence (Manuscript). Mrs. Fox was daughter of Richard Champion (1743–1791), the Bristol ceramist and friend of Edmund Burke. After the Treaty of Versailles, Champion emigrated to America where he died.
18. BL, vol. 2, pp. 340–44.

19. John Russell, 6th Duke of Bedford (1766–1839): Succeeded to title on death of brother, 1802. Was elected President of Royal Jennerian Society, February 17, 1803.

20. W&H, p. 104.

21. Samuel Parr (1751–1813): Educator and classical scholar. Prependary of St. Paul's 1783. Strong Whig and friend of Priestley.

22. BL, vol. 1, pp. 31–33.

23. George Shaw (1751–1813): Doctor turned botanist. M.D. Oxford 1787. Asst. Keeper, Natural History Section, British Museum, 1807 until his death.

24. WL, p. 71.

25. BL, vol. 2, p. 342.

26. Ibid., vol. 2, pp. 346–47.

27. James Dalloway (1763–1834): Distinguished topographer and scholar. Editor of *Biglands Gloucestershire*. Born in Bristol, son of a Stroud banker. Attended Cirencester Grammar School. M.A. Trinity College, Oxford 1784. Came under patronage of Duke of Norfolk 1792. After taking medicine degree (M.B.) at Oxford 1794, was appointed Chaplain and Physician to British Embassy, Constantinople.

28. Sir Richard Phillips (1767–1840): Journalist and publisher. Republican as a youth, he continued to befriend all liberals even after he was rich and established. Friend of Priestley and Henry Hunt.

29. Capel Loft (1751–1824): Barrister. Translated Virgil and Petrarch.

30. RB, p. 172.

31. Ibid., p. 173.

32. BL, vol. 2, p. 39.

33. GRO (Sherborne Court Baron), 1805.

34. BL, vol. 1, p. 344.

35. Richard Colley, 1st Marquis Wellesley (1760–1842): Governor-General of India and elder brother of Duke of Wellington.

36. BL, vol. 2, pp. 23–27.

37. Ibid., pp. 37–38.

38. Ibid.

39. Rev. James Plumtre (1770–1817): Friend of Lettsom with whom he had vast correspondence relative to vaccination. Claimed that the drama was a vehicle for the uplifting of moral values. M.A. Cambridge 1795.

40. Sir Isaac Pennington (1745–1817): F.R.C.P. 1779. Harveian Orator 1783.

41. BL, vol. 2, pp. 43–44.

42. Allardyce Nichol, *A History of the English Drama* (Cambridge, 1952), vol. 3, p. 298.

43. GRO (Sherborne Court Baron), March 1805.

44. Cheltenham Borough Archives. Deeds.

45. Ibid. Messrs. Horsley's Cheltenham Sale Circular, 1892.

46. Ibid.

47. FJ, p. 286.

48. GN&Q, vol. 1, p. 228.

49. Harriot Mellon (1777–1837): Born in London of Irish mother, deserted by father. First appeared on stage at Ulverstone, Lancashire, at the age of ten. Married 9th Duke of St. Albans, 1827.

50. DG, p. 242.

51. Lady Crewe (1742–1818): Wife of John, Lord Crewe, M.P. for Cheshire. He was created peer in 1806.
52. FD, vol. 2, p. 96.
53. BL, vol. 2, p. 56.
54. Ibid.
55. W&H, p. 98.
56. BL, vol. 2, p. 53.
57. Samuel Manning (d.1847): Executed memorial to Warren Hastings in Westminster Abbey. No other work of importance.
58. Anker Smith (1758–1819): An extraordinarily busy artist. Worked on illustrations for Bell's *English Poets*, Bowyer's *Humes History of England*, Baydell's *Shakespeare*, and many other standard works. Engraved the Royal Academy's Da Vinci cartoon the "Holy Family" 1798. A.R.A. 1797.
59. John Raphael Smith (1752–1810): A Derby linen draper turned painter. Mainly a miniature painter. De Wint was one of his pupils.
60. James Northcote (1746–1831): R.A. 1787. Pupil of Reynolds.
61. WL, p. 157.
62. BL, vol. 2, p. 77.
63. Sir William Russell (1773–1839): Scion of one of Cheltenham's oldest families—the Prynnes. M.D. Edinburgh. Created Baronet by William IV 1832 after a life of practicing in the East and Russia.
64. John Latham (1761–1843): Physician to Radcliffe Infirmary 1787. Middlesex Hospital 1779–1783, St. Bartholomew's 1793–1802. Medical scholar.
65. TC, vol. 2, p. 270.
66. BL, vol. 2, pp. 351–53.
67. Robert Willan (1757–1812): A dermatologist famous for his *Description and Treatment of Cutaneous Diseases*, issued in parts between 1798 and 1808.
68. FD, vol. 3, p. 81.
69. The book referred to was *A Reply to the Anti-Vaccinists* by James Moore (London, 1806).
70. FD, vol. 2, p. 35.
71. Grant David Yeates (1773–1836): Born in Florida. M.B. Oxford 1797. M.D. 1814. F.R.C.P. 1815. Private physician to Duke of Bedford when Lord Lieutenant of Ireland.
72. BL, vol. 2, pp. 60–62.
73. William Rowley (1742–1806): Known as "the man-midwife." L.R.C.P. 1784. M.B. Oxford 1788.
74. W&H, p. 118.
75. Leslie Blanche, ed., *The Game of Hearts. Harriot Wilson and Her Memoirs* (London, 1957), p. 31.
76. GJ, Sept. 13, 1806.
77. William Wilberforce (1759–1833): A loyal supporter of Jenner in addition to his anti-slavery activities. Died on the eve of the Abolition of Slavery Act, 1833.
78. Sir Thomas Bernard (1750–1818): Graduate of Harvard and son of the penultimate governor of colonial Massachusetts.
79. FD, vol. 2, p. 35.
80. Ibid., p. 36.

81. Sir John Barrow (1764–1848): Private Secretary to Lord Macartney, Governor of Cape of Good Hope. Founded Royal Geographical Society.
82. BL, vol. 2, pp. 84–85.
83. WL, p. 72.
84. BL, vol. 2, pp. 55–56.
85. Ibid., p. 440.
86. PhJ.
87. TC, vol. 2, pp. 178–79.
88. FD, vol. 2, p. 48.
89. BGS, vol. 57, p. 91.
90. Thomas Tregeana Biddulph (1763–1838): M.A. Oxford 1787. Fundamentalist preacher.
91. John Dawes Worgan, *Select Poems etc.*, with a preface by William Hayley (London, 1810), pp. 3–10.
92. Ibid., p. 12.
93. BL, vol. 2, pp. 77–78.
94. Ibid., pp. 354–56.
95. Ibid., p. 356.
96. GH, p. 272.

Chapter VI

1. Autograph letter in catalogue of Messrs. Kenneth Randall Inc. (Somerville, Mass.), pp. 26–27.
2. GC, autograph letter.
3. BL, vol. 2, p. 95.
4. Ibid., pp. 86–90.
5. WL, pp. 102–6.
6. Proctor commanded the disastrous British attack on Plattsburgh, N.Y. in 1814.
7. BL, vol. 2, p. 105.
8. Worgan, *Poems*, pp. 42–44.
9. Published by Ruff "for Phillips and others," Cheltenham, 1807.
10. FJ, p. 313.
11. Richard Payne Knight (1750–1824): Wealthy writer on numismatics and classical curiosa. Vice President, Society of Antiquarians. Left his collection to British Museum. M.P. for Ludlow 1784–1806.
12. Sir Anthony Carlisle (1768–1840): One of Hunter's last pupils. Surgeon to Westminster Hospital 1793–1840. Professor of Anatomy at Royal Academy 1808–1824. Knighted 1820.
13. Tiberius Cavallo (1749–1809): Born in Naples but settled in England as a young man. F.R.S. 1779.
14. Nathaniel Marchant (1739–1816): One of the leading medallists of his day. R.A. 1809. Engraver of gems to George IV.
15. Sir John Saunders Sebright, 7th Baronet (1767–1846): Famous agriculturalist. M.P. Herefordshire 1807–1835. Neutral in politics but leaned toward Whigs.
16. GN&Q, vol. 1, p. 226.
17. BL, vol. 2, pp. 69–70.
18. RB, pp. 173–74.
19. Ibid., pp. 60–61.
20. Ibid., p. 56.

21. Ibid., p. 60.
22. "Deep in Cheltenham's hallowed bowers————the poet here may court the shade." Anonymous lines that appeared in eighteenth-century guide books.
23. RB, p. 100.
24. Ibid., p. 368.
25. Ibid., p. 369.
26. PWL, vol. 6, letter 2370. (Thursday night, March 19.) The Duke of Clarence wrote to the Prince of Wales from Bushey House: "Mrs. Jordan was brought to bed with Amelia: Mrs. Nixon in charge." Mrs. Jordan had been in labor since seven o'clock that morning.
27. AA, p. 64.
28. Lady Hester Stanhope (1776–1839): Daughter of 3rd Earl of Stanhope, a brilliant man who bitterly opposed his brother-in-law, William Pitt the younger. M.P. for Chipping Wycombe, 1780. An eccentric, he eventually disinherited all his children including Lady Hester.
29. GJ, Sept. 6, 1807.
30. PWL, vol. 6, letter 2425, p. 217. The Prince was apparently just as disenchanted as his hostess. In a letter to Lady Hertford he wrote: "Pray remember me to him with every regard and affection. I am now undergoing martyrdom, from the mistaken attention and bourgois and insufferable vulgarity and ill-breeding of the Maestra de La Casa."
31. FD, vol. 4, p. 222.
32. William Carr, Viscount Beresford (1768–1854) was the bastard son of the Marquis of Waterford who was married to an aunt of Jenner's friend Bentinck.
33. Sir Rowland Hill, later Viscount (1744–1803) served under Hutchinson in Egypt.
34. BL, vol. 2, pp. 114–15.
35. Ibid., p. 115.
36. Ibid., p. 112.
37. Worgan, *Poems*, p. 98.
38. GJ, March 21, 1808.
39. BL, vol. 2, pp. 107–10.
40. George Rose (1744–1818): An expert in international finance.
41. *Wales' Chronology* (London, 1840), p. 680.
42. EL, p. 240.
43. Worgan, *Poems*, p. 99.
44. AA, p. 68.
45. Mary Ann Clarke (1776–1852): Left her stonemason husband when she went on the stage. Tried for libel 1809. Imprisoned 1813.
46. BL, vol. 2, p. 140.
47. FD, vol. 5, pp. 71–72.
48. William George Maton (1774–1835): Physician to Westminster Hospital 1800–1808. Vice President Linnaean Society. M.D. Oxford 1801. F.R.C.P. 1802.
49. BL, vol. 2, p. 156.
50. Thomas Pettigrew, *Medical Portrait Gallery* (London, 1821), vol. 2, p. 4.
51. Rev. Edwin Sidney, *Life of Rev. Rowland Hill* (London, 1834), pp. 225–26.
52. John Cox Dillman Engleheart (1783–1862): Member of celebrated family

of miniature painters and engravers that included the brothers **George** and Thomas and their nephews, John and Francis.

53. BL, vol. 2, p. 119.
54. Worgan, *Poems*, p. 112.
55. Ibid., p. 126.
56. Henry Moore (1732–1802): A Unitarian hymn writer.
57. Worgan, *Poems*, pp. 120–27.
58. BL, vol. 2, p. 76.
59. CC, July 27, 1809.
60. PWL, vol. 7, letter 2568, p. 367.
61. FD, vol. 4, pp. 114–15.
62. WL, p. 157.
63. Medico-Chirurgical Society of London, *Transactions* (1809), vol. 1, pp. 263–68.
64. Ibid., pp. 269–75.
65. Sir Lucas Pepys (1742–1830): First Baronet. Physician Extraordinary to George III 1777. Attended King during period of insanity. Physician in Ordinary 1792. President Royal College of Surgeons 1804–1810.
66. BL, vol. 2, p. 120.
67. CC, Aug. 20, 1809.
68. BL, vol. 2, p. 120.
69. Ibid., p. 143.
70. Ibid., p. 144.
71. FD, vol. 6, p. 4.
72. CC, Feb. 6, 1810.
73. BL, vol. 2, p. 370.
74. Ibid., p. 144.
75. Ibid., p. 145.

Chapter VII

1. PhJ.
2. JG, p. 92.
3. CC, May 18, 1809.
4. CC, July 20, 1809.
5. CC, Aug. 17, 1809.
6. CC, July 6, 1809.
7. A surgeon named Freeman is listed in *Shenton's Directory* (1800), but nothing further is known of him.
8. FJ, p. 304.
9. W&H, p. 98.
10. AA, p. 151.
11. Ibid.
12. Ibid., p. 152.
13. Ibid., p. 156.
14. CC, Sept. 17, 1810.
15. Williams, *Sacred Allegories* (London, 1810), pp. 147–48.
16. Ibid., p. 137.
17. Ibid., p. 147.
18. Ibid., p. 141.
19. FD, vol. 6, p. 179.

20. JG, p. 515.
21. BL, vol. 2, pp. 371–73.
22. Ibid., pp. 373–75.
23. FD, vol. 5, p. 109.
24. BL, vol. 2, p. 367.
25. Letter in possession of Mrs. Whyte Boycott of Malvern, Worcestershire.

Chapter VIII

1. TCh, preface, pp. i–ii.
2. BL, vol. 2, pp. 13–14.
3. Ibid., pp. 363–64.
4. TCh, p. 100.
5. Ibid., preface, pp. i–ii.
6. CC, April 29, 1811.
7. BL, vol. 2, p. 158.
8. Sir Thomas Plumer (1753–1824) was already well known to Jenner. Assisted in defense of Warren Hastings and of the Princess of Wales in 1806. F.R.S. Master of the Rolls 1818.
9. GC, 12302. *Minutes of evidence given before the Committee of Privileges to whom the petition of William Fitzharding Berkeley claiming as of right to be Earl of Berkeley was referred* (London, 1811), p. 851.
10. Ibid., p. 857.
11. Ibid., p. 851.
12. GC, 12300.
13. FD, vol. 7, p. 2.
14. BL, vol. 2, pp. 413–14.
15. GC, autograph letter with seal of the Countess of Berkeley.
16. CC, July 30, 1811.
17. BL, vol. 2, p. 282.
18. The Gloucester Music Meeting was established in the city in 1724 for the benefit of widows and orphans of the diocese (Gloucester, Hereford, and Worcester).
19. Angelica Catalani (1779–1849): Probably the most esteemed soprano of her time. She succeeded Billington in dominating the English concert stage and is said to have raised three million francs in charity performances. Died of cholera in Paris.
20. FD, vol. 7, p. 35.
21. Daniel Lysons, *History, Origin and Progress* . . . . *of the Three Choirs of Worcester Hereford and Gloucester* (Gloucester, 1812), p. 301.
22. AA, p. 203.
23. Ibid., p. 204.
24. Ibid., p. 203.
25. FD, vol. 7, p. 57.
26. BL, vol. 2, p. 306.
27. FD, vol. 7, p. 57.
28. GC, autograph letter.
29. BL, vol. 2, pp. 175–78.
30. FD, vol. 7, p. 35.
31. Thomas Pettigrew (1791–1865): Son of a surgeon. Very precocious. Came under patronage of Duke of Kent. One of the founders of Charing Cross

Hospital. Co-founder of Bristol Archaeological Society. Librarian and surgeon to Duke of Sussex. F.R.S. 1827. Included biography of Jenner in his *Medical Portrait Gallery.*

32. JCL, p. 127.
33. Thomas Cogan (1736–1818): M.D. Leydon 1767. Accoucheur in London 1772–1780. Lived in Holland 1780–1795.
34. CC, Nov. 16, 1811.
35. FD, vol. 7, p. 62.
36. BL, vol. 2, pp. 376–78.
37. Printed by D. Walker of Gloucester, February 1812.
38. Richard Raikes was the son of Robert Raikes founder of the Sunday School Movement.
39. Hannah More (1745–1833): One of the most famous of the bluestockings. Born at Stapleton, Gloucestershire. Pioneered female education. Mrs. Hester Lynch Piozzi (1741–1821): Friend and confidant of Dr. Johnson.
40. WL, list of verses known to exist, pp. 134–36.
41. JG, pp. 541–42.
42. Ibid., pp. 329–32. Goding gives the whole Lefevre saga in detail.
43. John Birch (1745–1815): Perhaps the most able of Jenner's opponents.
44. Cyrus Redding (1785–1870): Made international reputation as a journalist. Edited *New Monthly Magazine* 1820–1830.
45. Cyrus Redding, *Fifty Years Recollections,* 3 vols. (London, 1858), vol. 1, p. 44.
46. BL, vol. 2, p. 82.
47. CC, August 6, 1812.
48. BL, vol. 2, p. 379.
49. FJ, p. 289.
50. Thomas Moore, *The Works of Lord Byron with his Letters, Journals and Life* (New York, 1900), vol. 13, p. 91.
51. BL, vol. 2, pp. 379–81.
52. Ibid., pp. 381–82.
53. James Maitland, 8th Earl of Lauderdale (1759–1839): Opponent of Pitt who turned Tory in late life. Privy Councillor, 1806.
54. Joseph Grimaldi (1779–1839): Famous clown, subject of Dickens's biography.
55. CC, Nov. 16, 1812.
56. CC, Dec. 8, 1812.
57. Sir Alexander Crichton (1763–1856): M.D. Leyden 1785. Physician to Westminster Hospital 1794. F.R.S. 1800. Physician in Ordinary to Alexander I of Russia.
58. BL, vol. 2, p. 183.
59. Ibid., pp. 185–87.

Chapter IX

1. FJ, p. 210.
2. The deeds of Athelney House (Dr. Fowler's), in possession of the Misses Rotunda of that address, refer to Jenner's ownership of number seven.
3. PhJ. The existence of a dissection vault in the garden of number six would indicate this.
4. FJ, p. 20.

5. CPL. The prospectus, printed by Ruff of High St., lists fifteen pages of subscribers.
6. Dr. Robert Robinson. Burke gives us no more information than the fact that his daughter and heiress married Lord Ashtown on May 25.
7. CC, March 18, 1813.
8. Ibid.
9. CC, March 25, 1813.
10. Ibid.
11. BL, vol. 2, p. 385.
12. CC, April 15, 1813.
13. BL, vol. 2, p. 265.
14. William Wright (1736–1819): Spent first eleven years of his professional life in Jamaica. Accumulated a famous natural history collection relating to that island. M.D. St. Andrews. F.R.S. 1778. A close friend of Banks's, he was more botanist than physician, but became President of Royal College of Physicians, Edinburgh, 1801.
15. CC, April 15, 1813.
16. BL, vol. 2, p. 391.
17. Ibid., pp. 392–94.
18. Ibid., pp. 389–91
19. John Mackie (1748–1831): Educated Edinburgh University. Had influential clientele during long residence on the Continent including royal houses of Holland and Spain.
20. CC, July 22, 1813.
21. BL, vol. 2, pp. 391–99.
22. John Kidd (1775–1851): Physician to Radcliffe Infirmary 1808–1826. Regius Professor of Physics, Oxford 1822–1851. Pupil of Astley Cooper.
23. BL, vol. 2, p. 390.
24. Ibid., pp. 217–18.
25. B&C, Feb. 16, 1814.
26. JG, pp. 531–32.
27. John Cooke (1756–1838): M.D. Leyden. Physician to London Hospital 1784–1807.
28. BL, vol. 2, pp. 192–93.
29. CC, June 2, 1814.
30. BL, vol. 2, p. 206.
31. CC, June 2, 1814.
32. FD, vol. 7, pp. 246–53.
33. BL, vol. 2, p. 206.
34. FTh, pp. 219–42.
35. BL, vol. 2, pp. 291–92.
36. FJ, p. 282.
37. BL, vol. 2, p. 195.
38. Ibid., p. 196.
39. Ibid., p. 197.
40. CC, July 21, 1814.
41. BL, vol. 2, p. 212.
42. RCS Manuscript (see Le Fanu p. 136).
43. CC, May 18, 1814. John Lingard (1771–1851): Lingard had given up his clerical duties in 1811 to concentrate on his *History of England*. Many

of the great libraries of England were placed at his disposal, and in 1817 Cardinal Gonsalve, Jenner's powerful ally in Rome, threw open the archives of the Vatican for the historian's use.

44. John Augustine Birdsall (1775–1837): Son of a wealthy grocery magnate, was mainly responsible for the establishment in permanent form of Ampleforth College. Abbot of Westminster 1830.

45. FJ, p. 281. Fosbroke's words—"He was acquainted with an immense number of the eminent characters of the time"—suggest the social picture as it appeared to the young partner.

46. CC, June 9, 1814.

47. CC, Aug. 11, 1814.

48. JG, p. 542.

49. CC, Oct. 13, 1814.

50. WL, p. 147.

51. BL, vol. 2, pp. 215–17.

52. CC, March 2, 1815.

53. CC, Sept. 22, 1815.

54. CC, Nov. 10, 1815.

55. BL, vol. 2, p. 295.

56. PWL, letter 27444. Only three months before her death, Amelia wrote to her brother the Prince of Wales: "Baillie's skill I believe to be great but his manner is unpleasant. I am sure Pope understands me better than anyone else."

57. CC, March 9, 1815.

58. TC, vol. 2, p. 232.

59. Sir Francis Freeling (1764–1836): Born in Bristol. F.S.A. 1801. Baronet 1828. When Principal Secretary of the Post Office, Wellington describes him as "the best in the world."

60. Manuscript letter in possession of R. C. Alcock, Esq., Charlton Kings, Gloucestershire.

61. CC, Feb. 7, 1815.

62. Sir Arthur Brook Faulkner (1779–1845): M.D. Edinburgh 1803. M.D. Oxford 1806. F.R.C.P. 1808. Physician in Ordinary to Duke of Sussex. Knighted for his development of the quarantine system during the Plague in Malta 1815. Settled in Cheltenham; became friend of Lord Brougham.

63. FJ, p. 275.

64. Boisragon's son, Conrad, became a noted opera singer under the name of Conrado Borrani. Celebrated for his role in Balfe's *The Enchantress* at Drury Lane in 1845.

65. Robert Southey, *A Tale of Paraguay* (London, 1825), canto 1, stanzas 1–3.

66. RS, p. 26.

67. CC, Sept. 28, 1815. Borington received an assassination threat two months before receiving his earldom.

68. CC, Sept. 18, 1815.

69. FJ, p. 290.

70. BL, vol. 2, p. 230.

71. Ibid., pp. 394–96.

Chapter X

1. Segrave was a courtesy title permitted to Col. Berkeley after the peerage trial.
2. GC, 9092. *Trial at Large of John Perry (and 10 others) for the wilful murder of W. Ingram (Gamekeeper to Col. Berkeley) at Catgrove in the parish of Hill, Gloucestershire, etc.* (Gloucester, 1816).
3. CC, June 27, 1816.
4. BL, vol. 2, pp. 414–16.
5. Mrs. William Hicks Beach, *A Cotswold Family* (London, 1909), pp. 351–57.
6. Faulkner later moved to Evington, an estate six miles out of town between Gloucester and Tewkesbury, but was resident in Cheltenham for the period of Jenner's life.
7. CC, April 4, 1816.
8. CC, May 30, 1816.
9. Full text of the report as reprinted in pamphlet form by Griffith is given in the appendix.
10. CC, June 17, 1816.
11. CC, July 4, 1816.
12. CC, June 6, 1816.
13. CC, July 25, 1816.
14. Later Louis Philippe, King of France.
15. CC, July 18, 1816.
16. R. W. Chapman, ed., *Jane Austen's Letters* (Oxford, 1952), p. 133.
17. CC, July 11, 1816.
18. CC, Aug. 8, 1816.
19. CC, July 25, 1816.
20. Sir Stamford Raffles (1781–1826): A leading colonial administrator as well as scientific pioneer. Entered East India Company's service, Penang 1805. Procured purchase of Singapore Island 1819. First President of the Zoological Society.
21. Sophia Hull wrote Sir Stamford's biography.
22. BL, vol. 2, p. 188.
23. Maria Foote, later 4th Countess of Harrington (1797?–1867).
24. Wood's *Cheltenham Guide* (Bath, 1816).
25. BL, vol. 2, pp. 222–23.
26. Lord Dunalley was uncle of Lord Ashtown, patron of Cheltenham Dispensary.
27. FD, vol. 8, p. 88.
28. GC, autograph letter 349.
29. Ernest Augustus, Duke of Cumberland (1771–1851): Later King of Hanover.
30. CC, Dec. 12, 1816.
31. JG, p. 543.
32. GH, p. 172.
33. CC, Jan. 21, 1817.
34. BL, vol. 2, p. 402.
35. Ibid., p. 266.
36. John James Chalon (1778–1854): Born in Geneva. Historical and genre painter. R.A. 1841.

37. BL, vol. 2, p. 223.
38. FD, vol. 8, p. 167.
39. Farquhar had been in semi-retirement since 1813.
40. GC, 3959. *Papers and Correspondence Relating to the Election of 1818.*
41. BL, vol. 2, pp. 418–19.
42. FJ, p. 267.
43. BL, vol. 2, p. 419.
44. Ibid., pp. 417–18.
45. FJ, pp. 295–96. Young Fosbroke refers to Jenner's "desultory habits."
46. WL, pp. 77–78.
47. William Cobbett (1762–1835): Farington had a very poor opinion of Cobbett. He wrote (FD, vol. 8, p. 118): "Sir Thomas Lawrence confirmed the report that William Cobbett, the *Sedition* Publisher, having left England—it was agreed, that Cobbett, by his publications, had caused the evils which occasioned the suspension of the Habeas Corpus Act."
48. Benjamin Rush (1741–1813): Earliest United States physician of international celebrity. Born in Philadelphia and educated Edinburgh (1768). Pioneered yellow fever research.
49. Cobbett, *Rural Rides* (London, n.d.), p. 33.
50. JG, p. 525.
51. CC, Oct. 1, 1818.
52. BL, vol. 2, p. 422.
53. James Phipps who was vaccinated in 1796.
54. BL, vol. 2, p. 305.
55. FD, vol. 8, p. 205.
56. Ibid., p. 207.

Chapter XI

1. Robert James (1705–1776): A noted physician in his day. M.D. Cambridge 1728. L.R.C.P. 1745. Patented James' Powders 1746. Friend of Dr. Johnson.
2. R. Gell and T. Bradshaw, *Gloucestershire Directory* (Gloucester, 1820).
3. W&H, pp. 215–16.
4. JG, p. 344.
5. DNB, vol. 14, p. 108. Pettigrew vaccinated the princess with lymph taken from Lettsom's grandchild.
6. FD, vol. 8, p. 237.
7. WL, p. 79.
8. FD, vol. 8, pp. 223–24.
9. CC, Sept. 2, 1819.
10. CC, Sept. 30, 1819.
11. FJ, p. 275.
12. Barry Edward O'Meara (1786–1836): Eulogized by the poets Moore and Byron.
13. FJ, pp. 169–70.
14. Despite their differences, Jenner and Fewster corresponded with each other as late as 1816. Le Fanu lists letters from Jenner on April 27 and July 10 of that year, pp. 124–25.
15. FJ, p. 271.
16. Ibid., p. 151.

17. Ibid., p. 170.
18. Ibid., p. 158.
19. BL, vol. 2, p. 306.
20. GC, manuscript letter 6.5.62.
21. Henry Peter, Baron Brougham and Vaux (1778–1868): Educated Edinburgh. One of the founders of *Edinburgh Review*, 1802. Lord Chancellor 1830.
22. FJ, p. 293.
23. Ibid., p. 295. Jenner acquired "sufficient knowledge of human nature to disregard ingratitude."
24. John Nichols (1745–1826): Voluminous writer and printer. Close friend of Lettsom. Managed *Gentleman's Magazine* 1792–1826.
25. BGS, vol. 37, pt. 1, pp. 152–53.
26. John Smythe (1567–1641): Author of *Lives of the Berkeleys 1066–1618*. Steward of the Household, Berkeley Castle.
27. BGS, vol. 37, pt. 1, p. 157.
28. Ibid., p. 158.
29. WL, p. 82.
30. FJ, pp. 207–8.
31. Baron erroneously states that the circular letter was first printed in the Devizes newspaper. There was no paper in that town until five years later.
32. CC, Jan. 16, 1821.
33. BL, vol. 2, p. 422.
34. Nichols, the editor, did not mention that the letter had already appeared in the Cheltenham *Chronicle* however.
35. BL, vol. 2, pp. 424–27.
36. WL, p. 86.
37. William Armfield Hobday (1771–1831): An industrious portrait painter who regularly exhibited at the Royal Academy. After Drayton's humble drawing Hobday's is probably the most exact image of Jenner.
38. Thomas, 1st Baron Denman (1779–1854): Barrister 1806. M.P. Wareham 1818. Secured withdrawal of Lord Liverpool's Bill of Pain and Penalties against Queen Caroline 1820. Lord Chief Justice 1832.
39. W&H, pp. 187–88.
40. CC, Sept. 18, 1821.
41. FD, vol. 8, p. 304.
42. FJ, p. 288.
43. BL, vol. 2, p. 290.
44. Ibid., pp. 431–32.
45. Ibid., pp. 292–93.
46. BGS, vol. 37, pt. 1, p. 159.
47. GJ, Aug. 21, 1823.
48. Robert William Sievier (1794–1865): Sculptor and stipple engraver. Executed bust of Prince Albert and exhibited at the Royal Academy. F.R.S. 1840.

INDEX

LIBRARY OF CONGRESS CATALOGING IN PUBLICATION DATA

Saunders, Paul, 1908–
  Edward Jenner, the Cheltenham years, 1795–1823.

  Includes bibliographical references and index.
    1. Jenner, Edward, 1749–1823.   2. Physicians—
England—Cheltenham (Gloucestershire)—Biography.
3. Smallpox—Preventive inoculation—History—
19th century.   4. Vaccination—History—19th
century.   5. Cheltenham (Gloucestershire)—Biography.
I. Title.
R489.J5S28   614.5′21′0924   [B]   81-51607
ISBN 0-87451-215-8   AACR2